Glorify Yourself

—

BY
ELEANORE KING

—

WITH TWELVE COMPREHENSIVE LESSONS ON BEAUTY AND
CHARM INCLUDING FACIAL RADIANCE, SKIN AND MAKE-UP,
POSTURE AND RELAXATION, HOW TO DRESS, DIETING,
EXERCISE, HAIR AND MORE.

D1248474

British Library Cataloguing-in-Publication Data
A catalogue record for this book is available from
the British Library

MEET THE AUTHOR

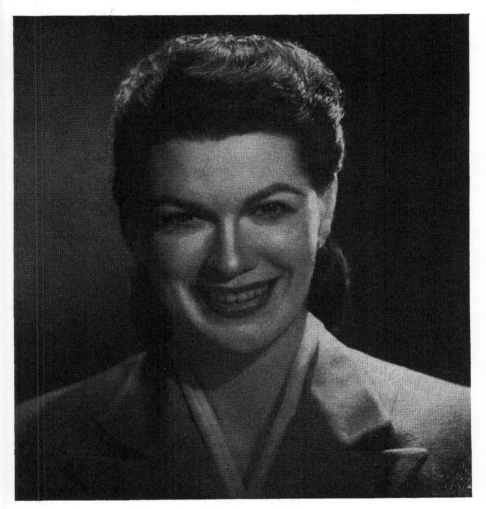

Eleanore King
Beauty Consultant to Famous Film Stars
also Teacher of Charm and Beauty to 83,000 Women

Who is The Author of "Glorify Yourself"?

Eleanore King is a famous Hollywood Beauty Instructor and Consultant. Lovely Virginia Mayo, Constance Dowling, Lenore Aubert . . . these and other leading Film Stars have been assisted in their beauty training by Eleanore King.

In this Course Eleanore King takes you behind the scenes at Hollywood. She reveals in "Glorify Yourself" the secrets of some of the world's most beautiful women.

In addition to being Beauty Consultant to famous Hollywood Actresses, Eleanore King has taught over 83,000 women of all ages and in all walks of life how to make better use of their charms and talents and to acquire grace and beauty.

She has also taught charm over the radio and trained smart airline hostesses.

Hundreds of Previously Unthought-of Beauty Secrets
Now Revealed for the First Time

In "Glorify Yourself," Eleanore King reveals to you the actual beauty secrets of many leading Film Stars and also gives the concrete, practical techniques she has used so successfully in her private classes—all of which you can adopt to express your own individuality to enhance your personal charm to the best possible advantage.

Formerly, only those living in a few large cities could enjoy the benefits of this beauty training as given by Eleanore King.

By the invention of special scientific methods, this same type of training is now made available for the first time by post.

Now you can put all this knowledge on charm, all the beauty techniques and the personality secrets to work for you in the privacy of your own home. By following Eleanore King's glamour guides you can easily achieve a fascinating personality.

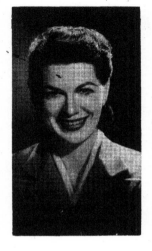

ELEANORE KING

Beauty Consultant to Famous Film Stars and to over 83,000 women of all ages and in all walks of life

Dr. C. C. CRAWFORD, Professor of Education, says:

" The Course has a definite and worthy mission : to make women more interesting, attractive and skilful in their personal contacts.

Miss King has had much experience in training women in personal effectiveness. In various business and teaching situations she has helped thousands to make better use of their charms and talents or to acquire qualities of grace, beauty and leadership which neither they nor their best friends suspected they could acquire.

Her work in the film studios has been equally spectacular in its success and in the general acclaim or approval expressed. Her Course gives a wider scope to this work."

" Glorify Yourself " has been specially designed to fill a great need. Thousands of women who have enrolled for the Course have been simply fascinated by it. Many Experts on Beauty throughout the country have praised it. Newspaper writers, radio and film directors and others equally as important have also joined in praising this new and unique method of acquiring radiant beauty, irresistible charm and glowing personality.

The Course, " Glorify Yourself," is now known throughout the world. Just as it has helped others, it will help you.

Something Entirely Different

The beauty techniques and secrets you get in t ese twelve exciting Lessons are decidedly different from anything you have ever seen. They can **only** be obtained through this Course and are not to be confused with the usual stereotyped beauty information so often dispensed by so-called " Beauty Experts."

The extensive knowledge and experience gained by Miss King has been put into the compilation of this truly remarkable and fascinating Course.

The Lessons reveal to you the highly successful beauty secrets and charm techniques that she has developed over many years in acting as Beauty Adviser to leading Hollywood Film Stars and in personally teaching thousands of women of all ages and in all walks of life how to be more charming, more beautiful and more attractive.

Only a Few Minutes a Day

You will find every Lesson fascinating —no tedious drudgery. The skilful techniques are easily mastered. You waste no time, but concentrate on the things that will help you most.

Just a few minutes a day show how to throw off faults—free hidden charm— give poise, confidence and a new outlook on life.

The Academy of Charm and Beauty, Marple, Cheshire.

CONTENTS

Foreword

I LIKE this Course. I think you will, too. It has a definite and worthy mission : to make women more interesting, attractive, and skilful in their personal contacts.

If anyone thinks that isn't important, he or she especially needs to read the Course and to face realities.

" Survival of the fittest " prevails in the competition for favour as well as for food, and women who make a poor showing lose in the competition.

Whether in the office or in the drawing-room, or even across the breakfast table, appearance and behaviour make the difference between success and failure.

Perhaps these little matters of personal attractiveness are mere trifles when thought of separately, but collectively, they mean the difference between riches and poverty, marriage or spinster-hood, and wedded bliss or broken homes. And these differences are not trifles.

Miss King has had much experience in training women in personal effectiveness.

In various business and teaching situations she has helped thousands to make better use of their charms and talents, or to acquire qualities of grace, beauty and leadership which neither they nor their best friends suspected they could ever acquire.

I know her work best from having seen her in action in her class in Air Hostess Training at the University, where her enrolments for years have had to be limited because the demand was beyond what she could satisfy.

Her work in the film studios and in other lecture series for business and social groups has been equally spectacular in its success and in the general acclaim or approval expressed.

Her Course merely gives a wider scope to the work. If you can't take her direct training, you may at least study self-improvement at home .

Her style is quite informal and spontaneous. She doesn't labour her paragraphs into strictly parallel and balanced outlines.

She expresses herself on paper in much the same way as she does in the classroom, in the studio, or on the lecture platform. She continues between stiff covers an informal spontaneity which has won thousands of readers daily in her newspaper columns.

More power to her pen.

Dr. C. C. CRAWFORD.
Professor of Education

1

Introduction

Be His Leading Lady

Men's natures are alike ;
It is their habits that carry
them far apart.
—CONFUCIUS

YOU may never wish for a film star's million fans, but you do want to be leading lady to one man. You want to be happy through making him happy. Haven't you often thought that with a little of the Hollywood star's training, you could make him the proudest man you know ? You wouldn't be a woman if you hadn't wondered just what is involved in a star's metamorphosis !

Why, then, is there so little known of the actual grooming that actresses receive *before* they're presented to their public ? You see them radiant with success and confidence. You read thousands of words about their lives, their background. Yet how little you see of what to you is the most important phase of their careers—the grooming period. Why is this ?

For too many years producers were afraid that a star would appear less glamorous if she were presented in any but the most fairy-tale fashion. Like Cinderella, she had to become a princess overnight ! True, her success often comes overnight ONCE SHE " CLICKS " ! But what of the sacrifice and education that preceded this? You know the stories of the great ones : Helen Hayes, Ingrid Bergman, Rosalind Russell, Claudette Colbert, Greer Garson, Judy Garland —each served an apprenticeship. Even Shirley Temple at the age of five, when the public first saw her, had put in two years that would prove the undoing of most babies—to say nothing of their mothers !

Fortunately, to-day, the studios realize that the most absorbing phase of a star's life to her public is that preparatory stage, because it makes her a sister under the skin to her most discouraged fan. Her favourite's loveliness becomes the impelling force behind the woman who asks herself, " She's done so much for herself ; could I do something about myself ? "

Here, then, is your challenge. If Hollywood can take a photogenic girl, who speaks no English, and groom her for her first starring role in three months, then by mastering the same techniques, why can't you prepare yourself for your role in private life in twelve months ?

As a studio coach, it is my aim in this Course to present to you the technique used in grooming a star. Surprisingly enough, the majority of these skills and techniques are acquired as you go about your daily tasks. You learn through doing, just as a potential star does. You move gracefully until that is your natural way of movement. You

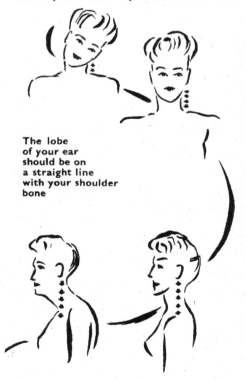

The lobe
of your ear
should be on
a straight line
with your shoulder
bone

Figure 1

3

incorporate only radiant facial expressions until they become yours. You practise tactful, gracious conversation until any other would be foreign to you. Soon your friends, your business colleagues even your family, notice first, a subtle change, then a remarkable one.

Then you hear his first, "You know, Jane, there's something different about you—I can't express it—I know I like it, though." After that, it's easy. You won't succumb to the pettiness and self-pity which are all too often the allies of those who justify their laziness with excuses. You will progress steadily forward to the ranks of happy, successful women.

Comparing the lives of happy women, you recognize a similarity in pattern. *That similarity is expressed in their qualities.* Analysing further, what is the basic structure of those qualities ? HABIT. If the quality that endears her to her husband and friends is her sincerity, then notice how that sincerity manifests itself ! Her voice *sounds* sincere, the things she says *sound* sincere, her eyes *look* sincere, her actions and deeds *proclaim* her sincerity. In other words, the combination of her habits declares her a sincere woman.

You are a combination of your habits, too. In fact, you are your habits ; your habits are you. Five thousand of them, good or bad, are you. Your habits of speaking, walking, thinking, eating, living, are moulding you day by day into the person you will be next year, five years from now, and fifty years from now.

Thus, the most glorious realization in life is that you can carve out a whole new world for yourself through formation of correct habits. Are you discouraged, hurt ? Are you on the wrong track ? Build anew ! Start afresh. You can be what you want to be. You can be his leading lady by mastering those skills and techniques that underlie the qualities which gracious, charming women possess.

I found, early in my coaching career, that I could suggest to my students many books that told WHAT they should do ; but they needed a Course to tell them HOW to do it. This Course is, therefore, dedicated to helping to fill the need for the HOW TO DO AND BE.

To make your transformation into the person you want to be as easy as possible, you will find that only the last few lessons require a certain amount of time in which to practise. All the rest you absorb and master through daily application.

List of Photographs

Contents of Lessons

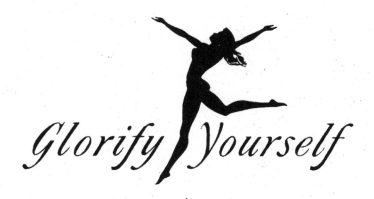

Glorify Yourself

★

A Complete and Up-to-Date Course on
Beauty and Charm by One of the
Most Famous Beauty Specialists
and Consultants in the World

Eleanore King

★

LESSON ONE

★

THE ACADEMY OF CHARM AND BEAUTY

MARPLE · CHESHIRE

STUDIO TALK •

Issued only for Students of the Eleanore King Course on Beauty. Charm and Personality.

Number One.

Dear Student,

Welcome to the Course on Charm, and Beauty and Personality.

In a very sincere spirit of friendship I greet you I invite you to come with me along the road that leads to a more attractive and fascinating personality.

In Part A of this first Lesson you will learn one of the most important secrets of charm and beauty - the cultivation of facial radiance.

You will be taught the correct posture for head and neck: you will be shown special techniques for making your facial expression irresistibly attractive. These special methods were formerly the closely guarded secrets of highly skilled Beauty Specialists entrusted with the task of grooming Hollywood Stars. Now they are yours: and I sincerely hope you will give them the attention they deserve.

"The eyes are mirrors of the soul" is an old saying in almost daily use. It may be trite, but it's true, you know. So an important part of this Lesson is devoted to consideration of the eyes; and you will be taught how to make them shine with compelling vitality and expression. Master this simple procedure, and you will immediately register on everyone you meet as a warm, friendly personality. <u>You will have begun truly to glorify yourself</u>.

Next to the eyes, the lips are perhaps the most important facial feature. Certainly, men often admit that they judge a woman's disposition by her lips.

So I have given Part B of Lesson One the title: "Inviting Lips", and in it I show you the simple techniques which will make your lips flexible, appealing and truly feminine. There is no need to worry if your lips are thin, undeveloped or weak. You will see from the Lesson that all these faults can easily be corrected.

Although I want you to follow conscientiously all my instructi is and suggestions I hope you don't think

that this Course is going to be hard work. In point of
fact rest and relaxation are two of the most powerful
aids to beauty. Perhaps you are a very busy person and
may not be able to relax as much as you would wish. I
have therefore included in this Lesson some hints on how
to extract the maximum benefit from short periods of
relaxation.

You realise, I am sure, that this is only your
first Lesson. You'll agree, I know, that just as you
cannot learn to swim or dance in a single lesson, neither
can you expect to acquire all the beauty secrets and charm
techniques in one lesson. But you have taken the first
important step towards doing so.

Yours sincerely,

Eleanor King

EK·1.

P.S. In our next Lesson you will learn how to take care
of your skin and how to use make-up to enhance its beauty or
conceal its defects.

Glorify Yourself

by

ELEANORE KING

★ ★ ★

Easy-to-Follow Instructions

This fascinating Course on the technique of developing personal charm and self-confidence tells you *how to be what you want to be*. Eleanore King, charm expert and personality coach to top Hollywood actresses, reveals glamour secrets that any woman can adapt to her own glorification. Simple, easy-to-follow instructions show exactly how to utilize each basic physical, mental and social skill to the best possible advantage.

Develop Personal Charm

The guides to glamour that really work :

*FACIAL RADIANCE
—how to have brilliant eyes, expressive lips, glowing skin, shining hair, a composed head.

*BEAUTIFUL BODY
—how to reduce or gain ; corrective diets, exercises.

*PERFECT POSTURE
—how to develop grace in every movement, whether walking, standing, sitting, or getting in and out of a car.

*FOURTEEN COUNT
—how to be well-dressed at all times, and how to assemble a smart wardrobe on a limited budget.

*POISED PERSONALITY
—how to meet people graciously, how to be at ease anywhere, hints for sparkling small-talk.

Guide to Glamour

Excellent photographs of popular film stars, supplemented by clever sketches, illustrate different points of attractiveness.

Comprehensive charts give weight and measurement tables, daily diet schedules, accessory ensembles and other valuable detailed information.

In a charming and effervescent style Eleanore King reveals dozens of unthought-of arts. For instance : blinking a lot gives life to the eyes ; tongue exercises will develop mobile lips, smiling at least once every sentence will give facial radiance and kill that " dead-pan " look ; sticking your neck and chest out won't get you there any sooner—you can't arrive until your whole body does.

Some " Do's " and " Don'ts "

Some emphatic " do's " and " don'ts " for attractiveness are : do dress your type and don't go beyond the fourteen count ; do carry your body with distinction ; don't be a " lump lander " ; do be vivacious, put vitality in your eyes and voice but don't lose the effect of a composed body.

Every woman is born with a certain amount of charm and beauty, but it is a clever woman and a determined woman who makes the most of her potentialities. By following Miss King's glamour guides faithfully and consistently, making them so routine that you never give them a thought, you can easily achieve a fascinating personality.

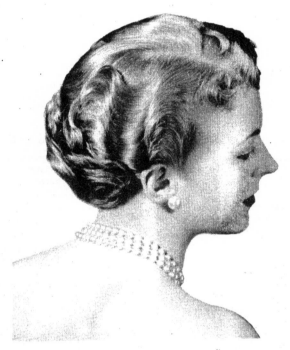

By Courtesy of Superma Ltd. London

LESSON ONE

Part A

Facial Radiance

O, she doth teach the torches to burn bright !
—SHAKESPEARE, *Romeo and Juliet*

YOU turn quickly to watch a woman. There's something compelling, distinctive about her. When you analyse what that " something " is, you realize it's the way she carries herself. A lot of it, also, is the way she carries her head.

Film stars differ in colour, features, personality ; but they all have one quality in common : they carry their heads magnificently. They learn early that the camera is an exacting master where heads are concerned. It picks up the least tendency towards slouching. The first principle you, too, must master in glorifying yourself is beautiful head carriage.

First of all, KEEP YOUR HEAD STILL ! A still head has power. There is no allure, no feminine grace, in a bobbing, restless head. You will never be without an occasional head movement ; no gesture can be more emphatic. But the average untrained woman uses her head too much. You ask her how to get to the City Hall, and she jerks and bobs her head on an average of three nods a second as she says, " Just a hundred yards down the road and then to the left." *Learn to put the vitality you waste in head motions into your eyes and your voice !*

For camera training, the prospective star is taught to move her head SLOWLY. About one-tenth as fast as she has been using it ! I wish I could tell you the name of the star-in-training who was so vivacious she simply could not control her head. Consequently, in spite of my repeated warnings, she ruined every scene on her first day before the camera. The director gave her four days to break the habit, explaining that he could " shoot " other scenes around hers. After that, they'd have to replace her. The next day she appeared with a peculiar upswept hair style. I said that I didn't think it was too flattering. She replied, " I know, but I have a little dinner-bell concealed in the top of it. Every time I bob my head the least fraction, it rings ! You'd be amazed the way people stare at me when it starts jangling." She had a well-poised, controlled head within two days ! You needn't be as

drastic as that, but do think about your head movements for a week. Ask a friend you can trust to help you, too.

Here's the simplest way to check your head posture. Stand or sit in what you consider your best posture. The lobe of your ear should be on a straight, vertical line with your shoulder bone. (See Figure 1.). Use a ruler or a piece of paper for your test. If your ear lobe is forward any distance from the shoulder bone, you know you are fostering a poor head position. Also, you can expect a dowager's hump on the back of your neck, and flabby chins in front.

No matter how poorly you are holding your head now, YOU CAN CORRECT IT. And you can correct it right on the job as you go about your daily work. Here's your programme.

1. Every few minutes, push your head back, thinking of that ear-lobe shoulder-bone test. Don't push your chin back so far, though, that you cause a double chin ; and don't antagonize others by carrying your chin too high.

2. Carry your head high by pushing up on the back of your neck. Stretch high and hard every few minutes. You can see how this stretching also helps those neck wrinkles.

3. To relieve neck strain, rotate your head. Drop it forward with a slow, heavy motion. Pause a second. Roll to the right. Pause. Open your mouth and let your head roll backwards as far as possible. Pause. Then complete the circle by letting it roll to the left. Repeat at least once an hour. (See Figure 2.).

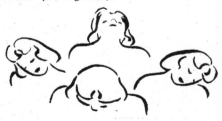

Figure 2

4. Since anything that affects your shoulders also affects your neck and head, guard against shoulder strain. Rotate your shoulders by pushing them up as close as possible to your ears ; then back ; and down. Repeat several times an hour. Rest and repeat often. Those around you won't object if you explain you're relieving tension, which makes you a better worker.

5. Carry your head balanced equally between your shoulders. *Carry it straight* ! Don't tilt it to one side or the other. A lateral head tilt weakens the appearance of even the strongest man, and it makes a woman appear giddy !

The cure. Suppose you already have that double chin and dowager's hump. The condition of your neck depends upon your general posture habits. It's easy to understand why our necks get old so early. Nature gave you sufficient flesh, tissue and muscle to hold your head erect. However, if, in your effort to get there faster, you constantly walk with your head leading,

You'll never get there—till your posterior is there! So why not slow down and wait for it ?

Keep your blocks stacked right

Figure 3

then you're sure to develop what posture authorities call a forward head. *You're never there until your posterior is there, so why not slow down and wait for it* ? (See Figure 3.).

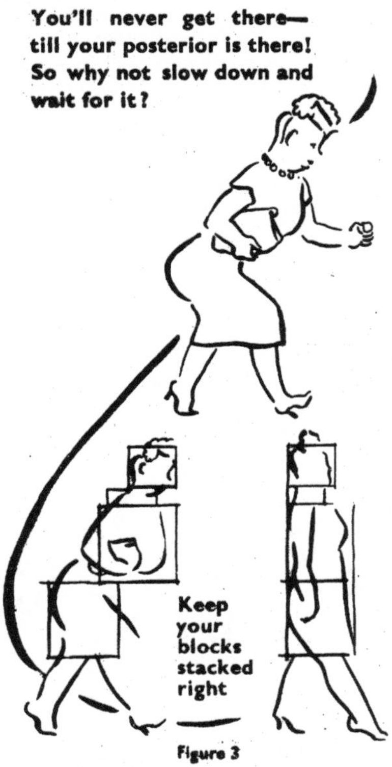

As your head strains forward out of position, the front muscles have no support and become flabby. Soon the skin of your neck looks crapy, too. The way to correct it is to get your head back, thereby strengthening those front throat muscles. You will also release the strain on the back of your neck and eliminate that dowager's hump. If you think your neck is really in bad shape, then turn to Lesson Six and do the posture exercises, because your whole body line-up needs correction. To help throat wrinkles and flabbiness, turn to Lesson Two on the care of the skin and make-up, but remember that there never will be a cream or lotion made that can do for your neck what good posture can do.

Once you have checked up the mannerisms of your head, then begin analysing your facial habits. Your expression changes continually, since your experiences vary from day to day. You may have been voted the most charming girl at seventeen. Two years later, strangers might classify you as bored or aggressive. What you did and what you thought during those intervening two years would tell in your face, UNLESS YOU REALIZE THAT YOU MUST BE CONSISTENTLY ALERT ABOUT FORMING AND MAINTAINING PLEASING FACIAL HABITS.

As you learn the outstanding rules for eye technique, you may think you have never been conscious that anyone whom you admire has been using them. But start watching your favourite actresses, lecturers or friends. They adhere to the same rules so openly that you will wonder why you never noticed it before and why you have not made use of the same skill yourself.

DEAD-PAN ALLEY

The MUST of every actress who has achieved distinction is the theory of *radiant, interested eyes in a very quiet, controlled head.*

It sounds so simple, but it is dynamic in its results. You've learned now how to master the posture of your head, and why you must keep it still most of the time. You've learned, too, that when you turn it, you must move it, oh, so slowly and smoothly. Now comes the startling contrast : THOSE LIVELY, ILLUMINATED EYES IN A QUIET SETTING.

What makes Ingrid Bergman's close-ups unforgettable ? Two expressive eyes in a serenely controlled head ! Nor is this law exclusive to women. Think of your favourite male stars. Without exception, they employ this same technique.

As an experiment, put two women side by side. One is beautiful, the other is moderately attractive. The former starts to speak, and talks all over her face with her head going as fast as her eyes. The other woman speaks with her eyes and lips *only* ; her head remains tranquil. Every man in the room will prefer the second woman. She has poise, allure. Perhaps this is one of the many indefinable qualities which men try to explain when they are asked, " What do you men *see* in her ? "

Here's another camera-timing trick that you can use. When you move your head and eyes, the eyes should move first and then the head follows. For example, suppose that to-day your set calls for you to be seated in an office when someone enters. Your eyes should lead out first to see who approaches and *then* your head should follow. *Most people use their eyes and heads together, thereby diminishing by half the power of their facial expression.* Fish move their heads and eyes together. You've heard people speak of that " fishy " look or stare. It took Walt Disney to put eyelashes on his fish and have them move their eyes *alone,* thereby creating tons of " come-hitherness."

FIT TECHNIQUE TO ROLE

In the theatre, this use of eyes and head TOGETHER is called " dead pan." It is employed only for character portrayal—for strange, eccentric, prim, vicious, or definitely typed parts. Yet many women attempt to play leading lady with a character actress's technique ! Then they wonder why they miss the boat !

Try it out for yourself. Go to a mirror and move your head and eyes together. Now, try letting your eyes lead first, and then your head follow. The latter is so much more commanding that there is no comparison. And the difference in time is but a second, if that. The first is dull, expressionless, flat ; the second is arresting, intriguing. This, then, is your first timing trick which fulfils two ultimate laws of poise-building : (1) You increase the restraint of your head ; and (2) you enhance the expression of your eyes.

Begin immediately to be conscious of this " timing " in your facial expression. (See One of the great disadvantages which

the inexperienced actor has to contend with in Hollywood is that often his eyes are not picked up by the camera. This is what the film critics mean when they say that the angles were poor. It means that the player seemed weak because his eyes were not seen clearly, and therefore his audience missed the necessary timing between head and eyes. You aren't at the mercy of one camera. You can be at your best all the time.

To help my students practise this timing until it becomes habitual, I have worked out a dead-pan exercise that you will find later in this Lesson on page 18

You may not be completely satisfied with the shape or colour of your eyes. Frankly, you can do little about either, although correct eyebrow, eyelid, eyelining and eyelash make-up will enhance their femininity.

Let me say at once that I think EVERY woman should use eye make-up, and she should use it day and night. Not enough to look artificial, but enough to make her eyes glamorous. You will find these skills discussed in detail in Lesson Two on Make-up. At present, I am more interested in talking about basic techniques for using your eyes.

You know that your thoughts register almost immediately in your eyes. " The eyes are mirrors of the soul " is almost a daily remark. Yet many women believe they can think unkind, unjust, malicious thoughts and not convey them to others.

I believe it would take many years' study to be such a proficient actress, and even then, those years could be so much better spent ! Improve your attitudes, and your eyes will immediately register warmth.

However, I do think it's possible to overdo this school of " Be a good girl and people will like you."

During the years I've been teaching I've made a study of the most dislikable women in my classes during the first sessions.

Then later, when I know those same girls and women better, I invariably like them. Usually they are women of fine qualities. Together we analyse their facial habits which repel those they meet for the first time.

Are you guilty of any of the same habits ?

First of all, when you talk to people, do you look directly into their eyes ? I am not advocating that you stare with such fixity of gaze that you embarrass people, as though to prove you're as good as the next one. But I do think while you are saying, "How do you do, Mr. Johnson?" that you should look as pleasant and steadfast as possible.

Learn to see people with an "overall look." You see their hair, clothes, gestures, without giving the impression of an appraisal. Some of the prettiest women become shrewish-looking because of their quick "once-over." This habit is especially repugnant to men. Clever men take a good look when a woman's back is turned.

Don't look at any imperfection in a person. For instance, some women stare at a mole on the chin or an obviously false tooth.

One woman told me that bald heads were her downfall—they fascinated her because she was constantly amazed at how much territory men covered with so few hairs ! *There is nothing about a person as important as the person !*

If you watched Gene Tierney meet and chat with a roomful of strangers, you would notice that her eyes seem to say, " I'll like you until you prove I shouldn't."

Many otherwise charming women make the mistake of looking at you right off with measuring eyes that ask, " H'm, what is it about you that you're hiding?" Usually they aren't thinking anything like this at all, but you *feel* that they are.

A trick every film star learns is to smile with her eyes as well as her lips. Watch Lana Turner's eyes. After her first test, her Cameraman said, "She lights up all over."

Think only pleasant thoughts as you listen to a friend or someone you've just met. THINK a smile. Smile with your eyes. You will be more flattering to the average person if you smile at his joke or anecdote and look directly into his eyes with understanding than if you throw your head back and laugh heartily as you look away.

This ability to smile with the eyes makes for true radiance. Frank Crowinshield, the famous editor of *Vanity Fair*, said of Clare Booth Luce : " I have seen her surrounded with more beautiful women, but there is a light and a radiance about her that gives her an individual glow."

Robert Quick, Paramount sound technician, told me of the day in Bermuda when the Duchess of Windsor first visited the sound set on which he was working.

He described briefly her simple dress, but spent considerable time explaining a quality of warmth that every man sensed immediately. He said, " It had been a long, hot day, and we weren't accustomed to the weather. A half-minute after she came in, and spoke to each of us, we forgot the weather and everything unpleasant. We sat back, relaxed, and frankly enjoyed watching her and listening to her.

" I've been in the film business for twenty-two years, and have worked with the most glamorous stars, but Wallis Windsor will always represent this quality of—well—radiance, I suppose it's called. She could have been dressed in sackcloth and she still would have had it." That, I think, is a tribute worth any woman's effort !

The most radiant, compelling eyes I have ever seen belong to Eleanor Roosevelt. I find that I watch them almost to the exclusion of listening to what she says.

Here's a way to tell how well your eyes register: Hang a mirror near your 'phone so that you can study your face from your eyes upwards. Can you honestly tell when you're happy ? Or are the little smile wrinkles around your eyes the only obvious indication that you're happy ?

In addition to guarding against wrinkling the area around your eyes as you *think* a smile, practise smiling as an actress does, without closing your eyes. If your eyes persist in shutting partially, hold them open with your fingers a few times. You see, if as you smile you close your eyes too much, you lose the most radiant feature you possess during the moments when you are happiest and should, therefore, share the most happiness with others.

June Allyson closed her eyes too much in her first picture, and although it was " cute," I notice that this was remedied in her subsequent films.

By learning to laugh with your eyes open, you can also avoid additional wrinkles around your eyes and soften those already there. It's worth the effort, isn't it ?

Directors often speak of " old, tired eyes." Unfortunately, they often have young owners. The actress knows she must guard against this bored, disinterested look.

Joan Crawford's eyes are as lovely and fresh to-day as the day she made her first picture.

Claudette Colbert's are, too. One important technique that an actress learns, to ensure young, animated eyes, is that of blinking. Simple as it sounds, the one surest and quickest way to bring back into your eyes that lustre and warmth which was yours when you were fourteen, is to begin *blinking*.

Watch the women you know. They blink only every *now* and *then*. Yet this is the one and only method Nature provided for relaxing the eyes during waking hours.

By blinking, then, you will not only be fulfilling a health function for your eyes, but you will look years younger. Try it. Blink. BLINK A LOT. I don't mean silly or cheap-looking batting of the eyelids—I mean intelligently registering your emotions and thoughts with your eyes.

You are missing one of your surest paths to fascination if you are overlooking the magical witchery encompassed in a pair of sparkling, understanding eyes under fluttering and animated eyelids. And don't forget the greatest captivation of all—look away quickly—or look down !

Many people have lost the muscular control necessary to blink. Any eye specialist will tell you what a common fault this is. Watch yourself in a mirror as you blink. Use only the *lids* for blinking.

If you make wrinkles around your eyes and on your forehead when you try to blink, then hold the skin firmly around your eyes with your fingers and put wrinkle plasters on your forehead as you practise blinking. The eye exercises in this Lesson will also help you to avoid making these squints and wrinkles.

Eyes, Barometer of Age

As one of the most powerful examples of the important part which eyelid movement plays in denoting age, I like to cite Helen Hayes' portrayal in *Victoria Regina*. You will recall that when Miss Hayes first comes on the stage as a young girl in her teens, and is told that she is the new ruler of the mighty British Empire, she is wearing long, dark lashes. And much of her enthusiasm and youthfulness is apparent from the manner in which she uses them, blinking repeatedly. Then you see her at about twenty years of age, enticing the man she wishes to marry. She is gay, vivacious, flirtatious, and again these qualities are demonstrated largely by her eye work. Her blinking seems to be timed.

Next follows her famous " boudoir scene " with her young husband. She registers every inflection of femininity with her eyes, even more than with her speech.

Every man who saw her was entranced with that particular scene. There is quite a jump in age sequence until you see her as the mother and busy wife. She is still charming, but there is a definite feeling of maturity. Her eyes have settled down, so to speak, blinking less and less, looking so much like those of thousands of women on buses and streets.

Finally, in the last act, as the ninety-year-old queen, she is wheeled on to the stage for the celebration of her birthday. To portray convincingly this age, Miss Hayes has her eyelids painted pink, her eyelashes powdered white, her eyes staring straight in front of her, and her eyes blink only about ONCE IN FIVE MINUTES ! You wonder how they could be controlled so well. She *was* old !

Here is one of the truly skilful actresses of our day. She uses only the most powerful weapons for her portrayals. She knew that in addition to voice, costume and make-up, her eyes would be the convincing agent in adding years to her character. And not the eyes alone, but also the movement of the eyelids. So, if you wish to play a role ten or fifteen years older than yourself, go right ahead ignoring your eyelids and your blinking !

Eyes Can Be Over-used

Perhaps I should pause here and warn you against the over-use of the eyes. Some women, in their endeavour to register interest, dilate their eyes unbecomingly. It's a habit like so many other unpleasant things. To effect a telling attitude with the eyes—and sometimes it is necessary to feel we are affecting one—think " I am interested, but I must not spoil it by overdoing it."

Don't consciously flirt with your eyes when you are in public. Nothing so embarrasses a man. There is a time for everything. Think how few times you have seen a well-bred man make a display of emotion in public.

Exercises for Schooling and Use of the Eyes

Here are a few eye exercises which you may do to help control the muscles around your eyes and prevent your forehead from wrinkling as you blink.

It is encouraging to realize that the eyes react to exercise faster than any other part of the body. I can always tell within a week if a student has been working with her eyes. Perhaps you know of an instance in which a friend of yours has been able to do without glasses partially or entirely, after wearing them for years, just by consistently strengthening the eye muscles through exercises, given under the direction of an eye specialist.

If exercise helps those really serious cases, think what you can accomplish for your eyes by just adding light and warmth to them.

Copy 'hese exercises on small, stiff cards, and put them where you will see them often in your car, on the door of your wardrobe or kitchen, in your handbag or purse. Practise until you can do them from memory whenever you are waiting for the children at school, for the dentist, or for your husband.

Remember, the first rule of all work in personal growth is this : *It is the thing which you do consistently every day for three minutes which is more beneficial to you than that which you forget for a week and then work on diligently for an hour.* And I repeat here that the colour and shape of your eyes aren't as important as how you use them !

1. Your first eye exercise is a simple one, but many of our most prominent players have used it. Do it twenty times daily, but I recommend that you start by doing it only once or twice. Open your eyes as wide as you possibly can, then shut them as tight as possible, contracting all the muscles around the eyes as you do so. Hold them tightly shut for a few seconds. Then open again, and repeat. If you get so that you can do this one with your face submerged in lukewarm or cool water you will get much more benefit from it. Don't practise it for the first time just before a date—you may get water in your nose and make it red !

2. These next two eye exercises are also intended to help control the eyes without over-using any other part of the face. The first one is called the " Spoke Wheel " exercise. (See Figure 4.) Imagine that your eyes are the centre of a large wheel. Check your head posture to be sure that your ears are on a straight line with your shoulders, and that your head is straight.

Now, look briskly up to the ceiling (Position 1) without moving your head. Blink smartly two or three times, and bring your eyes back to centre and blink again. Repeat in this direction six times.

Next, move your eyes to Position 2, blink two or three times, and come back to centre and blink

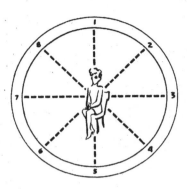

Figure 4

hard several times. Repeat this path six times. Then, look as far to the right as possible, or to Position 3, blinking and coming back to centre six times. Now, six times to Position 4. Next, down to the floor, or Position 5, head perfectly still, eyes blinking and coming back to centre six times. To position 6 ; blink, back to centre, blink six times, to the left as far as you can see, or Position 7, six times, without moving your head ; up to Position 8, blink, and back to centre six times. Keep blinking constantly.

Practise it until you can count quickly : One, blink (thus going from centre to first position) ; two, blink ; three, blink ; four, blink ; five, blink ; six, blink.

Be sure only your eyes are moving. You may have to hold your head to keep it still. Then on to the next position until you have completed the whole circle. Don't be alarmed if you feel this. Remember, you are just using a group of muscles which have been sluggish for years.

3. Your next routine is for adding more life to your eyes, and is called the " Eye Pendulum " exercise. (See Figure 5.). Think of an upper half-circle. Check your head posture again, and keep your head still by holding your chin in your left hand. Now, look to the left as far as you can. Then, with your right hand, trace a large upper half-circle and follow it with your eyes, going as far to the right as you can see without moving your head. Swing your eyes back to the left again.

Repeat this pendulum motion six times, blinking as briskly and as often as possible. Count : one (describe large half-circle), blink ;

two, blink; three, blink; four, blink; five, blink; six, blink. Get into the swing of it. Don't do it languidly.

When you have finished the upper half-circle, then repeat with a lower half-circle. Do these several times a day.

Try them lying down with your head lower than your feet, or your head hanging over the bed. Notice the little upward pull these eye routines give to that area which is inclined to sag around the eyes.

This is one of the very few things you *can* do to help tighten the skin there, once it has become loose or stretched.

4. Doctors who recommend eye exercises suggest that you look far away from what you are doing several times each hour, just for a second. If you are reading or sewing or doing exacting work in an office, then by all means form the habit of looking out of a window for a second at the farthest object you can see. If a window isn't near, then glance towards the farthest wall, and blink.

5. *Dead-pan exercise.* Check your head position, as you learned previously. See that your ears are on a straight line with your shoulders. Pull up strenuously behind the ears, and raise your chin in front just a fraction of an inch. Keep your head in this position.

Now, raise your eyes straight in front of you as far as you can toward the ceiling. Then let your head slowly rise so that you look up. Making your head stay in this position, look down at the floor with your eyes.

Now, lower your head. Lift up your eyes to centre front, and raise your head slowly. Look to the right as far as you can with your eyes

alone. Now, let your head turn. With your head in this position, look up to the ceiling with your eyes, your head slowly following again. Next, look to the floor with your eyes, your head following.

With your head still turned to the right, look over your right shoulder at the floor with your eyes alone. You may feel quite a muscular pull, but it is good for you. Now, lower your head. Stretch, stretch that neck and double chin. Look up at the ceiling still over your shoulder, your head following. Bring your eyes back to centre front and then your head.

Repeat the exercise, this time to the left. Practise this for several days. Make your head follow your eyes all day long and especially while you are with others. Your eyes will take on new interest because they are learning control, and you will be more poised because your head is still.

A STAR IS BORN

Many film stars have taken a course in visual eye education to help themselves withstand the glare of the studio lights. Often they do not need actual sight correction, but they value the ability to relax the eyes, which they learn. This relaxation also helps to relieve those wrinkles caused from tension around the eyes. Dr. W. H. Bates, a pioneer in the eye education field, describes one method of eye relaxation, or " palming."* He writes : " All the methods used in the eradication of errors of refraction are simply different ways of obtaining relaxation, and most people, though by no means all, find it easiest to relax with their eyes shut. This usually lessens the strain to see, and in such cases is followed by a temporary or more lasting improvement in vision.

" Most people are benefited merely by closing the eyes ; and by alternately resting them for a few minutes or longer in this way and then opening them and looking at a test card for a second or less, flashes of improved vision are as a rule very quickly obtained. Some temporarily obtain almost normal vision by this means, and in rare cases a complete restoration has been effected, sometimes in less than an hour.

" But some light comes through the closed eyelids, and a still greater degree of relaxation can be obtained, in all but a few exceptional cases, by excluding it. This is done by covering the

* Dr. W. H. Bates, *Better Eyesight Without Glasses* (London : Faber & Faber, Ltd.).

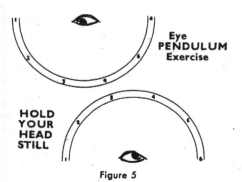

Eye
PENDULUM
Exercise

HOLD
YOUR
HEAD
STILL

Figure 5

closed eyes with the palms of the hand (the fingers being crossed upon the forehead) in such a way as to avoid pressure on the eyeballs. (See Figure 6.) So efficacious is this practice, which I have called 'palming,' as a means of relieving strain, that we all instinctively resort to it at times, and from it most people are able to get a considerable degree of relaxation."

Practise this " palming " method of relaxation between your other eye exercises. *It's not only splendid for the eyes, but it's also one of the most effective relaxation exercises I know for the whole body.*

It may take you five or ten minutes to memorize these eye exercises. After that, you'll find many occasions during the day to work them into your programme. You'll get such quick relief of tension from them that you'll enjoy them—to say nothing of the years that you'll take away from the appearance of your eyes !

"Upsy-daisy." The last eye technique but by no means the least important is the benefit of lying in an inverted position. Place two pillows under your hips and lie on the floor with your feet on the bed. Or lie on your bed with your feet up on the headboard. You'll get better results by lying on a board—an ironing board or a surfboard will do. Eventually, you'll want a board made up with a permanent stand padded and wide enough for comfort (See Figure 6), so that you can relax on it every available minute. If you have to wait to carry a board from behind the door, you won't use it as often as one which is a permanent piece of furniture. Let your friends raise their eyebrows at your peculiar chaise longue !

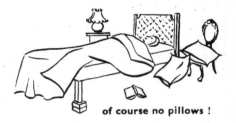

Begin with a two inch block then increase to a four inch block

of course no pillows !

Figure 7

The important thing is to try to lie with your feet about fourteen inches higher than your head, at least fifteen minutes daily. If you have a telephone cord that will reach your " upside-down " board, what could be a better position for your telephoning ? You can feel the blood rushing to your head and neck, and this extra stimulation is as beneficial for your eyes as for your hair and face. Haven't you noticed how often doctors recommend this position after an operation ? And have you also observed how much younger and rested a woman looks after even a strenuous period in hospital ?

You are getting a rest, too, from that severe pull of gravity. Dr. LeRoy Lowman, ortho-paedic specialist, says that lying with the feet higher than the head also tightens the abdominal muscles. It is, therefore, not only a beautifier but also a relaxer. Many stars owe their day-long sparkle to a few minutes' rest on the set in this position. In fifteen minutes you feel as refreshed as though you'd had an hour's nap, with none of the sleepy after-effects of the latter. You may get so that you sleep for a couple of hours this way.

Adhering to this same inverted principle of extra stimulation for the head and neck area, you may wish to put a peg or block under the foot of your bed. (See Figure 7.). Begin with a two-inch block, and increase it over a period of months to four inches. You'll look and feel younger and better for it ! AND, OF COURSE, NO PILLOWS !

With such potent aids as these for your neck and eyes, there's no reason why yours shouldn't be lovely, is there ?

Palming

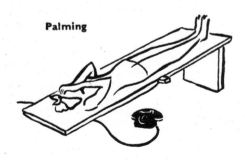

Figure 6

LESSON ONE
Part B
Inviting Lips

*Mouth ; In man, the gateway to the soul ; in
woman, the outlet of the heart.*
—*Devil's Dictionary*

MEN admit that they often judge a woman's disposition by her lips. Whether or not they have any basis for their judgment, they don't like women with thin, tight lips ! They're afraid she's selfish, calculating, cold. Phoebe Cary did us a lot of harm with her now-famous quotation, " And though hard be the task, keep a stiff upper lip." I think that no task is worth tight, compressed lips !

Look at your favourite film star's lips. They are full, soft, appealing. They are young lips. If with accomplishment a woman loses her femininity she ceases to attract. Thus, every attractive woman wants to incorporate a few techniques that will keep her lips feminine. Leave those firm executive lips to men !

Do master a professional lip make-up. Improve upon nature in colour and shape by learning to use a lipstick pencil. During World War II Winston Churchill in lifting the ban on lipstick said, " Scarlet stiffens the spine." In four words he practically waved lipstick into the necessity class. You will get complete details on lip make-up in Lesson Two. Right now, let's consider the lip techniques that keep our star's lips lovely throughout the years.

KEEP THEM FLEXIBLE

Your first rule is to keep your lips flexible. Rigid lips make your whole face tense, and this ages you.

The simplest and most effective exercise I know for flexible lips is to blow into them. Take a deep breath and blow against your lips until they flap. Blow hard. Alternate this blowing by saying the word " yawn " slowly. Stretch your lips as you say the " y," drop your jaw wide open on the " aw," and stretch them again on the " n."

After this stretching, blow again. You'll find a second or two for this several times daily—or hourly—if you really want to improve your lips.

Of course, you must discriminate between flexible lips and those which have a loose, flabby look. Also don't over-use your lips. Such over-use in the theatre is called " mugging." A stage actress may get away with a certain amount of it, but a film star has to guard against it constantly.

On the screen, a star's face is enlarged so many times its true life-size that every slight movement is magnified. To guard against any tendency towards " mugging ", she has learned to speak pleasantly without undue lip action. The jaw and lips are relaxed, but they needn't be stretched into unpleasant habits. You've seen the woman who " talks all over her face ! " Usually, she's the victim of poor speech habits.

One of my convictions about enduring facial beauty is the necessity for sound speech methods. So many women write asking why stars retain their beauty so long. They cite an actress like Irene Rich, who is as youthful and as vibrant to-day as she was twenty years ago. My answer is that *those high rounded planes on the face are the result of good speech training.* Ethel Barrymore's face at sixty-seven had no cruel downswept lines.

If these actresses had some secret cosmetic formula for everlasting youth, other women would soon know about it ! The vast cosmetic houses would find a way to make it available to women throughout the country. It isn't a question of cosmetics solely. There is no tutor who values more than I the importance of a corrective make-up. But the minute the face gets into action, the speech habits must be pleasing or they destroy the illusion of beauty.

It's a matter of common sense. Suppose that each time a woman says the letter " o " she drops her jaw an inch, at the same time rounding her lips into a perfect circle.

Since "o" is such a common letter in our alphabet, she says it dozens of times daily. Isn't it reasonable that this one speech habit deepens the hollows in her cheeks and the wrinkles around her lips? Add to this, other improper, ageing speech habits.

Go to the mirror and say "o" as I have described its formation here. (See Photograph 2.) See what I mean?

Since the beginning of sound Pictures, Hollywood has learned that *you can have pleasant-sounding as well as pleasant-looking speech.* For example, where the "o" is concerned, now hold your lips naturally and pronounce it.

The muscles inside your mouth round somewhat and do most of the job. I have written a book on the speech phase of beauty.

Here I should like to point out only the outstanding sounds which mar the appearance of your lips. They are the sounds of " oo, " " ee, " " p, " " h, " "w, " " g, " and " y. " Exaggerate the sounds of each in a mirror, and judge whether you are " mugging " as you say them.

Try these words : Who, green, poor, gay, yacht. With just a little practice, you can learn to pronounce them correctly and STILL KEEP THE LOWER PART OF YOUR FACE ATTRACTIVE.

This is an opportune spot to mention the unsightliness of lipstick on the teeth. Owners of thin lips have the most trouble in this respect.

An overdose of poorly applied lipstick may cause some of it, but on the whole, it is caused by forming the consonants "f" and "v" incorrectly. Watch yourself as you say fuss, friend, vacant, vanity. Do your upper teeth close on the FRONT part of your lower lip? Then it's easy to see why you get more than your share of lipstick on your teeth, isn't it? Instead, place your upper teeth on the BACK part of your lower lip, where there is no lipstick. Your "f" and "v" are just as well enunciated—and you've cleared the lipstick area !

USE A MIRROR

You needn't have special speech lessons to improve your facial habits. Put a mirror near your phone or near a spot where you can watch yourself occasionally as you talk with friends.

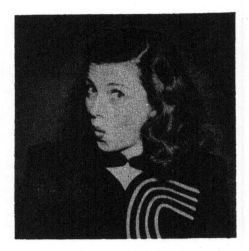

Photograph 2. Lenore Aubert illustrates what you should never do with your mouth.

You'll have your best critic right there.

Chiefly, it's a combination of knowing you're not appearing at your best, and of correcting the reasons for it.

Men, particularly, dislike seeing a lovely face twisted and "mugged" out of its loveliness. It's strange but true that women aren't as conscious of this fault as men.

This may be another reason why a plain woman who has facial poise is often more attractive to men than a handsome or pretty woman who repels or displeases with over-animation.

I trust that the emphasis I've placed on controlled use of the muscles of the face will not be confused with a heavy, dull expression.

Every lecturer has tried unsuccessfully to lighten the dejected countenance of some women in the audience.

The amazing aspect of this so-called "sourpuss" is, that she will often come up to you afterwards and tell you how much she enjoyed your talk. To look at her, however you would still think she heartily disapproved of you !

It would be interesting, some time, to make a study of mothers who have pleasant expressions, and to see whether or not their children also have them. I think that a charming parent is the best insurance for good start in charm !

Just as parents who speak well and who have good posture, usually rear children who speak well and have good posture.

Failing this parental advantage, go to a tutor or a friend whose judgment you respect and ask :
(1) Is my face USUALLY PLEASANT ?
(2) When I am pleased or enjoying the moment, do I look it ?

Try another experiment : Watch any twenty women close to you in the theatre. Presumably they are there because they felt they would enjoy the show. What do their expressions tell you ? Do they appear happy ? Or do some look bitter, some sceptical, some " you'll-have-to-show-me"? You'll be fortunate if you find two uninhibited faces.

I spend hours telling my students the necessity of facial radiance. I'd be satisfied with mere pleasantness. I have to admit that I get fewer results in this one respect than in any other phase of teaching. There is this exception : The girl getting ready for the screen, who KNOWS that she has to " deliver the goods ! " And she also knows she won't be given long to show what she can do. Those who attend the cinema don't pay good money to see another dull, down-in-the-mouth face !

By now you are asking, " Well, what do you want ? We musn't use our faces too much, we must look poised, yet we mustn't look un-pleasant." You've answered the whole problem of an attractive face yourself.

If the movements that quickly etch them-selves on your face are controlled *and* pleasant, you never need envy a beautiful face. You notice that I say little about actual beauty itself. This is because in writing about great beauties for my newspaper, the ones the public selects as beautiful usually are not beautiful. Their faces have warmth and appeal. Capitalize on this by concentrating on a pleasant expression.

Learn to smile, even when you're not smiling. You may recall your father singing the ditty of " The smile that won't come off." True, there is nothing more insipid than an empty, forced grin.

You can be serious, sombre ; but keep the corners of your lips up. Your lips may be together in moments of repose, but feel that they are relaxed. Don't clamp your teeth together

tightly and expect your lips to be relaxed. When you speak, show as much of your upper teeth as is comfortable.

Speak, for a moment, into the mirror. How much of your teeth do you show ? If your upper lip has already dropped to the extent that you can't see any of your teeth, then practise a few lip exercises, because a dropped upper lip makes you look fifty years older.

LIP EXERCISES

Here are two good lip exercises :

1. Turn your upper lip up. Try to touch your nose with it. Turn the lower lip down. The muscles of your lips may be so weak that they won't budge. Be patient. Use your fingers. Keep working with them. You'll soon get some control.

2. Raise your upper lip until you can see your upper gum. Push it up with your fingers if necessary. Don't let the muscles around your eyes push up, though ! Don't be alarmed if you feel muscles trembling on this.

You may be concealing your teeth because you feel that their irregularity is so ugly. You are losing more than you are gaining. You're hiding a few crooked teeth, and your whole expression is heavy and dull.

Doesn't it seem reasonable that a smile and a radiant, pleasing appearance will more than offset what you consider your defect ? (Of course, I take it for granted that you've done everything in your power to have your teeth as presentable as possible).

In speaking, the corners of your lips should strike what speech coaches call a neutral position —turned neither up nor down.

There is not one speech sound in English which calls for down-turned lips. (I wish I were enough of a linguist to check this fact in so far as other languages are concerned.). Since this is true why do we see so many turned-down expressions? I say : Most women don't KNOW.

I notice, in my classes, that when I discuss this seriously, each woman agrees about the importance of a pleasant face. But almost every woman there will be agreeing with an UNPLEASANT face.

Ninety-six per cent. of our adult women read the advertising campaigns against body odours.

INVITING LIPS

Seventy per cent. feel that these advertisements couldn't apply to them.

This same principle applies to women and their expressions. They think that because they FEEL all right, they show it ! Often, they don't. Make sure you aren't one of these women.

After you're satisfied about your eye techniques, put your mirror by the telephone, so that you see only your lips. Watch them as you talk, over a period of a week. You may receive a surprise. You may even realize that the habits you are criticizing in your daughter or friend are stamped right on your own lips ! Then instead of being discouraged, get busy forming appealing mannerisms.

When you smile, let as many of your upper and lower teeth show as possible. Study a smiling picture of Bette Davis or Esther Williams. You can practically see their molars !

When you were in your teens, you probably felt " toothy," and consciously tried to conceal some of your teeth. You may have succeeded so well that to-day you have a cramped, forced smile.

I heard of a large concern which employed a special tutor to teach salesmen how to smile. The salesmen were, at first, resentful ; but since this course was paid for during office hours, they had to attend. One by one the tutor impersonally showed the salesmen where they could improve the sincerity and " quality " of their smiles.

Soon, sales began to improve. The men admitted they felt surer of themselves. They seemed to get better receptions. Why shouldn't a technique that sells a star to millions be just as valuable to a professional salesman ?

One airline trains hostesses to smile ONCE EVERY SENTENCE. I thought that was overdoing it, but after talking with the chief stewardess, I walked from the airport thinking of her as one of the most charming girls I'd ever met. In trying to analyse her charm for my newspaper, I decided it was her engaging manner of smiling.

From time to time you see pictures of an actress snapped in some night spot with a society figure. The actress may be in her forties and the debutante only eighteen, but because the star is a technician in handling her lips and showing much vitality through her " lip break," it is she who looks young and vital, and perhaps

the young girl who looks bored and sullen with her lips together.

Here are some fundamental camera techniques for smiling :

1. Don't smile with your lips together. This gives you a pulled Cheshire cat grin.

2. Don't be afraid that smiling will cause wrinkles. (Lesson Two will explain in detail correct massage for preventing and softening wrinkles around your mouth.)

3. Don't close your eyes when you smile.

4. It's better to smile too much than too little.

You don't have to inherit a fortune to favour those around you with cheerfulness. I contend that it's all right for the poets to eulogize those rare smiles that break occasionally from grey skies ; but for everyday appeal put your faith in frequent smiles.

Personally, I don't know any other one quality that wins friends faster than the ability to smile and be pleasant when things go wrong. Remember how the men flocked to see Myrna Loy in the *Thin Man* series with William Powell ? She played the type of wife every man wants—the one who can be decorative as well as a real pal.

YOU CAN IMPROVE

As you read these lip techniques, you may be discouraged because your lips are thin, undeveloped, weak !

I wish you could follow me around for six months and see what my students do for their lips with practice and determination.

Although I never admit it, there are many times when improvement has surpassed my hopes.

I shall never forget the student who practically reshaped one side of her lips with exercise. She was about twenty-four, had never had a boy-friend.

A man in a drunken moment asked her why she sneered all the time. That did it ! Her doctor confirmed the fact that there was no reason for one side of her mouth to droop. He recommended lip exercises. Make-up helped too, and to-day her lips looks normal and she's happily married.

Often, self-consciousness will seemingly paralyse the lips. This tension, in turn, affects the action of the tongue and jaw.

Speech authorities, like Dr. Mario Marafiati, who was Caruso's teacher, will tell you that the personality of your voice is dependent largely upon the combined motion of lips, tongue and jaw. *This sound shaping, then, is not done mysteriously in the diaphragm or windpipe, as some speech teachers would lead you to believe.*

Therefore, when the lips are incorrectly manipulated, the tongue and jaw usually are also deprived of functioning to best advantage.

For instance, when an individual speaks with the lips held in a tight, unnatural position, or when the lips " over-mug " it is the tongue itself which is not being properly managed in the mouth. If the tongue is handled incorrectly, or if it is tense or too thick or too active, any of these faults may react on the work which the lips should do and cause the lips to make an adjustment by either overworking or underworking. Such an adjustment has not only a marked effect on your voice, but it also has a serious effect on the whole appearance and expression of the face. You look older, because any over-working of the facial muscles causes wrinkles.

Fortunately, the tongue may be trained and exercised just like any other organ of the body.

Actors know the importance of keeping their tongues flexible, relaxed and controlled, because they realize that a stiff tongue or one which blocks the tones or one which is over-active, can alter the sound produced.

We find that successful radio performers spend a few minutes a day going over tongue gymnastics. Some of our finest speech schools and coaches to-day present the International Phonetic Alphabet. In this system, the student is taught where to place his tongue for every sound spoken. With this knowledge much of the guess-work is removed, and the student soon gets release from tenseness because the tongue is handled correctly.

The position of the tip of the tongue is usually behind either the lower or the upper front teeth, which helps to keep the sounds forward in the mouth. Contrast these two basic positions with those all-around-the-mouth tongues you so often see ! Their owners sound as though they have a mouthful of plums. On the other hand notice how little action there is in Bing Crosby's tongue, or that of Frank Sinatra.

Often, too, a stiff tongue may " colour " tones, so that they seem those of a much older person. In fact, character actresses who must at times impersonate people much older, often make their voices sound older by tensing the tongue.

Many of our more mature radio actresses have voices as young as a girl in her teens. Most of them admit they do their " tongue-twisters " as faithfully as the dancer goes over her routines constantly to keep her body in first-class form.

Here are a few tongue and jaw exercises which will improve your facial expression, your voice, *and* help to eliminate a double chin.

Then, too, if your face is thin, these exercises will help to fill it in. If your face is fleshy, they help to reduce it. They're so important that I hope you'll find a second here and there to work them in.

TRY THESE EXERCISES

1. *Tongue flap to strengthen and limber-up.* Place the tip of your tongue behind your upper teeth and direct as much breath as you need to cause the tongue to flap up and down about an eighth of an inch. When you can do this success-fully, add voice to it.

Start your tone as high as you can, beginning with your tongue on the hard palate. As your voice lowers, your tongue will flap nearer the tooth ledge, which is that flat surface just behind your upper teeth. Come down the scale with your tongue roll and then go up again.

This is a real tongue exercise, so do it several times a day as you are driving, dusting, walking,

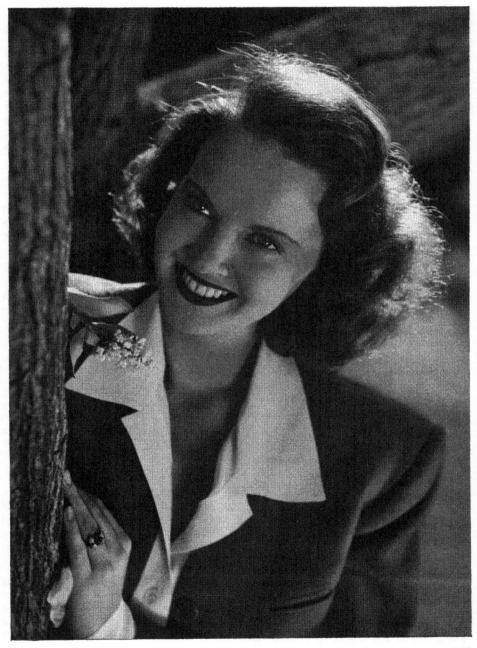

Photograph 3.   Lucille Bremer's radiant eyes bring added warmth to her attractive smile.

and so forth.

2. *Tip tongue roll.* If the tip of the tongue is tense, the lips and often the muscles around the lips try to assist with the tongue's work. This adjustment often causes premature wrinkles around the mouth.

You often see people who seem to have difficulty in speaking. This is not a real speech defect, but is traced to a tight tongue which is not performing its function and therefore produces this seeming handicap.

As mentioned, the greatest space that the tip of the tongue should move, in good English speech, is from behind the upper teeth to behind the lower teeth.

The faster the tongue shifts between these two positions, the clearer the sounds.

This particular exercise is designed to help this shifting motion. Separate your lips about three-quarters of an inch. Start the tongue off in position behind the upper teeth. Then rapidly push the tongue towards the outside of the upper lip and pull it into position again. Repeat this as fast as you can. Do it until you tire.

3. *Tongue trough.* A heavy, thick tongue which shapes unattractive vowels, can become more agile if properly exercised.

Push your tongue out of your mouth as far as you can. Hold it tense in this position while you count fifteen. Relax. This catches those unused under-the-tongue muscles.

Now push it out again as far as it will go, and pull the two sides of the tongue up to meet in the centre. If you can't manage this at first, put a long, thin object such as a knitting-needle along the centre of the tongue, and then push the sides up with your fingers.

Keep working with this until the tongue will accomplish it alone. When you can achieve the trough comfortably, here is your routine : Push the tongue out as far as you can from the trough position, and pull it back rapidly. Repeat twenty-five times.

4. *For tongue and jaw.* Separate your lips by the width of two fingers. Hold the two fingers there. With the tip of your tongue, touch the spot where your right upper wisdom-tooth is, or used to be.

Now, holding the jaw with one hand, so that it cannot move, shift the tongue over to the spot where the left upper wisdom-tooth is. Do this eight times.

Still holding the jaw still, touch the tip of the tongue to the two lower wisdom-teeth to the count of eight. Then make a tour of the two upper and the two lower wisdom-teeth, counting eight. The jaw will try to help you do this one, but you benefit only by insisting that the tongue do the work alone.

Since the muscles of the tongue are rooted in the jaw, it is desirable to keep the jaw flexible. Many tight, mechanical smiles originate in a tense jaw action. Say the letter " y " and let the jaw drop open, snapping it shut quickly. Repeat six times.

Practise these exercises regularly and you will find great improvement in your speech.

Self-Test Questions Based On Lesson One

Beauty of feature and clever make-up are not the only source of charm in a woman. You can attract by developing mobility of features, radiance, vivacity and poise. Every woman needs to practise at least some of the exercises in this first and all important Lesson.

After you have studied this Lesson you should be able to answer the following questions. If you have any difficulty in doing so, refer to the Lesson for further study and revision. Your answers should not be sent to the publishers of this Course.

1. What should you practise most if you wish to stand out in a crowd?

2. What should you master first in order to attain beautiful carriage?

3. How can you cure a double chin and dowager's hump?

4. What is a true smile? Have you practised this and followed out the suggestion in the Lesson?

5. What should you do to make your eyes alive and attractive?

6. What are the most effective of the exercises for resting the eyes and relaxing the whole body?

7. What is the first rule for cultivating inviting lips?

8. What is it essential to do correctly in order to avoid developing wrinkles?

9. What are the rules for an attractive face?

10. Have you arranged a mirror, as suggested, to enable you to watch your mouth and expression?

If you wish to determine the progress you are making, give yourself 10 points for each question you answer correctly. If the total comes to 90 or more, it is excellent; 80 or more, good; 70 or more, fair.

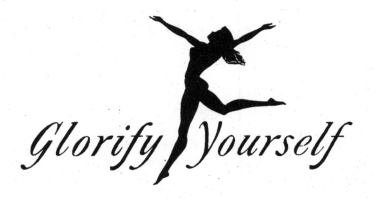

Glorify Yourself

★

A Complete and Up-to-Date Course on
Beauty and Charm by One of the
Most Famous Beauty Specialists
and Consultants in the World

Eleanore King

★

LESSON TWO

★

STUDIO TALK •

Issued only for Students of the Eleanore King Course on Beauty. Charm and Personality.

Number Two.

Dear Student,

You are about to commence your study of the Second Lesson in our Course.

Before we embark on the second stage of our journey, let us pause and look back at the ground we have already covered.

In Lesson One you were asked to master certain principles, and to practise a number of simple exercises. Don't be discouraged if you have not done as well as you expected to do. Remember what was said in the previous talk about not being able to learn to swim or dance in one lesson.

You should also remember that you learn much quicker and derive more benefit if you have a real interest in, and a genuine liking for the subject matter in hand. Of course, every woman is - or should be - interested in making herself more charming and attractive. You certainly must be, for otherwise you would not have enrolled for the Course. Nevertheless, it is a good idea for you to pause occasionally and think exactly what these Lessons can mean to you.

Your appearance and your behaviour can make the difference between success and failure. Personal attractiveness may mean the difference between riches and poverty, marriage or spinsterhood, happiness or a broken heart. Feminine appeal can be your most valuable asset: and in learning how to cultivate and exploit it, you will be adding not only to your own happiness and well-being, but also to the happiness of those with whom you come in contact.

Here's another vital point. We forget most readily just after new material has been learned for the first time. To combat this initial forgetting, you should go back now and then and re-read the previous Lessons, especially in the early stages.

May I suggest that you apply this important principle <u>now</u>? Before you go on to Lesson Two, re-open Lesson One, and go again over its most important teachings.

And when you come to Lesson Three re-read both Lessons One <u>and</u> Two.

By the way, there is no need for you to complete the Self-Test Questions unless you want to keep a permanent record of your progress; but they do help to bring out the highlights of each Lesson.

And now - forward to Lesson Two!

Yours sincerely,

Eleanore King

EK.2.

P.S. You can express your personality just by the way you stand! In Lesson Three you will learn how deportment can be an aid to glamour.

LESSON TWO

Part A

An Enticing Skin

I'll not shed her blood ;
Nor scar that whiter skin of hers than snow,
And smooth as monumental alabaster.
— Othello, SHAKESPEARE,

YOUR idea of a beautiful skin may not be "whiter than snow," but, as Shakespeare puts it, it should be " smooth as monumental alabaster." If there is one beauty standard common to the average man, it is that he likes and expects his ideal to have a nice complexion. Beautiful women through the ages have varied greatly in features and figures, but there is one common denominator that they all had and that is a beautiful skin. Or so we read ! *The encouraging element about a beautiful skin is that every woman can have one.*

Fortunately, fifteen minutes every day devoted to your skin will produce better results than a week of neglect and three hours of intensive steaming, massaging, packing and patting.

Make-up can do mysteriously magical things for you if you have a clear, smooth skin. In Part B of this Lesson you will learn the secrets of applying correct make-up. That is, make-up which will help correct irregularity of features, but first *you must have a smooth skin texture.*

How to care for your skin has been presented as such a complicated time-requiring subject that I find my students disgracefully confused about this whole phase of grooming. There are, no doubt, women who have leisure to follow elaborate schedules for taking care of their skin. But the busy mother, career girl, professional woman must make every minute count. Therefore, this Lesson on care of the skin will be designed for them and divided into the following phases : First, daily care of the skin schedule for (a) dry skin ; (b) oily skin ; (c) combination skin ; (d) teenage skin. Second, techniques for facial pick-ups. Third, care of blackheads and large pores.

Don't take a friend's advice for serious skin blemishes. You cannot afford to use wrong creams, lotions, emollients for an unhealthy skin. You may be doing the very thing which is harm-ful to it. *See a dermatologist.* A legitimate specialist is cheap in the long run. If you could see the number of ruined, scarred skins that have come to me for help, you would understand my urging you to be cautious about your skin condition.

On the other hand, I find that girls and women generally magnify their skin-condition faults. Hundreds of women with reasonably normal skins have come to me quite upset because they think their pores are too large—their skins too dry or too oily. They have instead, reasonably normal skins. You can consider yourself very fortunate if you have no blemishes, or really glaring skin faults. With a little care, a normal skin can become radiant, glowing, a definite asset.

Just as you would go to a dermatologist for serious blemishes, do consult his advice about removing moles and birthmarks. Also keep your face and body as free of hair as possible. It's normal to have some covering of hair, but any objectionable growth should be taken care of. Electrolysis is perhaps the most effective and lasting method. Be sure you go to a fully qualified operator. Many women bleach black hair, which makes it less objectionable. Every day you may have to yank out a few stiff, bristly hairs with your tweezers. Form the habit of looking for these ambitious sprouts each day, standing in front of a window where you have a good light. There are many depilatories in the form of waxes, and pastes on the market which will remove hair. Their results last from a few days to a few weeks. And rather than go around with repelling growths of hair, I would certainly recommend that you keep at all times a sharp razor which will, in an emergency, do a quick and clean job. By keeping plenty of cream and oil on these parts, you will avoid stiff bristles as the hair grows back in.

24-Hour Schedule

Before you consider your classification for dry or oily skin, let's talk about the fundamental basis for every lovely complexion : *bathing*. For a long time it was felt that a shower was as good for the skin as a bath. Today most authorities feel that a bath is more beneficial. You can make it as luxurious or sparkling as you wish. But *you should bathe five minutes once in every twenty-four hours when you are almost completely submerged in lukewarm water.* Work up a good, soapy lather and cover every part of your body. Rinse off, and use a body brush with the second lathering. Let the warm water out and add cooler water for the last half minute or so or duck in and out of a shower.

This is allowing minimum time. It's better if you can plan from fifteen minutes to a half-hour. Relaxation authorities feel that a bath has definite therapeutic value. If your feet burn, your back aches, or you are especially tired, add a couple of handfuls of Epsom Salts. *When* you take your bath depends on you. You may wish a bath at night and a quick shower in the morning. Let's suppose that you have taken a bath just before bedtime. Bathing is essentially for the neck down. Now let's concentrate on the neck and face.

Schedule for a dry skin. Research cosmeticians report that 87 per cent. of adult women's skins are considered dry, and they therefore require special care. Here is the type of 24-hour schedule which make-up artists like Jack Dawn, director of make-up at Metro-Goldwyn-Mayer Studios for twenty years, recommends for his contract players :

1. Don't go to bed without cleansing your face. THIS MEANS EVERY NIGHT.

The basis of all beauty care is skin cleanliness— this cannot be over-emphasised and it means not only washing the face with soap and water but the deep pore cleansing which results from using cleansing cream. Atkinson's cleansing cream is light and fluffy and liquefies very readily on the skin; it is excellent to use at the end of the day as it penetrates deep into the pores, clearing away not only the surplus dust and dirt which have been gathered during the day, but removing every trace of make-up, and that under-surface dirt which gathers under the skin and tends to make enlarged pores, even blackheads and pimples.

Apply the cream liberally to the face and neck and then massage in thoroughly, working up the neck to the chin line, then with firm stroking movements work along the jaw line, afterwards moving up the face to the cheeks, nose and forehead. Firm circular movements round the chin will help to clear away the little acid deposits which gather in this area, but you must be very gentle over the cheek bones and round the eyes, in the latter area in particular the skin should never be stretched as it is very fine and should be treated with extreme gentleness.

This massage should take approximately two to three minutes and then the surplus cream should be removed with little pads of cotton wool wrung out in warm water. The warmth of the water as well as the massage opens up the pores and helps the cream to do its deep cleansing action with great effectiveness. (See opposite page.).

Now you must think of softening your complexion—cover your face and neck with Atkinson's Night Cream or Skin Deep Nourishing Cream. The great benefits of these creams are that they soften the skin surface and help to round out the skin cells with both nourishing oil and health-giving moistures, so preventing dryness and deterioration.

The massage you use in applying it will help stimulate and tone your skin. Both the lubricating and massaging will postpone wrinkles, and will soften those you already have. A skin which is properly oiled and creamed always takes a more naturally radiant make-up, also.

Use plenty of cream. Massage it lightly into your face and neck. When you have finished the complete 24-hour cycle, you will find complete information and illustrations on massaging the skin. Right now, you're off to bed.

It's a pretty good idea to plan your before-bed duties in such a way that you can leave the cream on your skin while you rinse off your stockings, put up your hair, turn out the lights, etc. Even if it's late and you can't allow much time, do not omit the creaming drill entirely. Just before you doze off to sleep, wipe off the excess cream. It's a good idea, also, to form the habit of rubbing cream into your hands, elbows, feet, legs or any other part of your body that seems dry. Femininity is almost synonymous with softness. Your husband may have a distinct aversion to cream or " grease " of any kind, but you should try to win him to your way of thinking.

Creaming your skin is so important that you

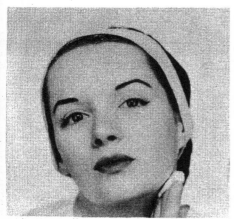

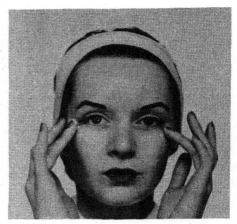

How to deep-cleanse —Be gentle, of course, and be generous, smoothing the cream into your skin with a circular, upward motion on the face and neck . . .

With the merest touch, pat the cream into the fine and delicate skin below the eyes, but with a firmer movement over the bridge of the nose, and around the nostrils . . .

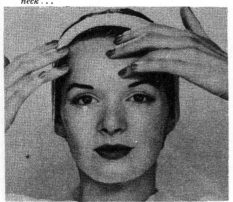

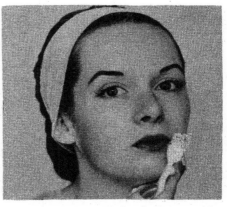

Then upwards and outwards from between the eyebrows across the forehead . . .

Remove the cream with a pad of cotton wool squeezed out in warm water, remembering always to use the same upward movement.

should give a great deal of attention to it. One screen star I know had the habit of applying a coat of castor oil to her whole body once a week, the night before the bed linen was changed. She tells of a time she stayed in a hotel with a linen shortage, and slept five nights in her castor-oil scented sheets. *Be sure you oil your body before exposing it to the sun.* BUT ANY WOMAN OVER TWENTY-FIVE SHOULD NOT EXPOSE HER FACE OR NECK TO THE SUN FOR MORE THAN THREE MINUTES

AT A TIME. She can get all the healthful benefits she needs from the sun by lying with her face and neck under an umbrella or in the shade but with the rest of her body exposed. If there isn't any other protection for the face and neck around, spread a bandana, handkerchief, scarf, or anything you can find, over your face and neck. The sun's reflection is strong enough to give you an even tan. You may feel that I am over emphasising the importance of lubricating the skin, but remember, dryness causes wrinkles, wrinkles make you look old, and a wrinkled skin soon sags and becomes loose. Do you recall Shakespeare's quotation from Henry IV ? " My skin hangs about me like an old lady's loose gown."

2. *Comes the dawn.* Your morning's skin schedule will depend upon your activities—upon whether you leave your home immediately after breakfast, or whether you stay at home and get your family off. But whatever your day is to be, cleansing must be your first consideration.

Wash your face and neck with a mild soap and warm water. Atkinson's Skin Deep Complexion Soap is ideal for this.

The most beautiful skins I have ever seen have been washed thoroughly at least once every twenty-four hours with soap and water. Don't use water that's too hot. Don't let anyone steam your face. Have two face flannels ; one for your face and neck, and the other for your body. Rinse and wring your flannels out well between usings, and hang them where they will get light and air. Many a girl owes her pimples to face cloths that hang on the *inside* of her wardrobe door. Bacteria flourish away from the light.

For lathering or soaping your face, use your hands and work a light lather into neck and face. Rinse this off. And then give a second soaping. Massage the lather well into the skin taking particular care of those areas where most of your blackheads and largest pores are. Use firm circular movements all over your neck and up into the hairline. (Incidentally, one of the characteristics of a great beauty is her clear-cut hairline, and this daily treatment will help accentuate yours). As you dry yourself, train your hair-line so it won't look wispy. Rinse this second soaping off with warm water and you may wish to use your flannel to help rinse your face at least for half-a-minute with cold water. Don't use ice on your skin. Dry your skin well. Then apply Atkinson's Toning Lotion; it is mild but very effective, closing the pores, bracing the skin, tissue and muscles and preparing the skin for make-up. (See opposite page.).

FACIAL PICK-UP

There comes some time during the day when you want to freshen up or change your make-up. Watching the habits of many famous beauties, it seems to me that part of their technique is taking the time to freshen up several times a day. If you've had your make-up on for six or seven hours and you want to look your best, you must start from scratch. The time element will determine how elaborate your schedule is.

Two-minute Facial Pick-up.

1. Cleanse your face and neck with cleansing cream. Wipe off.
2. Pat in Skin Toning Lotion.
3. Blot skin dry. (See opposite page.).

Fifteen-minute Facial Pick-up.

1. Apply cleansing cream and wipe it off.
2. Apply Skin Deep Facial Mask and rest with feet elevated. (See page **9** .).
3. Shower.
4. Pat in Beauty Mask Tonic.
5. Blot skin dry.

Thirty-minute Facial Pick-up.

1. Apply and remove cleansing cream immediately.
2. Apply softening cream.
3. Ten-minute bath.
4. After bath, apply Skin Deep Beauty Mask and rest for a few minutes. (See page **9** .).
5. Use Beauty Mask Tonic and blot skin.

24-HOUR SCHEDULE FOR OILY SKIN

Although you women with oily skins have the problem of shiny noses, and sometimes large pores and blackheads, you do not have to worry about premature wrinkles. Because of this excess oiliness, your skin will remain young-looking longer than any other type of skin. You need to take scrupulously good care of your skin, however, so that it will look fresh and feminine. Excess oil in the face looks dirty. To avoid this you will need to follow a simple but effective daily routine for the care of your particular type of skin.

Here is a simple one which many of our stars find successful. Before retiring, wash your face with lukewarm water and soap. The lukewarm water will give a good lather and you can then massage it into your face and neck like a cream. Rinse your face and then apply Cleansing Cream as for the Dry Skin routine. This double cleanse is most helpful in keeping the greasy skin in good condition. Further use the Skin Deep Beauty Mask about once a fortnight. It will refresh your complexion and help make-up to last (Continued on page 8)

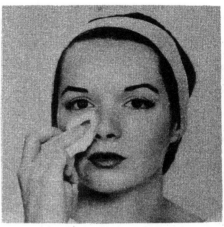

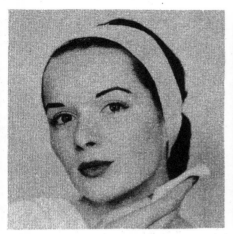

After cleansing your skin in the morning, soak a piece of cotton wool in Toning Lotion and pat it briskly in upward movements along neck and jawline . . .

And cheeks and forehead, not forgetting your nose, which especially wants attention.

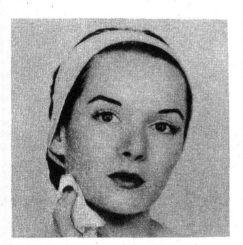

Now pat dry with a face tissue.

How to make the mask

Get a flat piece of cotton wool that's about 8 inches by 6 inches. Cut holes for eyes, mouth and nostrils, allowing quite large spaces for the eyes.

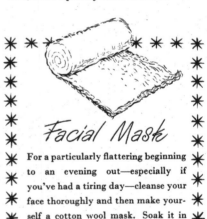

Facial Mask

For a particularly flattering beginning to an evening out—especially if you've had a tiring day—cleanse your face thoroughly and then make yourself a cotton wool mask. Soak it in toning lotion, secure it round your face with crepe bandage or a long strip of linen, and leave it on for ten minutes while you relax with your eyes closed.

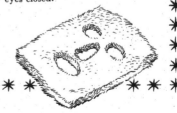

much longer.

If you are over thirty years of age with this type of skin, then start massaging a softening cream around your eyes and into your neck before you go to bed. Atkinson's Night Cream is beautifully balanced and will not add too much lubricant to your skin. Leave it on a few minutes while you roll up your hair or clean your teeth, and blot off the excess. Many times women do not use cream at all for fear of increasing oiliness, thus allowing their necks and the areas around their eyes to become wrinkled and crapy. Often, too, an oily face and very dry neck go together. To look young and unlined, a neck needs a lubricant daily, especially if its owner is over thirty.

In the morning wash your face again. You are the fortunate type who can wash your face as often as you wish and not have to worry about having your skin becoming flaky and causing your powder to cake. Any time during the day you wish to change your make-up, you do not have to go through a long creaming process in order to get your skin clean, either. *You must be meticulous, however, in changing your make-up often.* You should really change your make-up at least every four hours if you wish to compete with the fresh appearance of the girl whose skin is dry.

NORMAL SKIN OR COMBINATION SKIN

Women have written me asking what to do about skins which are a combination of oily or dry. Some complain that their noses and the middle area of their faces are oily and the rest of their skin is dry. *All of these women will be wise in following the routine for a dry skin given here.* You may wish to observe one exception. Whereas the woman whose skin is definitely dry should wash it only once a day with water, you, who fall into the half-and-half group may try water twice a day ; say, at night and upon arising. The minute your skin becomes a bit rough, though, you will know you must cut down on the extra washing and supplant it with cream cleansing. You can also be very liberal with Toning Lotion down the centre panel of the face, patting in the refreshing liquid quite firmly. (Refer to page 7.).

TEEN-AGE SKINS

Also, many teenage girls have asked what care they should give their skins. The routines given

here are so safe and sensible that even young girls may follow them. And I warn you young girls again to be careful that you do not leave cream or oil of any kind around those spots where the blackheads flourish. *If you are troubled with skin eruptions of any kind (and what teen-age girl isn't ?)* include as much fruit and vegetables in your diet as you can and take care to see that you don't let any dandruff from your hair fall on to your shoulders or touch your skin after touching your hair as infection can be set up in this way.

A clear, soft skin makes a bigger hit with the men than any other one single thing, girls!

You teen-agers can take sun baths for longer periods at a time than your older sisters. The sun alone clears up many pimples and blackheads.

HOW TO MASSAGE YOUR SKIN

How long should I massage my face ? Is it true that massaging one's own face is harmful ? These and many other questions confront the woman who wants to know how to take care of her skin. First of all, it is reassuring to realise that the woman who massages her own face and neck daily for perhaps five minutes will have a better chance of good results than the woman who neglects her skin most of the time and then strenuously tries to revive it for an occasional appearance. Massage as long as possible. But the important thing is to be positive that your massage is focused correctly and scientifically, so that each stoke is beneficial. Here, then, are the laws which our studio beauty consultants recommend :

1. Before beginning a massage, pin your hair up on top of your head. Tie a band around it for protection. A crepe bandage or an easily laundered cotton square is excellent.

2. *Do not rub your skin with a heavy movement.* Think of a feather being rubbed over your face, and try to make your movements imitate its lightness. Even though you feel your wrinkles are deep and definite, don't attempt to banish them by rubbing hard. Your fingers should slip over your face and neck *lightly* but firmly.

3. Patting movements can be very helpful under and on the chin and sides of the nose, but they must never be heavy.

4. Don't ever rub downward on your face

For special occasions –
Skin Deep beauty treatment

BEAUTY CREAM MASK

Whenever you want to look your loveliest have this wonderful beauty pick-up —Skin Deep Beauty Cream Mask. (Try it every few weeks, anyway—it's a wonderful tonic!) It soothes away tired lines and brightens dull complexions. The Cream Mask is ready to use in sealed sachets containing just the right quantity.

After thoroughly cleansing your skin, spread a thin layer of the Beauty Cream Mask over your face, chin and neck. Leave the area around eyes, lips and nostrils clear. Now place damp pads over your eyes and completely relax for a quarter of an hour. Rinse off the mask with warm water.

BEAUTY MASK TONIC

After the Cream Mask comes the finishing touch—the gently stimulating Skin Deep Beauty Mask Tonic. It makes your skin so fresh and radiant. Give yourself a Skin Deep Beauty Mask treatment whenever your complexion needs that little extra stimulus to bring out its true beauty.

Dry your face after you have rinsed off the Beauty Cream Mask, and then gently pat in the stimulating Beauty Mask Tonic. Now your skin is in the most perfect condition—and it looks it! Put on your evening make-up and go out looking absolutely wonderful.

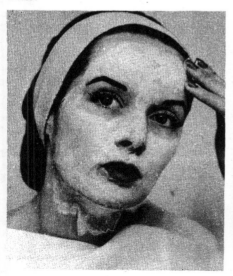 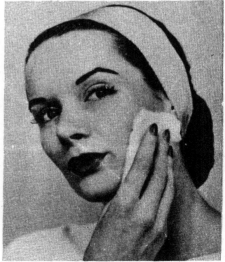

or neck. Your movements must always aim to counteract the downward tendency of sagging muscles. In other parts of this Course you learned posture exercises for your head and neck to further encourage this upward lift. Begin first by massaging the back of the neck. Place the fingers of both hands on the part of the spinal column at the back of the neck called the " dowager's hump." This is the one spot where you can rub rather firmly. Pull your fingers up your neck to the hairline. (See page 11). Repeat this stroke several times. Push your head back with each stroke to help you relax.

5. Then massage the sides of your neck by placing the palms of the hands on either side of the neck and rubbing up to the ear. (See page 11). Repeat this several times. It is much lighter than that used on the back of the neck. Next start on the front of the neck. Place the palms of your hands crosswise on the base of your neck, and lightly rub up the chin line. (See page 11). Repeat the same motion with the other hand, practising until you alternate the hands rapidly and lightly. Repeat several times.

Patting under the chin with the backs of the hands can break down the weight in the face, dispersing the fatty tissue.

6. Now, you are ready to massage the *face*. Begin with the chin line and gradually work up towards the forehead. in order to make your fingers as light as possible, place your elbows on your dressing table and cup the inside of your wrists together. Then your fingers are free from arm and elbow weight. With the inside of the wrists together, bring the finger tips together on the chin. Outline the jawbone from the chin to the ears by having the second, or index, finger of each hand underneath the bone and the other fingers above it. The second finger beneath will press a little harder than the ones above. Make this motion from chin to earlobe several times. Some specialists advise a moulding movement here to be alternated with massage. This is the part of the face where weight usually collects first and your aim is to keep the jawline as clear as possible.

7. With even lighter strokes, describe a line from your chin up to the middle of your ears. Then lift the fingers from the face and repeat

this same upward-line motion several times,

8. This time describe a line from the chin to the top of the ears, covering more of the cheeks each time. Repeat several times. Never make a return trip, however, with your fingers : that is, *don't bring them down from the tip of the ears to the chin.*

9. You are now ready to work on the expression lines around the mouth. Again, start at the base of the chin, bring the fingers in a light stroke to the corners of the lips. (See page 11). And then around the upper lip to the cupid's bow and press the two ridges of the bow together. Lift fingers and repeat this several times. If you have vertical wrinkles forming around your lips, look up the lip exercises I gave you in the Lesson on lips. *Massage alone cannot do the whole job.* Also, lightly describe little circles about one-half inch in diameter around your lips to eliminate these lines. (See Figure on page 11).

10. Another good massage trick for overcoming the downward turn at the corner of the lips is to place your thumb in the cupid's bow at the top of your lips, place your index finger at the corner of the mouth, and massage from the corner to the centre, lifting the lip tissue each time. Repeat as often as you wish ; and shift to the other side of the mouth, this time reversing the position of thumb and forefinger. Pinching the cupid's bow ridge of the upper lip together helps, too.

11. The next massage stroke begins at the corners of the lips and with little circular movements continue to the sides of the nose, the fingers meeting on the bridge of the nose. Repeat several times. This helps smooth out the " laugh line " which forms early from the nose to the corners of the mouth. You might. then put these last two motions, 10 and 11 together by starting at the chin, going to the corners of the mouth, up along the laugh line to the nose, and out over the cheeks to the ear. All the time using circular movements in an upward direction.

12. The wrinkles around your eyes get your attention next. *Here your strokes should be feather-light :* for once this skin is stretched, it can never regain its elasticity. Close your eyes, place two fingers on either side of the nose,

near the tear duct. Press rather firmly here to relax muscle tension. Then lightly move from the centre across the lid, around the sides of the temples, under the eyes, and back to the tear duct region again. (See Figure opp.). Thus your stroke is over the lid, around and under. Repeat several times. Do NOT massage under your eyes from the centre OUT toward the outside temples. *This is contrary to every rule of good massage and does much harm.*

There is another version of this eye massage technique. Place the third finger of your right hand on the outside corner of your right eye and with the third finger on your left hand, start at the outside temple of the eye, massage under the eye, pressing at the tear duct area before going up over the lid. The advantage of this is that the finger eliminates any tendency to stretch the skin under the eyes.

13. Crow's Feet. Flatten the skin with two fingers of one hand, and with the second and third fingers of your other hand make round circles over the wrinkle area. Be sure you don't stretch the skin in your attempt to flatten the wrinkle. By this time you are weary of hearing me say, use light strokes and don't stretch the skin. But unless you obey these two commands you are courting trouble.

In connection with prevention of wrinkles around the eyes, tinted glasses are very helpful as a protection against sun glare; they give the face a more composed appearance and can be very becoming.

14. You still have the forehead wrinkles to work on. They form both vertically and horizontally. These, again, are formed to some extent by exaggerated facial expression and your habit of frowning, and worry and sorrow add their share. Your strokes on the forehead may be stronger than on the rest of the face. For the up-and-down wrinkles caused by scowling unnecessarily, place your fingers at the bridge of the nose and work out towards the temples with a firm stroke. Repeat several times.

For the wrinkles which form crosswise, describe small circles about an inch in diameter over the entire brow and continue for two minutes. (See Figure opp.). Link this massage with the very effective eye exercises given in Lesson One, Part A.

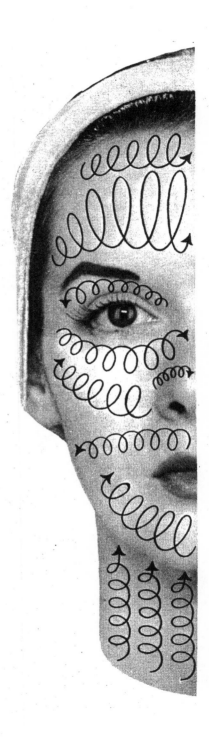

No matter how neglectful you have been in the care of your skin, you can get results if you faithfully adhere to a few correct massage strokes. You young women who do not have wrinkles can postpone them indefinitely with the same technique. Add to this, a determination not to allow every reaction you have to leave its impression on your face. Allow your facial expression to remain happy and serene.

You'll recall that I have stressed the importance of lying with your feet elevated higher than your head to stimulate the circulation.

How to Massage Your Hands and Arms

At night while you are creaming your face, put generous amounts of cream and oils on your hands, arms and elbows. Start with the finger tips and massage toward the knuckles. Stroke each finger separately as though you were trying on tight gloves. Then stroke up the arm from the wrist to the shoulder. Use a rotary motion in massaging the elbows. If they have become rough or inclined to show goose flesh use a soft nail brush, soap and warm water.

Plastic Surgery

As I have said before, many of my students have had their noses, breasts, chins changed by plastic surgery. As a result, there is often such a noticeable psychological change for the better if a competent plastic surgeon is engaged.

On the other hand, in checking with dermatologists about plastic surgery, I found them most conservative and while some results are excellent, others alter appearance without adding either beauty or charm. On the whole, most women are content if they can have trim, graceful figures, know what to do about their make-up, hair styling and clothes. Tampering with nature's expression areas is dangerous. Where there are birthmarks, scars, burns, and bruises, you certainly have a legitimate excuse to seek out the finest plastic surgeon and see what he can do for you.

In summarising this long Lesson on care of your skin, may I emphasise again three points :

1. Consistent daily care.
2. Control over use of the face in talking.
3. Being the kind of person you're proud to be, so that you are not etching unpleasant expressions on your face.

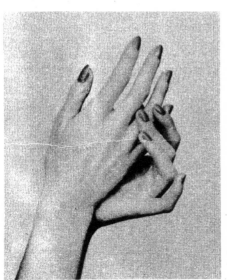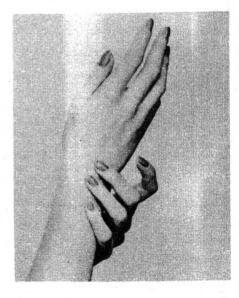

Your hands can be the loveliest, most expressive things about you—indeed many people notice your hands as soon as your eyes or your smile. Are your hands cared for? They can be, even if you do many jobs about the house, pound a typewriter, dig in the garden or drive a car.

44

LESSON TWO

Part B

Corrective Make-Up

The outward forms the inward man reveal—
We guess the pulp before we cut the peel.
—O. W. HOLMES, *A Rhymed Lesson.*

THE term make-up is unfortunate, because it implies that which is "made up," or artificial, whereas the most successful make-ups are natural-looking. They enhance your own natural colouring. Occasionally, you see a woman get away with an extreme or exotic make-up. This is only *occasionally*. Most men prefer you to look like yourself. Your aim is to be an artist in making the most of yourself.

Hollywood discovered very early that correct photographic make-up could do wonders for a star whose features were not perfect. They could make a nose look longer or shorter. They could make chins look larger or smaller, as desirable, and they could make any shape face look almost oval, the classically recognised standard for facial beauty. *Make-up artists do this with the use of highlight-and-shadow make-up.*

Just what does this mean? If you want to look larger, you wear white, or light colours. If you want your hands or feet to look smaller, you wear black, or dark shades. Clever women everywhere are applying this same technique of illusion to their faces by imitating the make-up artist's highlight and shadows. True, for social use, you can't use the extremes of very white or very dark make-up, such as is permissible in black-and-white screen photography. You can however, apply this principle within reason.

IS YOUR BASE DARK ENOUGH?

Here is how you work it.

Decide, first, the colour of your base. (And, incidentally, every woman should wear a powder base or foundation). Be sure that it is correct, neither too light nor too dark but a near match for your own skin colour. So many otherwise well-dressed and well-groomed women make this mistake with their foundation cream that it is worth giving very careful consideration to the point.

Once you have determined upon this base colour, then you are ready to decide what there is about your face that needs to be made larger or smaller. Before we go into the different types of faces let's consider the different types of bases on the market.

1. *There is the untinted cream base.* It adds no colour to the skin but forms an excellent foundation for face powder. It is particularly suited to the fine-grained skin or the complexion which needs care and help. Skin Deep, for example, keeps the skin in beautiful condition, softening and helping the complexion all the time it is worn.

2. *There is the tinted cream*, a foundation cream coloured so that it actually transfers a tint to the skin. These are made in very attractive shades. Atkinson's base, for example, has four delightful shades, and the great advantage of these products is that they give the skin an even tone. It matters little whether the skin is blonde or brunette provided that it is smooth and even in colour. It is blotchiness and patchiness which make a complexion look unattractive.

3. *You may prefer a liquid-type base.* This type used to be called "Liquid Powder" and was used for the arms and neck exclusively. The new bases, however, are of a much heavier consistency, and have enough oil to give the face a flattering sheen and finish, and are easy to use. Many women use all three types of bases. I do. Some women feel that make-up is harmful to the skin. This is not so. If it is carefully selected and applied it serves as a protection against the extremes of climate—heat, cold, wind, rain, etc., and will prevent dirt and impurities entering the pores while it softens and conditions the complexion. But it is absolutely essential that the skin is thoroughly cleansed and creamed, as was described in Part A, and that make-up is not added on top of make-up in layers.

Our screen stars have the most exquisite skins I have ever seen, and they live long hours under heavy grease paint. Fortunately, most of the foundations to-day have the same lubricating essence as the grease paint. The stimulation you give your skin in applying them and taking them off, is also very helpful.

I KNOW NO OTHER MAKE-UP STEP WHICH GLAMORISES THE AVERAGE WOMAN AS MUCH AS THE CORRECT BASE.

Remember that artificial light tends to take the colour out of make-up, so you can safely use a deeper toned foundation cream at night than in the day. A good way of selecting the shade is to match it to the shadows between your fingers. Your face should be at least as dark. Remember that a base always goes on lighter than it looks in the jar. After you have applied the base carefully and evenly, you may find that you need no further highlight or shadow. Most women need to take great care in the application of their foundation cream round the eyes, taking it well up to the lower eye lids in order to mask any shadows which may lurk there.

The advertisements always tell you not to apply your base too heavily. *Yet every woman I know used too much base when she first started.*

The advertisements also tell you to apply only the smallest amount and blend it thoroughly. Let the skin absorb the cream or liquid making quite sure that there are no streaks or smears of cream.

HOW TO MAKE UP YOUR NECK

BE SURE YOU MAKE UP YOUR NECK WHEN YOU MAKE UP YOUR FACE.

Your neck will age faster than any other part of your body. Applying and taking off your neck make-up will add just a little protection, and the stimulation involved will help forestall those early wrinkles. You may object to neck make-up because it discolours the collars of your clothes, but this is probably good because then you will send your clothes to the cleaner more often. *My experience with some of our*

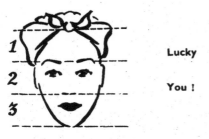

1

2

3

Lucky

You !

Figure 8

finest women is that they do not do this often enough. No girl was ever any the worse off for smelling good !

DO YOU NEED HIGHLIGHT OR SHADOW?

At this point, you may be wondering how you can tell whether or not your face needs highlight and shadow. Check with your rules for a perfectly proportioned face. Here they are :

The distance from your hairline in the middle of your forehead to the top of your nose bone— at a place level with your eyebrows—should equal the distance from the top of the nose to the bottom of your nose. And each of these two measurements should equal the distance from the bottom of your nose to the bottom of your chin. (See Figure 8.). Your face should have a more or less oval shape. In other words, it should be more oval than round, or square, or triangular. If your face almost meets these oval standards, you are ready to go on with your rouge and other make-up and forget the highlight and shadow. Very few women, however, are so fortunate. The rest of us are anxious to know how to create the illusion of that oval face. So we borrow some natural contouring with the help of highlight-and-shadow technique. In other words, we " share the beauty plan."

HOW TO APPLY ROUGE

Before we go into the different types of faces that need corrective make-up, let's scan the rules for doing a good rouge job. The best over-all principle to apply to your rouge is, that you look *unrouged.* Blend the outside borders of the rouged areas until you cannot tell where the rouge starts or ends. This isn't easy, but once your skin has been moistened with a foundation, you will find the procedure simplified. It's worth the time you spend learning to be skilful because too much rouge, poorly blended, of the wrong colour, is ageing.

For most skins, the *cream* type of rouge is best, because it blends easily, giving a lasting effect for six or eight hours. Select a cream rouge which goes on smoothly. If it won't rub or slide through your finger tips, it's too heavy to put on your face ! Powder rouge is useful touching up make-up in case you have not applied enough cream rouge to begin with ; also to renew make-up during the day.

The lighter the colour of your skin, the lighter should be your rouge. *Match your rouge*

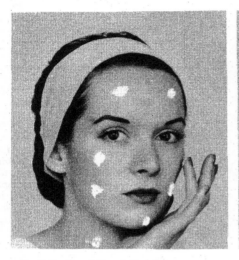

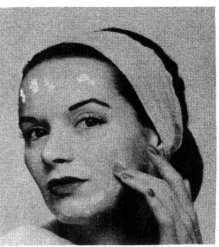

Put little dots of Tinted Foundation on your face and neck . . .

Gently smooth it in, lightly and evenly with little upward strokes . . .

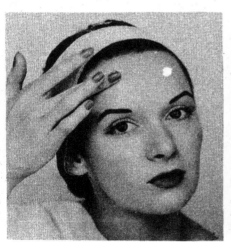

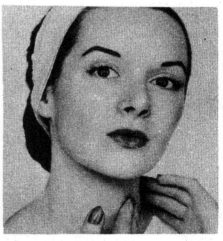

Take care to go right to the hairline . . .

And right down to the base of the neck.

Many people prefer not to make up that tiny area just below the lower eye-lashes. The skin there is extremely thin and is not supported by bone, so the less it is pulled about, the better. Always wait for a moment after putting on your Tinted Foundation and before powdering. This ensures that the film of Foundation is quite set and won't darken your powder.

to your skin, more than to your eyes or hair—and one shade range is sufficient for every costume. Very often, a dusky-skinned blonde will have to use almost a brunette rouge to get the best effect. If you have very fair skin but dark hair and eyes, your rouge will be almost as light as a fair-skinned blonde's. On the whole, keep your rouge a soft and natural pink or red. Be wary of the freakish off-colours.

If you are using a cream-type rouge, then apply it just *after* the base. Should you be using a powder rouge then apply it *after* the face powder.

There are important do's and don'ts in rouge application.

1. Don't apply rouge over any part of your face which might be classed as a hollow. The rouge accentuates these spots and makes them seem deeper than they are.
2. Do apply rouge on the prominent or high places of your cheeks. Study your face until you are sure.
3. Don't put any noticeable amount of rouge on a wrinkle. Here again, the rouge accentuates the line you are hoping to disguise. Sometimes you can't avoid rouging a wrinkle ; then, be sure you blend it well.
4. Don't apply your rouge lower on the cheeks than the region opposite the bottom of your nose, especially if you are over thirty-five. Rouge placed lower than this gives a dragging-downward effect.
5. Don't allow rouge to run into your hairline at the sides.
6. Don't place rouge closer to the nose than that area which would be on an approximately vertical line with the middle of your eyes. (See Figure 9.) You will

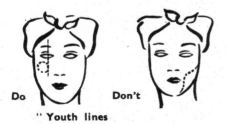

Do   **Don't**

" **Youth lines**

slant upward "

Figure 9

find other suggestions for using rouge in the paragraphs on the shape of face most like yours.

Should your face have any noticeable irregularity, such as a too prominent nose or receding chin, be most sparing in the use of rouge. After you have applied your rouge, you should have it so well blended that your friends will say, " But I didn't suppose you used any! " The modern trend in make-up is : a good base, very light colouring on the cheeks, with accent on the eyes and lips. In case you are still smearing lots of bright pink or red rouge on your face and neglecting your lips and eyes, you are dating yourself as a woman who learned make-up ten years ago. When you go around white and wan, without ANY rouge, you hark back to the days before Technicolor.

In applying rouge, it's wise to put a little bit on the palm of your left hand, and use it direct from there instead of from the container—very much as an artist works from his palette. This prevents your getting too much at a time on your fingertips. It's easy to keep adding a bit more, but hard to rub off successfully the bit too much.

Apply your rouge in four diamond-shaped dabs, to the centre of the area you wish to colour. Blend carefully.

With more than thirty years behind you, here's a studio trick for giving your whole face a blended, smooth appearance. After you have placed your rouge, describe very lightly a little track extending from the cheek bones to your eyes, about one-half inch lower than the eyes' outer corners. *You must blend it so cleverly that the trail cannot be detected.* This " trek " serves as a bridge whereby you can make the white or the dark circles around your eyes less obvious. It unites the more or less unattractive plane around your eyes with the more appealing colour sphere of your cheeks.

Several times during the day you may wish to give your face a lift. Use a dry or cake rouge in the same place you applied the cream variety. Never try to apply cream rouge *after* you are once powdered. Dry rouge requires even more expert handling than the other types. Apply just a little and blend it in well, with your powder puff. The trouble is, as you rub it over, you move the colour from the middle area where you intended it. It's much better not to use it at all than to try to do a good job hurriedly.

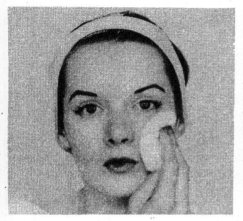

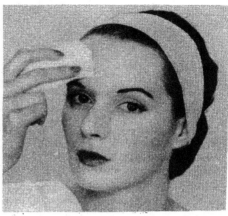

With a swansdown puff or piece of cotton wool press powder liberally all over your face and neck. Being generous with powder here is an economy—this way, you'll find it lasts hours longer.

Now, gently dust off surplus powder, taking care to brush away every trace from hairline and eyebrows—use a little make-up brush, or cotton wool.

Remember that where rouge is concerned, the least bit goes a long way. It's better to have on too little than too much !

How To Powder

Use powder after your base and your rouge, but be sure your technique is expert. You want to look natural and lovely when finished. Select a powder about the same shade as your powder base. Take a fresh powder puff or piece of cotton, and pat on quantities of powder.

When I first began studying corrective make-up, I once watched the late Monte Westmore, famous Hollywood make-up artist, powder Vivien Leigh for her exquisite Technicolor scenes in *Gone with the Wind*. He used a piece of fresh cotton about five inches in diameter and very thick. He recommended that powder be *shaken* on to the puff to prevent its " packing." (This often happens when a woman presses the puff down into the powder box day after day for months. Transfer your powder to a talcum powder box, to a talcum powder jar or an old-fashioned salt shaker). Miss Leigh's hair was concealed, and every *n*th degree of skin on her face, neck, and behind her ears was thoroughly patted with powder. As he patted, he lightly pressed the powder into the skin. He often spent eight to ten minutes on this phase of her make-up alone. He insisted that there be no rubbing or smearing.

Then he brushed her face and neck lightly, but thoroughly, with a powder brush. This is a brush made especially for this purpose. You brush in the direction the hair grows on your face, and continue until no one can see that you have used a trace of powder. You will notice that the brush bristles have a way of getting into wrinkles where the ordinary puff cannot reach. Once you have tried this almost magical powder technique, you can never be persuaded to go back to the old hit-and-miss method, with its conspicuous and unattractive results. And you won't have to powder very frequently during the day, either.

How To Camouflage Wrinkles

Since any type of face is apt to have wrinkles, let's discuss means of camouflaging and softening them with make-up. You already have massage and facial exercises to help you. Here is a clever trick that a photographer uses to soften a wrinkle, but it needs considerable practice, so don't try it for the first time immediately before going out. The following spots are most apt to line first :

(a) at the corners of the lips, (b) from the nose to the lips, (c) between the eyes and on the forehead, and' (d) around the eyes. Let's leave the eyes out of it for now, and consider them a little later. After you have applied your base, apply to your wrinkles a foundation cream of a lighter shade, smooth it in with extreme care making sure that it does not smear. A wrinkle is a crevice or depression, and registers as such to others, unless it is lightened—or " evened " as the professional make-up artist calls it, and this second application of a lighter coloured foundation can do just this if it is carefully applied.

HOW TO MAKE UP A LONG FACE

Let's study first how to make up the long face by means of highlight and shadow ; and then work on the other types. Remember, each step is designed to make your face SEEM shorter.

1. Apply your main foundation first. Blend it all over your face and neck, according to suggestions already given.

2. Usually, it's the chin which is too long in this type of face. How can you tell ? Well, go back to the measurements given here. If the distance from the base of your nose to your chin is longer than the distance between the top of your nose and the base of your nose, or greater than the distance between your hairline and the top of your nose, then you will want to shade off some of your chin. So use your shadow base—at least two tones darker than the main foundation—applying it over the other on your chin. (See Figure 10.) If your chin is, for example, an inch longer than the ideal measurement, then apply the shadow base lightly over your chin for an inch in length and all the way across. Don't bother now about blending it in ; just put it on. This shadow has seemed to shorten

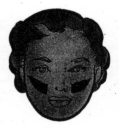

Round Face

Rouge should be applied high on the cheeks and near the nose, keeping the outer edges of the cheeks clear. This will minimize the roundness of the face.

Figure 11

your face, we'll say, about an inch.

3. Now, you need to broaden your face, also. Use your highlight, or the lightest base, and apply it carefully to the sides of your face. This extra white application will make your face look broader and fuller. Start the highlight at the hairline about one-half inch above the eyebrows ; bring it down close to the outside corners of the eyebrows, down even with the eyes and out to the hairline again, just above the cheekbones. If your face is broad enough above the cheekbones, then skip the highlighting application here and concentrate on that area below the cheekbones.

4. Are there some hollows on the sides of your cheeks ? Then whenever you see this so-called " sunken-in " area, apply the highlight again. Even if there are no hollows, apply the highlight to the sides of the cheeks for breadth. Start your blending just below the cheekbones, out to the middle of your cheeks and back down, close to the jawbone. (See Figure 10.)

To be sure that you have the right spots, study Figure 10 regarding the long face. By shadowing (using a *darker* base) you have made the face shorter. By applying highlight (a *lighter* base) to certain areas you have given the illusion of breadth.

5. Then apply your rouge, following the general rouging instructions in this Lesson. Use a cream rouge, so that it will blend with the bases, and keep your dry cake rouge for touch-up jobs during the day. You apply the cream rouge cross-wise, high on the cheekbone, again cutting your face length. (See Figure 10.)

Now that you have the highlight, shadow, and rouge all on the correct spots, start blending, TAKE PAINS WITH IT, AND BLEND SO SKILFULLY THAT IT IS DIFFICULT TO TELL WHERE THE HIGH-LIGHT OR THE SHADOW BEGINS OR ENDS. USE

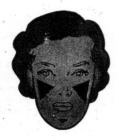

Long Face

A good tip is to smile and apply rouge to the cushions of the cheeks, keeping it well away from the nose. A touch of rouge on the chin helps to shorten the face.

Figure 10

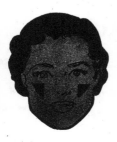

Square Face
Shape the rouge in faint triangles on the outer part of the cheeks, with the upright side of the triangle in line with the nose and the points towards the ears. This softens a too-strong outline.

Figure 12

YOUR FINGERS IF THE BASES ARE LIQUID OR CREAM TEXTURED : A SPONGE, IF THE BASES ARE DRY. *Never apply highlight and shadow to the same area.* It takes lots of time at first but, like all skills, you reduce the time factor, with practice.

HOW TO MAKE UP A ROUND FACE

If your face is round or inclined to be fat, you must pay especial attention to the way you apply your powder base. By using two shades of powder base, you can give your face the illusion of more oval proportions.

1. Apply, first of all, a base to your face and neck, according to suggestions in this Lesson.

2. Next, study your face in the mirror, and block off with your hands that part which you think makes it look too round. Have a clear idea of how much less face you think you should have in order to make it conform to the standard oval shape. Then select a powder base of several shades darker even than that which you put all over your face and neck, and use this darker base as your " shadow." The shadow is to be used on the part of your face which you would like to shade off. In the average round face this shadow is applied about one and one-half inches along the sides and jaws. However, you may not need to cut off quite so much.

3. Apply the shadow quite generously, blending it carefully along the inner line, so you can't tell where one base begins and the other ends. Before you begin to blend the base, stand several feet away from your mirror. Your face actually *does* seem longer and narrower. This is the principle of studio make-up. In case your chin is small, highlight it.

4. If your base is of cream or lotion texture, you will do the blending with your fingers and will apply your rouge after the base and shadow are on. Follow the suggestions for your rouge. (See Figure 11.) Have the deepest colouring

to the centre, blend it outward, following the rouging instructions in this Lesson. Observe that this rouge placement is carefully worked out to further elongate your face and take away from its width.

HOW TO MAKE UP A SQUARE-SHAPED FACE

Usually, this face is so classified because of square jaws. You want to create an illusion of less squareness. Here's how :

1. Apply a base on your face and neck. Blend it well, and be sure it isn't too heavy-looking. (Follow suggestions in this Lesson for application of base).

2. Sit in front of a mirror and, with your hands, cover the part of your face that you feel makes it look too square. This is approximately the area that you should shade off. For this shading or shadowing, use the darker base. Apply it rather heavily and blend it well over the jawline. Be particularly careful on the upper borders of the shadowed area.

3. Use very little rouge on your cheekbones, and create a definite circle. Be sure you blend it so well that you do not leave a hard, cheap circle line. Again, follow general rouging principles explained in this Lesson.

HOW TO MAKE UP A DIAMOND-SHAPED FACE

1. Apply a base on your face and neck. Blend it well, and be sure it isn't too heavy-looking. Follow base application instructions in this Lesson.

2. Highlight chin and forehead to help proportion extra breadth through the cheekbones.

3. Next, shadow the cheekbones out towards the temple.

4. Use only a little rouge, in accordance with rouging instructions in this Lesson. Apply in a circle approximately an inch in diameter.

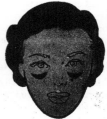

Oval Face
Apply the rouge in a half circle near the eyes. This accentuates the classic shape of the face.

Figure 13

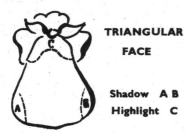

TRIANGULAR FACE

Shadow A B

Highlight C

Figure 14

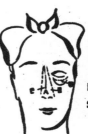

Shadow top of puffs D

Highlight small nose A

Shadow C—B

Figure 16

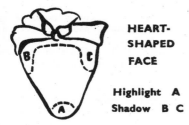

HEART-SHAPED FACE

Highlight A

Shadow B C

Figure 15

How To Make Up a Triangular Face

Since this type of face is broader at the jawline than at the cheekbones, and even smaller across the forehead, your make-up aims to do two things : (1) play down the jaw area ; and (2) emphasise the cheekbones and forehead. Here's how :

1. Apply a base on your face and neck, according to suggestions given here. Blend it well, and be sure it isn't too heavy-looking.

2. Put on the jaw area a darker base than that used on the rest of your face. (See Figure 14, Areas A and B). Use a lighter base on the forehead, temples, and cheekbones, Area C. Let the applications dry or become absorbed, and then blend well.

How To Make Up a Heart-Shaped Face

This type of face is really an inverted triangle, being broader at the top than it is at the bottom. Your aim is, first, to broaden the jaw area ; and, second, to diminish the forehead spade. Try this :

1. Apply a base on your face and neck, according to instructions on base applications

given here. Blend it well, and be sure it isn't too heavy-looking.

2. Apply a lighter base to the jaws and chin. (See Figure 15.) This is Area A. Next, apply your shadow, or darker base, to your forehead, temples and cheekbones, Areas B and C. Let the skin absorb the bases, and then blend well.

Add or Subtract

With any of these definite classifications mentioned, you may still want to add or subtract from the following features :

How To Make Your Nose Seem Longer

Use a powder base several shades lighter than your first base for a coat right down the middle of your nose, or Area A. (See Figure 16.) It will average about three-quarters of an inch in width across the bridge of the nose. This is called " highlighting," by the studio make-up artist. Then, on either side of the nose (Areas B and C, Figure 16) use a shadow, or darker base, thus creating the illusion of the classic feature

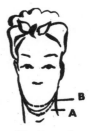

Shadow A

Highlight line B

Figure 17

52

which has a natural light down the centre with accompanying shadow to the sides.

How To Make Your Nose Seem Shorter

If your nose is too long, do this : After you have applied the powder base all over your face and neck, then use a base several shades darker—the shadow. Apply it across the bridge of your nose, and on the very end. These two darker applications will break the length of your nose. Just smear it on and prove it to yourself. Some women whose noses compete with Jimmy Durante's, should shadow the whole nose.

How To Make Your Forehead and Chin Seem Shorter or Longer

For enlarging : After the base is on your face and neck, apply the highlight to your chin or forehead. Yes, all over it. Let it settle a minute, then blend it.

For making your forehead or chin shorter or smaller, use darker base or shadow to these areas. (See Figure 10 and Areas B and C in Figure 15).

How To Shade Off A Double Chin

After the main powder base, apply the shadow to the sagging portion. (Area A Figure 17.) Your double chin isn't half as conspicuous, see ? You might further create the illusion of a clearly defined jawline by drawing a highlight with

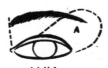

Blend shadows from mid-lid to temple on Areas A

Figure 18

" Natural Browline "

Brow even with tear duct.

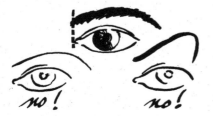

Figure 19

light base all along the jawbone, to Area B. (See Figure 17.)

How To Camouflage Bags Under The Eyes

Concealing puffiness under the eyes is one of the most difficult of all tasks. First, of course, the foundation must go on. Then, where the puffiness is most definite, apply a shadow, or dark base to Area D. (See Figure 16.) *This makes the puffiness recede.* You'll get best results for this correction around the eyes if you use a clean lipstick brush for the shadow application. Be careful that you don't put the shadow on a wrinkle or line, because it would intensify them. Place the shadow on the puffs *only.*

How To Shade Off Prominent Cheekbones

Many authorities think you can do this best with rouge. Personally, I have always felt that rouge calls attention to the area. Therefore, I would suggest that you use a base all over your face and neck. Then apply a darker base right over the prominent part of the cheekbone.

Eyes Bright, Eyes Light !

Your skin and hair may change, but your eyes remain much the same, year after year. *The wise woman will capitalise on this knowledge and enhance the beauty of her eyes.* You can make your eyes larger, brighter, and more expressive with a clever eye make-up. This includes (1) the eyebrows ; (2) the eyelids, and (3) the eyelashes.

How To Make Up The Eyebrows

The most beautiful eyes are spaced so that the distance between is equal to the length of either eye, measuring from corner to corner of one eye. (See Figure 18.) Using your fingers, measure to see how closely your eyes conform to this classic proportion. If they are not quite as far apart as you would like to have them, remember that you can create the illusion of widely spaced eyes by the manner in which you pluck your brows and apply your eye shadow. Your eyebrow should begin at a point above and level with the tear duct. (See Figure 19.) You may have to take out an eighth of an inch of brows on either side of the nose to get the effect. But don't pluck them too thin in other places.

The smartest women to-day have a natural brow line, because they know that the eyebrows, more than any other feature, give expression to the face. The shape of your eyebrow should follow generally the upper curve of your eye. Avoid points on your brows. They are apt to give you a perpetually surprised look ; they focus interest away from your eyes, and are unbecoming to most faces.

Have an eyebrow brush almost the size of a toothbrush for your home brushing, and carry a smaller one in your bag. Brush your eyebrows up toward your forehead first and then brush them out toward your temples.

Use a black eyebrow pencil only if your brows are definitely black. Otherwise, a light brown for blondes or a dark ·brown for in-betweens and redheads is much more flattering. When you colour your brows, have a sharp point on your eyebrow pencil. You may prefer to use a regular carbon drawing pencil. Use small strokes about the length of a normal eyebrow to fill in or add to the desired line. (See picture opposite.)

One of the most cruel things a woman can do to her face is to draw one continuous, hard line through the brows. It stands out grotesquely and dominates the whole face. Practise these small, shaped lines until you are expert. If your eyebrows are very light or faded, apply mascara to them before using the eyebrow pencil. This gives a natural and lasting effect.

Most women must extend their brows about a quarter of an inch to the side, so that the brows give the appearance of framing the eyes. (See Figure 19.) Be careful not to extend your brows down at the sides of your eyes, because any downward line is ageing. If your brows grow that way, naturally, you may find it wise to pluck a few of the lower ones and extend the pencil strokes out to the sides for correction.

How To Make Up Your Eyelids

Select an eye shadow to flatter your eyes. For dark hazel, brown, or green eyes, use a blue-green eye shadow. For light hazel or grey eyes, use a blue-grey shadow ; and for blue or grey eyes use either blue or blue-grey shadow depending upon the colour of your clothes. Use the shadow sparingly. Apply it two-thirds of the way along the upper lid, just above the lashes, and extend it up to the eyebrows and even out beyond the eyes to the temples, to enlarge the eye area. (See Figure 18.) Never place shadow closer to the nose than I have indicated if you want to create the illusion of widely spaced eyes.

You may be that one woman in a thousand whose eyes are too widely spaced, so that you wish to shadow to the tear duct, to decrease this condition. Blend the shadow carefully so it is not apparent, having the darkest amount near the lashes. If you have plucked your eyebrows, and there is a white space where the hairs used to grow, be sure to soften these spots with shadow. Should your eyes be inclined to bulge, use quite a 'bit of shadow regardless of eye colouring, to make this tendency appear less prominent. During the day, you may only need an eyelid pomade such as Atkinson's Naturelle eye shadow. (See picture on opposite page.)

This gives the eyelids a groomed slightly shiny appearance and takes away any powdery or dusty look, but it does not add colour. But for evening experiment more boldly. If cleverly applied, eye shadow can be most glamorous. Some women when they have applied their eye shadow as described add a deeper line of colour just above the eyelashes. This they carry outwards and slightly upwards at the outer corners and it gives quite a devastating effect.

If you haven't been using an eye shadow begin with very little and as you become accustomed to it, add a little more. Carry some in your bag, since it won't last much longer than four or five hours and is a real pick-up.

How To Enlarge The Eyes

One of the most delicate bits of make-up to master is that of outlining the eyes with an eyebrow pencil. This is usually the same shade as you use on your eyebrows. Just as an etching often is improved by good matting and framing, so the eyes take on an interesting depth and apparently more size, when they are outlined. This will not show if it is done on that ledge of skin where the lashes grow. Do not put it *above* the lashes for then it will be too noticeable. Start your outlining at the middle of the upper and lower lids and extend out to the sides. By tracing a few dot lines in the form of a triangle from the corners of the eyes out towards the sides you can add still more size to the eyes.

How To Make Up The Eyelashes

Before you begin glamorising your lashes, be sure you have brushed out all traces of powder. You will need to apply your mascara faithfully to both upper and lower lashes if they are very light, but otherwise concentrate on the upper lashes *only*. The colour of mascara to use will depend upon your general colouring, and you

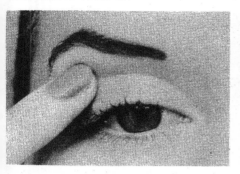

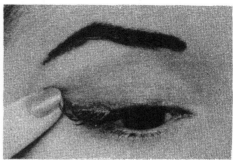

EYE SHADOW—With your finger-tip, apply the eye shadow to the outer half of the eyelid only, blending it upwards and outwards towards the temples until it fades completely.

For evening, put a thin, emphatic line immediately above the eyelashes—it looks exceedingly pretty.

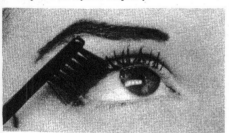

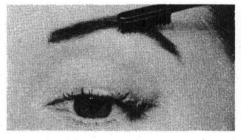

MASCARA — EYELASHES—Use Mascara on upper eyelashes only, brushing lightly upwards with a dryish brush. Two thin applications are much more efficient than one thick one. After two applications let the mascara 'set' for a moment and then brush the lashes gently with a clean, dry brush to groom them thoroughly.

EYEBROWS—With your brush feather in little strokes along the natural line of your eyebrows, slightly darkening and emphasising, but not altering the real shape. Long, strong, sweeps of the brush will not look natural, so be very light in your touch.

should be careful not to use too dark a shade. Most blondes and redheads look best with dark-brown mascara. Preferably, only the darker brownheads and brunettes should use jet-black lash colouring. Some authorities say, " If the eyebrows are black, then and *only then* use black mascara."

Keep the mascara brush spotlessly clean AND NOT TOO DAMP. Dampen the brush and mix some mascara evenly into the brush bristles. Apply it to the lashes from the base to the tips. If your lashes are naturally dark, but perhaps sunburned or light at the tips, then apply the mascara to the end only. Avoid an artificial beady look by separating the lashes carefully. When you remove the mascara make quite sure that the lashes are left scrupulously clean. A little Vaseline or cream on the lashes helps to keep the lashes soft and stimulates their growth.

HOW TO MAKE UP YOUR LIPS

Be sure that your methods for applying lipstick are modern and up-to-date. Some people prefer to use a lipstick brush for applying lipstick. Others get on better with the stick itself, but whichever you decide on, use small, feathery strokes to make sure that the lipstick clings well to the lips. While wholesale re-shaping of lips gives an unnatural appearance, skilfully effected minor changes can be very becoming.

In the accompanying sketches you will notice the different types of lips. (See Figure 20.) Select the picture which most nearly approximates your lips. The dotted line shows how they can be improved. Here are some rules which studio make-up artists recommend.

1. Don't try to alter the shape of your mouth too much. Every hair's breadth makes a

lot of difference. Begin by simply outlining the shape of your lips.

2. Select for the first coat a lipstick that is reasonably light in colouring. Brownheads or brunettes use a darker red than blondes and redheads.

3. If you are going to use a brush get a genuine camel's-hair lipstick brush. Ask for a professional's brush with a long handle for home application. Then, for your bag carry a smaller one with a cover to protect the brush.

4. Have your lips perfectly dry.

5. To create an upward lift to the corners of your mouth, part your lips and begin applying colour at the inside of the upper corners. Have your brush saturated with the lipstick.

6. Using small, curving strokes, gradually colour toward the centre of the upper lips. When you have completed one side of the cupid's bow, start at the other outside corner of the upper lip and work toward the centre. Notice that in the sketches all types of lips have rounded upper curves. Once you have established the upper line, then fill in the rest of the upper lip. Use plenty of lipstick. Brush it with up-and-down strokes, also to fill any crevices.

7. Now begin on the lower line. Again, start at the inside of the corner of the mouth. Then continue along the natural line of the lower lip. Colour every bit of lip, and fill in as you did on the upper lip. Some make-up artists recommend that you show the bow on the *lower* lip.

8. Let all the lipstick remain for a minute or

so. Next, press a cleansing tissue between your lips and blot off as much surface colour as possible. Blot three or four times. This keeps some definite colouring on your lips all day or evening—one film you can't eat off! (See illustrations.)

9. Suppose now, that you are wearing a dress with orange colour in it. Then select a lipstick which has a definite yellow or orange tone. If your costume has a purple tone, select a lipstick with a cyclamen note like Atkinson's Tomboy. In other words, match your lipstick to your fashion shades with pastel colours. I think the softer tones of pink look delightful but with clear reds, dark brown or greens a true red lip colour is essential. You must, therefore, keep several lipsticks of different shades, not just one colour to go with all your dresses.

This whole technique takes a few extra minutes, but once you're finished you have a make-up which will stay fresh-looking for hours. It needs to be retouched only when you eat, or every four hours, so you needn't constantly be daubing at your lips.

Now, Start Alterations. After you have mastered the art of making up your lips like a professional, then begin altering them, but remember only slightly. If your lips are too small, or thin enlarge both upper and lower lips a tiny bit at a time. (See Figure 20.) You will be surprised to find that the stain of the lipstick will soon fill in the skin above your actual lips until a new line seems to be formed. After a few months you won't be able to tell which is your original lip line and which has been filled in.

Many women think that their lips are too large when actually they are most flattering and feminine. Full, soft, lip lines are much more beautiful than small, thin ones. But if you are sure that your lips are too large, here is the way to shade off a bit of their size. When you apply your powder base put a generous amount on the corners and outer edges of your lips. Do the same when you powder. Then, when it comes to lipstick, don't go all the way out to the corners, or to the edges, but stop at the line created more or less by the base. You will find that the continued disuse of colour to that area which you wish to decrease will gradually make the part of the lip line almost extinct.

Don't worry about whether your lower or upper lip should be the larger. Follow the

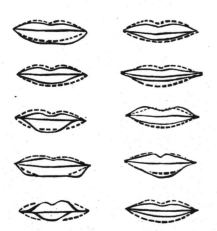

Figure 29

CORRECTIVE MAKE UP

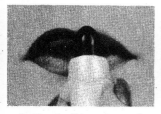

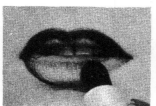

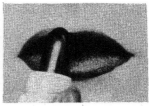

Outline the lips, going to the extreme edge of your natural lip line if your lips are a little thin. .

Staying just inside the margin if they are slightly too full. (Never make an outline that is right outside or right inside your own lip line—it looks false and hard.)

Fill in, smoothing lightly and surely over your lips.

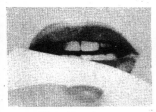

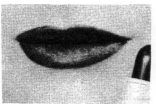

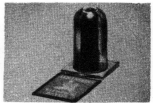

Blot with a tissue.

Now one final layer—let it 'firm' —and you're all set for hours.

Here's the Atkinsons Lipstick Refill. It makes the job of putting in a new lipstick so simple —so clean—you don't have to handle the lipstick at all!

Two-Tone Lipstick Technique. . .

Apply *two* lipsticks sometimes. You can match dress shades exactly this way, and you can get delightful. translucent effects. Try a darker shade over a paler one, a rosy tone over a tangerine. natural contours of your lips for this, so that you keep your lips individual. AND KEEP SMILING !

How To Make Up The Hands And Arms

In concentrating on your face, don't neglect your hands and arms. They age and discolour so much faster than the face and neck, anyway. Here's a pretty good plan to follow :. First, make a habit of wearing old gloves soaked in cream at least one night each week. This will add to what you have already learned about the care of arms and elbows. (See Part A of this Lesson). Every time you wash your hands during the day, apply a hand cream or lotion. If your sleeves are short, put some lotion on your arms and elbows also. Be sure that the cream or liquid that you are using is actually softening. If, as you use a hand lotion, you find your hands becoming drier and drier, that's the cue that you'd better change. As hand softeners, like other cosmetics, vary with individuals, your favourite softener may not help your sister at all. Rub on generous amounts. Blot off excess. Then, too, *do use a liquid powder, the shade of*

your hands, on your hands. Used over the softener it is not drying, and it gives them a beautiful finish. Again, if you are wearing short sleeves or no sleeves, use the liquid powder to cover the entire arm area. Backless evening dresses need a little attention, too. Just be sure your base is the correct colour. If you go in for an elaborate sun tan, you must ask for professional colours. There are several such liquid preparations on the market which will not rub off. Some are of lighter texture than others, so experiment before buying. When your elbows are exposed, and especially if you have thirty years behind you, rub a little cream rouge on the elbows. Blend it in thoroughly, to " cut " the drake's-tail look that your mother cautioned you against !

This has been a long, involved Lesson. I would never be one to tell you that make-up does not require time. But show me anything which does a girl more good than a skilful make-up job. One last reminder : It's all right to re-colour your lips quickly or powder your nose ; BUT don't forget to be an " under-cover " girl about other make-up details.

Notes:

Self Test Questions Based On Lesson Two

Even the plain woman may cultivate an enticing skin; this, with health, vitality and radiant personality can give the illusion of beauty, making the lucky owner an attractive and fascinating person. A good skin is the only sure way to perfect make-up Begin to cultivate your enticing skin by following the advice in this Lesson; your correct make-up will then reward you fully.

After you have studied this Lesson you should be able to answer the following questions. If you have any difficulty in doing so, refer to the Lesson for further study and revision. Your answers should not be sent to the publishers of this Course.

1. Quote two ways in which you may cultivate a beautiful skin.

2. What is the essential condition which you must possess before you can benefit 100% by correct make-up ?

3. What is the value of day and night creams on the face and neck, and oils on the body ? How important are they and how often should they be used ?

4. If you want to look your best at any time during the day, what should you do ?

5. What are the three important points to remenber in this Lesson on care of the skin ?

6. Describe the method the author recommends for applying the base when doing your make-up.

7. What is the test of whether your rouge is applied correctly ?

8. Describe shortly the best method to use when powdering.

9. How may you enhance the beauty of your eyes ?

10. Have you decided which of the sketches most closely resembles your lips ?

If you wish to determine the progress you are making, give yourself 10 points for each question you answer correctly. If the total comes to 90 or more, it is excellent; 80 or more, good; 70 or more, fair.

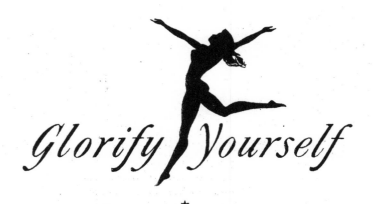

Glorify Yourself

★

A Complete and Up-to-Date Course on
Beauty and Charm by One of the
Most Famous Beauty Specialists
and Consultants in the World

Eleanore King

★

LESSON THREE

★

STUDIO TALK •

Number Three.

Dear Student,

You are now about to commence the study of Lesson Three in which you will be shown some of the secrets of good posture.

Good posture is a **very visible asset.** It makes you appear confident, poised -- and _youthful_. It streamlines your appearance and gives grace to your every movement; and it is a great invisible asset too, for it is one of the basic essentials of good health.

Part B. of Lesson Three deals with legs -- and it may surprise you to learn just how important legs are. It certainly surprised me when a leading Hollywood Publicity Expert told me about the vast amount of money the major studios spend each year on photographs which emphasise the leg appeal of their stars.

Perhaps you don't want to make your name in show business. But it is still vital for you to master leg technique if you want to look your best when you are in the public eye.

Fortunately, it is easy to make the most of beautiful legs and to effect a wonderful improvement in legs which are not quite so beautiful. All that is required is a little thought and careful practice of a few simple routines which will be fully explained to you in the Lessons.

By mastering them you will have laid the foundations of a graceful carriage. If your feet and legs are graceful the chances are that your whole body will be equally attractive.

Yours sincerely,

Eleanore King

P.S. Good deportment is of such vital importance that we shall continue the study of this fascinating subject in Lesson Four.

LESSON THREE

Part A

Body Line-Up

Oh, wad some power the giftie gie us
To see oursels as ithers see us !
—ROBERT BURNS, *To a Louse*

EACH year as I watch the Motion Picture Academy Awards winners, I am impressed with the restraint and flexibility which they invariably possess.

During the years I've been covering these banquets for my newspaper, I've watched Bette Davis, Vivien Leigh, Ginger Rogers, Greer Garson, Jennifer Jones, Ingrid Bergman and Joan Crawford acknowledge their victories. These artists represent many types : tall, small ; blondes, redheads, brunettes. *But every one of them carries herself with great distinction.*

I recall the year Ingrid Bergman's name was announced. As she glided down the centre aisle of Grauman's Chinese Theatre like one of the ancient Greek goddesses, a man near me said, " Gad, that girl moves with the grace of a panther ! "

Posture is such an essential quality in a graceful woman that you don't have to " sell " it any more.

However, not so many years ago women generally associated posture with unpleasantness. I believe this came about because the early crusaders for good posture represented it as something stern, rigid—almost military.

Today, good posture means almost the opposite: litheness, flexibility, gracefulness. Posture is that control of the body which allows it to function most normally.

One of the greatest authorities on good posture, Dr. Charles LeRoy Lowman, says : " Good posture is correct body alignment, and may be defined as the correct relation of the body segments to each other and to their external environment. All of the ' bearings ' or joints should be in proper relation, so that the muscle will pull in a normal line."

You notice that he stresses the importance of how one part of the body is carried in relation to other parts. Therefore, you think of your body as made up of hinged parts, all working towards a pleasing, efficient co-ordination.

Another enlightening idea about posture that many women are not aware of is that *efficient* body carriage is also the most *graceful.* Thus, each moment that you carry yourself gracefully you are also incorporating valuable health rules.

Before we get into this subject further, I should like to stress the fact that you don't need to take a lot of time to acquire good posture. You don't have to go across town to a teacher or a gymnasium. You don't have to spend a penny. You don't have to wear special exercise clothes.

Here is one of the most valuable assets you can possess. And it's yours IN YOUR OWN TIME. You have to stand, walk, sit, turn every hour, anyway. Why not stand, walk, sit, turn so that you are a joy to those around you ?

Let's list some of the concrete values that you acquire through good posture :

1. You appear confident. Because correct posture is tangible. You see it. It expresses positive qualities of courage. Mr. Samuel Goldwyn, President of Samuel Goldwyn Motion Picture Studio, says : " There is no such thing as an inferiority complex—just poor posture. If a player walks on the sound set the first day looking sure of herself, the whole picture gets off to a good start. No matter how capable she is, if she LOOKS unsure of herself, she conveys that feeling to the whole crew. It may take hours to undo the harm."

If posture is important to film stars, it's certainly important to you.

2. Good posture makes you appear poised. You seem equal to your tasks. Thus it helps you to inspire others.

Show me a great leader with poor posture. Even the infamous dictators were wise enough to command respect through the weapon of great bodily forcefulness, which is just another way of saying they carried themselves like leaders.

3. Good posture makes you look young. Did you see Ethel Barrymore in " The Corn Is Green " ? She was almost seventy, yet as she

made her entrance in a schoolteacher's costume of the 1800's, she seemed—oh, maybe thirty-five, maybe forty! Her carriage and movements were superb. Correct posture enhances the natural exhilaration associated with youth.

4. Good posture helps to distribute your weight, so that your figure looks better pro-portioned. You look streamlined. Gravity doesn't appear to be dragging you down and getting the better of you. You don't have "the sags." Have you ever thought what a negative word "sag" is? Everything that even rhymes with it is bad—try it: nag, hag, lag, rag, tag, BAG!

5. Good posture helps to build good health. You are helping Nature to put correct stress at the correct spots. After all, your two hundred muscles must hold up your skeleton.

Just try making a skeleton stand on its own! It has to have support, doesn't it? The better the support, the more efficient the skeleton appears. You are your skeleton's only support. How efficiently you take care of your task is your own responsibility.

You might pay the finest posture teacher in the world a fortune to teach you correct posture. *However, you would have to do the actual support job yourself!*

Fortunately, posture is simple. There's nothing difficult about it. Even if you've been holding yourself incorrectly for years, you can begin improving immediately.

There's a glorious challenge about posture, too; because if you correct only the smallest fraction of an inch each day for thirty days—see what you have accomplished at the end of a month?

Don't worry what your Aunt Sophie should be doing about her posture. You take care of your own. Each person is an individual case. You may have to concentrate on your shoulders and she may have a hip problem.

To start off correctly, get a good over-all picture of yourself. Take off your clothes. Go to a full-length mirror. Stand so that you can see yourself from the side. STAND AS YOU USUALLY DO. What is the general tilt of your body? Do you lean forward from the hips? Do your hips protrude? (Sh! They probably do!)

Since you've been working on the technique for head posture presented in Lesson One, Part A, I hope you see improvement there. Or is your head still too far forward? How about

Draw a

vertical

chalk line

on your

mirror

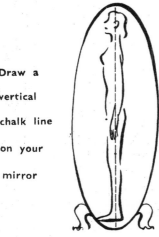

Figure 21

your shoulders? Are they pushed forward? Too tense? Do you carry them too high? And your abdomen. Does it protrude? What is the position of your feet? Do they point straight ahead? Chiefly, is your back almost straight? This gives you an over-all idea of how you appear to others.

Now, let's think of you as you would like to be. You should be standing relaxed, natural. If a person were to draw a line from your ear-lobe to the floor, the line should fall opposite your shoulder-bone, down your torso, opposite your hip-bone, and a little in front of your ankle-bone. This is the "plumb-line" you hear so much about when posture is stressed.

Although I have taught the gravity-line principle for several years, still I find its application is vague to the student of posture.

If there isn't someone to tell you how far you deviate from the "plumb-line," here's a practical test that you can make. Draw a chalk line on a full-length mirror. Stand sideways a foot away from this line, which you can consider your centre of balance. Stand so that the line cuts the ear-lobe vertically in half. (See Figure 21.) Following the chalk line down your body, it should be directly opposite your shoulder-bone, hip-bone, and in front of your ankle-bone.

If any part of your body is either too far behind or too far in front of this line, that is the section you want to work on chiefly. For instance, if the

66

line falls in front of your hip-bone, then you are carrying your hips too far back. Should the line fall opposite the *front* part of your knee area, then you know you are holding your knees too rigid, and your body weight is thrown too far forward.

This plumb-line is where you should be carrying your body weight. You know that there is one point at which any object can be supported by a single upward force. Think of this line as the centre for supporting what to you is the most important object of all—your body. It also gives you a clear idea of how important one part of your body is in relation to another. You can't correct one segment without proper alignment of ALL the segments.

Therefore, think of the chief segments of your body in this simple way : Your hips must be balanced over your feet, your chest area balanced over your pelvis, and your head must be balanced evenly over your chest. This isn't such an easy feat when we realise how much more weight the head, chest and hips have in comparison with the legs and feet ! No wonder we get out of line occasionally !

STACK YOURSELF UP

In order to understand more deeply just how much you can go about controlling that mass of muscles, joints and bones that is YOU, let's take up in their order each of the following essential parts of the body so far as posture is concerned. I've seen Rita Hayworth very visibly line herself up before each " take " in this manner !

(1) Feet and Knees.
(2) Pelvis and Buttocks.
(3) Abdomen.
(4) Chest.
(5) Shoulders.
(6) Head and Neck.
(7) Arms and Hands.

1. *Your feet and knees.* Stand with your feet about two inches apart. Point your toes straight ahead. Each leg and foot should carry half your body weight.

Therefore, upon each foot falls the task of balancing at least half of your body. Your weight should fall just in front of the ankle-bone, as just mentioned.

How you carry your knees has a direct bearing on how you carry your weight. Try this test. Stand with your knees rigid or " locked." Your weight falls to the front of your feet, almost on

your toes, doesn't it ? Notice what this does to the rest of your body : your rear pushes out behind and your head forward in front.

It's that old principle of compensation at work. Dr. Eleanor Metheney, Head of the Women's Physical Education Department at the university, explains this principle very simply in her classes in Body Mechanics. She says, " If you're stacking a pile of blocks, you will put one directly on top of the other. Should you make a mistake and put one block a little to the right, then, to balance it, you will have to put the next one to the left. That is what you do in your body line-up, too. One part carried too far forward causes another part to be carried too far to the rear." That's reasonable, isn't it ?

Now, bend your knees a lot—maybe several inches. Where is your weight ? It's on your heels and your whole body slumps.

This time let's relax the knees just slightly. For example, as much as you relax your elbows. This third time does the trick, because your " easy " knees bring your weight just in front of the ankle-bone where you want it.

In the next Lesson, we'll speak of what happens when the weight is carried to the *inside* of the feet. Right now, let's get on with the complete body line-up.

2. *Pelvis.* The average woman thinks of hips and buttocks when she thinks of the pelvis. And to hear most women talk, you'd think this is the seat of all their troubles.

Nature intended a woman to be padded at the hips, but perhaps not to the extent noticeable to the most casual observer.

It is, therefore, a comfort to realise that a correctly lined-up pelvis will make her seem inches slimmer.

I don't care who the woman is : she can't look anything approaching her best or be graceful as long as her buttocks and abdomen protrude.

One of my students confided, " I always feel there's something following me ! " She was right, too ! A large portion that should have been under her *was* bringing up the rear, and she has lots of company, judging from what you see on every street corner.

The very first lesson I present to a student, therefore, is the theory of pelvic rotation, the medical term for carrying your pelvis correctly. Posture experts often use less technical terms, such as " getting your tail under you," " the tuck under," " penny pinching," or " coccyx under."

Let's see why the correct line-up of the pelvis is so important in our study of good posture and grace.

The strong bone beneath your stomach is the pubis. You know that at the very end of your spine is a bone called the coccyx. The part of your body that you call the " back of your hips," on either side of your lower spine, is another strong bone called the sacrum. All of these bones take on the formation of a bowl or basin. This whole area is called the pelvis (meaning, " basin") The hip-bones form an arch called the pelvic girdle. This pelvic girdle with the pubis makes up the front and sides of the pelvis. The sacrum and coccyx form the back.

Thus, the pelvis is one continuous strong joining of bone, and is capable of great strength. The average woman must learn to make use of this great strength through correct position.

Don't tip the pelvic basin in such a way that its top slopes towards the front. Its top must be kept flat. The least tilting and your hips shoot out behind and your abdomen sags in front. This gives you some idea of why the pelvis must be carried correctly. If it isn't, the whole body is thrown out of balance, since the pelvis is the base of the torso and also the area where the legs join the torso. It is the crucial spot.

Check to see exactly how well lined up your pelvis is. Stand with your feet four inches away

from a wall, but with your head, shoulders and hips touching it. Does ALL of your spine touch ? (See Figure 22.). Even the small of your back ? *If there is more than an inch of space between you and the wall you need to do a few posture exercises to help you to get your pelvis area in the correct position, so that the rest of your body can function smoothly and gracefully.*

You will find these exercises in Lesson Six, Part B. Don't do them, however, until you have a complete picture of how your whole body should be aligned.

Do this posture exercise so that you can begin to FEEL the way you should be lined up. This may be the only one you'll need.

Stand away from the wall, with your feet about ten inches apart, toes straight ahead. Bend your knees and keep them bent during the exercise.

Place one hand on your coccyx (the end of your spine) and one on your pubic bone. Rock your whole pelvic area forward. Count : " Rock one, relax ; rock two, relax ; rock three, relax ; rock four, relax."

Only you needn't have any tension.

As you rock forward, knees bent, do you notice how your hips seem to fold down and under you ? Your buttocks play a part, too. (See Figure 23.) They press together.

Many teachers of deportment have their students stand and walk with a coin between their buttocks, feeling that this is the fastest

**Does
all of
your
spine
touch ?**

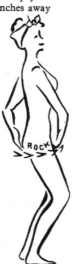

Figure 22

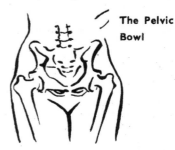

The Pelvic Bowl

Exercise

Coccyx under

Stomach in

Rock one, relax, rock two, etc

Figure 23

approach to the " tuck under." If it helps you, all well and good ; because when you contract the buttocks, you do get correct bone rotation, too. *I caution you, however, against any continued tension in the gluteus muscles of the buttocks.*

This pelvic rocking with your knees bent should make the whole lower area of your body more flexible. When you get a definite forward pelvic motion with your knees bent a lot, then try it with your knees only slightly flexed.

Go over once more to a wall. Try this pelvic rocking, or rotation, again. As you straighten your knees and keep your hips folded under you, see if you can get your entire back to touch the wall.

Now step away from the wall, trying to keep your hips and back in the same position as they were in when against the wall.

Let's review your standing position thus far : feet straight ahead, about two inches apart, four inches from the wall. The weight of your body just in front of your ankle-bones. Your knees flexed slightly. Your coccyx pushed forward until your back is as straight as you can get it. So far so good.

3. *Abdomen.* As your buttock muscles tighten when you push your coccyx forward, do you notice that your abdominal muscles contract also ? They do and your abdomen looks flatter.

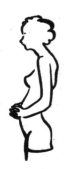

Figure 24

The abdominal and gluteus muscles can work together. Your abdominal muscles pull up and in as your buttock muscles contract together and push down.

Here is the best method for ensuring a flat abdomen that I know. It's one you can do without anyone noticing, too. You will find exercises for reducing the abdomen in Lesson Seven, Part B.

4. *Chest. Carry your chest high* ! No matter how many times your mother slapped you on the back and said, " Throw your chest out," DON'T DO IT ANY MORE. You can see that as you push your chest forward, you push forward the whole rib cage. This, in turn, increases whatever tendency you may have

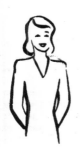

Figure 25

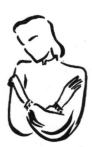

Figure 26

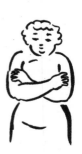

Figure 27

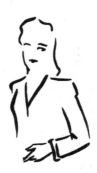

Figure 28

69

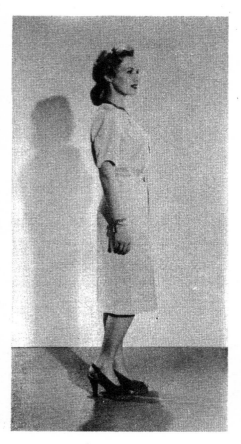

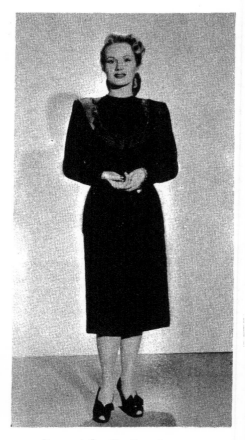

Photograph 4   Perfectly balanced posture
is demonstrated by graceful Virginia Mayo.

Photograph 5   Miss Mayo shows proper
position if hands are held in front of you.

toward a " sway-back."

In deportment circles, it's called " lordosis."
Raise your chest until it hurts. Then slowly
relax the chest muscles until you feel comfortable,
but your chest is still high. Notice, too, that as
you raise your chest, your abdominal muscles
flatten. So far, your chest is over your pelvis,
and your pelvis is over the balls of the feet.

5. *Shoulders.* Your two collar-bones (clavi-
cles) in front and your two shoulder-blades
(scapulae) behind make up the shoulder girdle.
Since so much of the shoulder girdle is attached
to your trunk chiefly with muscles, you can
understand the importance of developing those

muscles correctly.

You do that hour by hour in the manner in
which you carry your shoulders.

Carry your shoulders relaxed, broad and low.
NEVER BACK ! That old command, " Throw
your shoulders back," has ruined many an
otherwise good body line-up, because the body
must compensate for shoulders thrust too far
backwards by pushing the abdomen forward and
the buttocks to bring up the rear. Try it. You
have to see the body as a whole—and not in
unrelated parts.

Here's a simple test for your shoulders. Chest
high. Rotate your shoulders up as high towards

your ears as you can get them, back a little, and then let them drop.

This last position is approximately how you should carry your shoulders. Guard against shoulder tension. Not only does it cause undue fatigue for you, but it conveys tension to those around you. Haven't you noticed that if your hostess is tense, with high, tight shoulders, you have difficulty in being at ease yourself?

Every star learns the importance of a high chest-line and a correspondingly relaxed shoulder line. Inexperienced actors and actresses realise that if they can master the art of an easy, natural shoulder-line, they will appear much more poised. High strained shoulders make you look self-conscious, too.

6. *Head and neck.* We've already discussed these two important parts of the body in Lesson One. Let's relate them to our complete body line-up here. By now, are you beginning to see that your rod-like spine has quite a duty to perform in balancing the weight of your heavy head, which has about one-tenth of your total weight? Military authorities tell you to keep your chin in and your head up. If that helps you, do it; but don't do it so vigorously that you show off any tendency you may have towards a double chin.

It was months after my first teacher of deportment told me to think of pushing my neck up behind my ears, that I had any actual feeling of doing that very thing. Even telling you to think of standing, sitting, and walking upright may not help you. If all these suggestions fail, at least push your neck back and think of carrying your head balanced straight on your neck. Your head is then over your chest, your chest is over your pelvis, and your pelvis is balanced over the balls of your feet.

Is this line-up beginning to sound like a limerick? That's my idea! (See Photograph 4.)

7. *Arms and hands.* Your arms are related to your shoulders, neck and chest. Correct posture for one helps all the others. Let your arms fall relaxed and free. Your elbows are always slightly bent.

An actress or model is trained to let the *palms* of her hands touch her sides. See how this knocks off about three inches on either side of your hips? Your thumbs should be at your side seams (or where your side seams would be), and your fingers should fall relaxed behind the thumbs.

It's a good idea to know several poised positions for hands and arms in addition to this classic one, because hand-control has an influence on general poise.

As one student writes, "Always inclined to get nervous and flustered in strange company, I have had the utmost difficulty in controlling my hands which betrayed my nervousness.

In having my photograph taken, interviewing employers, and in countless other situations, I have been bothered by those two floppingly unmanageable appendages. I was surprised to find how very simple a thing hand poise can be, once mastered. Your simple formulas to suit every situation did the trick!"

You'll get hand positions for walking and sitting in later Lessons. Let's concentrate now on some helpful ones for standing:

1. DON'T stand with your hands clasped across your abdomen. (See Figure 24.) This is one of the most unbecoming gestures you can assume. It not only outlines any extra pounds you have on your stomach—almost like " X marks the spot "—but it pulls your head and shoulders forward and your chest down. When I have a student who simply insists on this pose, I send her out to the zoo to watch the big chimpanzees slouching around with their hands across their paunches. One visit is enough! The habit is dropped ON THE SPOT.

2. DO clasp your hands behind your back if you think your fingers are twitching. (See Figure 25.) Clasp them firmly together for moral support. Don't relax your elbows too much, because this broadens your body. Besides, it's masculine.

3. DO fold your arms over your chest only if you're the extremely smart type. (See Figure 26.) Usually, you succeed in looking like an aspiring executive; or just plain dumpy! (See Figure 27.)

4. DO keep your hands at your waist-line if you like to keep your hands in front of you as you talk. (See Figure 28.) Don't let them break up your bust-line. This looks coy and affected for small women, and makes a tall woman seem awkward. Turn your palms up and put the thumb of one hand in the palm of the other. Relax your wrists and your fingers will be relaxed. (See Photograph 5.)

You'll find exercises for loosening up, relaxing and beautifying hands in Lesson Seven, Part B.

I hope this Lesson has helped you understand

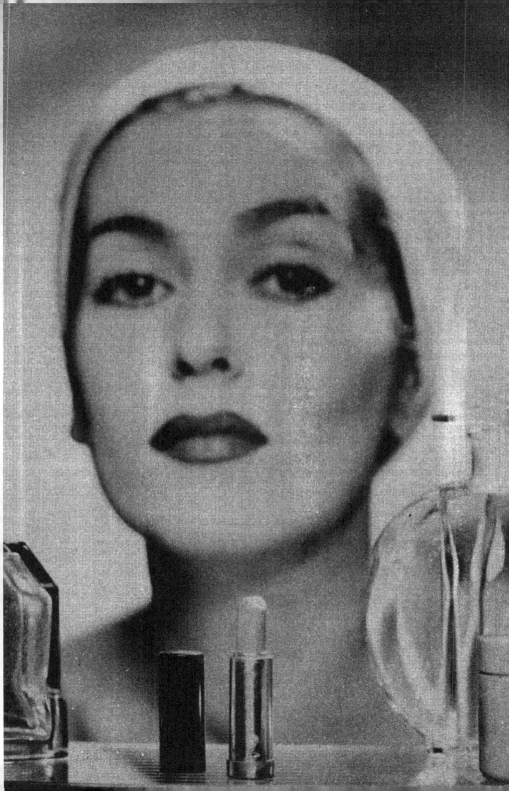

BODY LINE-UP

HOW you should carry the important parts of your body. You can't slump and slouch through your week with every part of your machine working contrary to its normal function and expect to offset this during two hours' strenuous exercising. Don't make a fetish of good body line-up, thereby getting tense and upset. Just do it in an easy way, without attracting attention. Of course, the longer you've let yourself slump, the harder it will be to " pull yourself together." This is what you'll say to yourself dozens of times each day to make sure you're looking your best and feeling your best. Toes straight ahead, weight on outside of feet ; knees slightly relaxed, so that weight falls in front of ankle-bone ; coccyx under ; abdomen flat ; chest high ; shoulders relaxed and broad ; neck back ; arms easy ; thumbs at side seams, fingers relaxed, palms in.

Say it, do it, think it, over and over and over and . . . over . . . and . . .

Notes:

LESSON   THREE

Part B

Attractive Legs

Down flow'd her robe, a tartan sheen,
Till half a leg was scrimply seen ;
And such a leg ! my bonny Jean

Could only peer it ;
Sae straight, sae taper, tight an' clean,
Nane else cam near it.

—ROBERT BURNS, *The Vision*

HAVE you ever seen a film star with an un-attractive leg position ? Maybe two or three times in fifteen years. If the star herself forgets, then it's the cameraman's job to get a flattering angle. Or if both of them slip up, then the cutter knows that the first scenes to come to his cutting-room floor are those with awkward legs.

Not every star has perfect legs—just as not every woman has. BUT EVERY STAR KNOWS SHE MUST HANDLE HER LEGS SO THAT THEY SEEM PERFECT ! Beautiful legs still make up 90 per cent of her " sure-fire " publicity. Many a girl has climbed to stardom with pictures of her appealing " pins." Once she's proved she has other talents and possibilities as well, she refuses to pose for what is called " cheese-cake."

" Cheese-cake " is the expression used for pictures where the model's legs are photographed as the centre of attention.

The model wears shorts, bathing suit or lingerie. Her face may be beautiful, but interest is focused on her legs. Do you think the time and money spent on these thousands of poses are solely to publicise some model or actress ? No. *The publicity agents know that nothing will attract the average man's attention so quickly as a pair of pretty legs.*

I've found that women like to look at them too ! Only they look for reasons other than admiration, sometimes wistfully, sometimes hopefully.

How about applying this principle of leg appeal to yourself ? The average woman is interested chiefly in her face. Then vaguely her figure. If she thinks about her legs, it's because she likes nice hosiery. She doesn't realize that anyone sitting a few feet away from her is as conscious of what is apparent from her knees to the floor as from her neck to the top of her head—or the area between her neck and her knees.

Judging from my fan mail, I'd say the average man is *more* interested in a woman's legs when he first meets her than he is in any other feature !

If a star doesn't have nice legs, she must have a great deal to make up for this lack. Even then, she is thoroughly schooled in leg technique.

Before she's allowed to pose for her first " stills," she learns how to make the most of what she has. She launches out on a very definite campaign of " leg philosophy." It's as important for your morale as it is for hers. Here it is :

1. *Know exactly why your legs are not perfect.* I'm constantly amazed at the women who say, " I know there's something the matter with my legs, but I'm not sure just what it is ! " Legs are classified as normal, bow, heavy and thin.

(a) Normal legs, or ideal ones, are straight, and they touch at the ankles, calves, knees and thighs. (See Figure 29.)

(b) Bow legs do not meet at the calf, and some-times do not touch at the knees or ankles. The knock-kneed leg, where the knees overlap and the ankles do not come together, may also be bow or heavy. Often, too, knock-knees and " knock " ankle-bones are found together.

(c) Heavy legs have too much weight. They can be straight " piano " legs or bow also.

(d) Thin legs touch at the ankles and knees, but may not meet at the calf or above the knee because they are so slender. They are, however, definitely straight.

2. *Do everything known to correct your leg im-perfections.* Don't take the attitude, " Well, they're skinny and there's nothing I can do about them."

Hollywood has proved time and again that you CAN REDUCE FAT LEGS, DEVELOP THIN ONES,

ATTRACTIVE LEGS

IMPROVE IMPERFECTIONS CAUSED BY INCORRECT POSTURE AND MUSCLE DEVELOPMENT.

Even bow legs can be improved. True, you can't change bone structure, but here's the approach we use in the studios.

Suppose there's a two-inch space between your calves. Then you develop the muscles on the inside of each calf three-quarters of an inch. The remaining half an inch isn't so very noticeable. You will find in Lesson Seven Part B effective exercises for every type of leg problem, but don't turn to them until you have read the earlier Lessons first.

3. *Don't use your leg imperfections as a topic of conversation.* You should not mention the good or bad points of your legs to anyone. Two Rules to keep in mind about *any* physical deviation which you may have are :

(a) Learn to do everything possible to correct your deviation—do it faithfully and consistently.

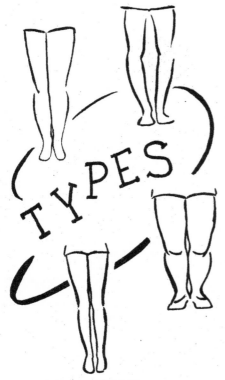

Figure 29

(b) Never refer to it or mention it. Women who would consider it most conceited to say, " I have such lovely blue eyes," will tell you when you've just met them, " You know, I have such big feet," or " My hands are always in the way," or " I'm always forgetting something," as though these things were conversational topics or as though they were proud of them. This is just another form of egotism. They feel they can't say the nice things about themselves, so since they *must* talk about themselves, they tell about their " failings."

Men especially dislike this belittling of oneself, for they feel called upon to come to your rescue. And after all, what can they say but, " Why, Jane, I never noticed your feet were large," and then for ever after, when they see Jane, think of those big feet ? They may come to your defence graciously once, but not more than that. If they want to say something nice, they want to do it of their own volition and not be goaded into it.

4. The last phase of your leg philosophy, but by no means any the less important, is this : *realize that plain legs handled gracefully are more glamorous than average legs handled awkwardly.* If you have legs anywhere near normal, you can handle them so that they appear positively ravishing !

I wish I were professionally free to mention to you the lovely stars who do not have perfect legs by any means but whom you consider the essence of fascination. You can easily learn to assume foot and leg positions that will disguise your deficiencies, too.

Earlier in this Lesson you learned how to line up your body correctly. You learned that you should stand with your body weight distributed between both legs. THIS IS THE CORRECT AND HEALTHFUL POSITION FOR YOU TO ASSUME WHEN YOU ARE WORKING. It is your " attention " position. But it is not particularly glamorous, especially if your legs deviate a bit from the normal. Legs placed side by side exaggerate flaws.

You should master an unusually flattering position for your feet and legs. These need not violate, to any extent, correct posture or the laws of body mechanics. Remember, too, that you need not employ them for any length of time.

STANDING INVITATION

A leg and foot position is called a stance. A model or star is taught that she must have a flattering leg position when she pauses for just a second or two, and another, more stable foot position for those moments when she is standing for any length of time " in the public eye," so to speak.

Let's list a few occasions when you, too, are in the public eye.

1. When you stand at the door before joining or leaving a group of friends or business colleagues.

2. When you stand to give a report or your opinion at a meeting.

3. When you enter a store or shop.

4. When you enter a theatre, dining-room, or club.

5. When you walk into your own living-room.

6. When you walk into your own office or your superior's.

Can't you see how this list could go on and on ? Another way to decide when you're in the public eye, is to list the times during the past week that you've felt timid or self-conscious. You might not have thought of these occasions as public appearances, yet they are *your* test just as a stage is for the actress.

Cornelia Otis Skinner, the talented actress, wrote of a " complete overhauling job," done on herself. She said she found that the less self-conscious she became when she looked at herself naked in the mirror, the more confidence she had when dressed in front of her audiences.

When the mirror showed a woman grown heavy and fat in places, she was timid and ashamed of herself, even when she was alone. When her body became slender and graceful once more, she felt no self-consciousness at all. She thought only of her role or her audience.

She mentioned a fundamental principle involved in all self-improvement. *Once you remove the cause of your timidity, or replace that timidity with the positive quality of confidence, you can forget yourself completely.*

Here's a challenge : Make a list of the times during one week that you felt self-conscious ; then learn how to stand so beautifully that you never have to think of your feet, legs or body.

Following this accomplishment, make another list of moments of self-consciousness for a period of a week. You've reduced your list by

half ! Of such tender stuff is our ego fashioned.

Let's consider first a position for your feet when pausing. Make a test. Walk around the room and pause frequently. Notice what your feet do when you stand still. If your feet are graceful, the chances are that your whole body looks attractive. If your feet look awkward, so do you.

A graceful position for pausing must do two things for you : (1) Show your legs off to their best advantage during the pause ; and (2) have your weight distributed so that one foot is ready for action. (See Photograph **6**.)

You've seen women who look as though they're going to set sail every time they begin to move. Their hind quarters heave up and down, or back

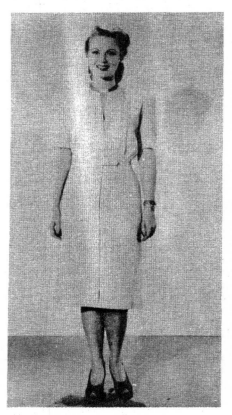

Photograph **6 .** Virginia Mayo reveals how to pause gracefully when you are walking.

77

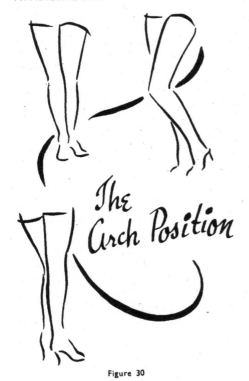

Figure 30

and forth. *Regardless of how large your buttocks area is, if your weight is smoothly distributed as you go from a stationary position to a walk, you will seem graceful.*

THE ARCH POSITION

To smooth out this weight-shifting transition, the first position I teach a student is the so-called " arch." (See Figure 30.) It's a model's expression, meaning essentially a foot position that leads, or creates the arch, from standing to walking. You will use it constantly, when you realize how many times a day you pause. Here's how you do it :

1. Put the toe of one foot level with the arch of the other. Suppose you put the toe of the right foot level with the arch of the left foot, or half-way back.

2. Put the weight of your body on the left foot, that is, the front one.

3. Lift heel of right foot so that only the ball of your foot is on the floor. (Not just the toe,

since this looks affected.)

4. Bend the right knee quite a bit.

5. Right knee touches the left knee.

6. Turn right toe out (or away from the centre of the body) about two inches, so that one foot won't look pigeon-toed.

There you are in the first " grace " position you must learn before you can move beautifully. They don't look like your legs, do they ? You've doubtless seen this position often in pictures and advertisements. This is, however, for our purposes only a *pause* position.

In other words, you have your stance which is far more flattering and natural-looking when you know you will be standing for a little while, but this " arch " is just to get you from your walk into your stance. You should practise it just as any starlet does for her first arch lesson.

Take a step and count, " Step, arch ; step, arch ; step, arch." (See Figure 30.) Practise this back and forth across the room until you achieve a certain amount of ease.

Suppose you start off with your right foot— all right, step with right foot and bring left foot into arch position. Glance in a mirror to be sure you have each part of it. Now, this time your left foot has no weight on it, so you take your next step with it, and bring the *right* foot into the arch position. When you have learned this thoroughly, you will have made a definite step toward developing body rhythm and poise. Practise it until you can do it with a book on your head—oh, so smoothly and without a break anywhere. Step, arch ; step, arch ; step, arch ; step, arch ; step, arch.

If you are a good-looking girl and reasonably graceful, you could do modelling with just this one step to help you get by. It is as important as that. Without it, you could do very little. Your movements would not be smooth and thus would detract the customer's attention from the costumes you were modelling.

Some of you may be thinking : " Well, why all this talk about modelling ? I never intend to model one stitch." No, nor does the great majority of my students, but *if you know the model's technique,* you can handle your body under any circumstance with the same ease and confidence.

78

THINKING ON YOUR FEET

You often hear this term with respect to public speakers, but since each of you has a public to please, you, too, must learn to think on your feet. You must know automatically what to do with your feet. You must *consciously* make your feet fall into these routines usually for about twelve weeks. After that, habit being what it is, they will fall into these positive patterns more naturally. And there in a nutshell you have a concrete, specific road to true poise.

Here, then, is your model's second lesson. This time you will pretend that you are showing a garment to every chair in your living-room or wherever you are working.

The more chairs the better. Walk up to your customer, or chair, stand directly in front, and arch. You notice I say directly in front of the chair. Make this a habit at once. So many people, both men and women, live their lives " on the bias." Their bodies are never positive-looking. Yet if we analyse their trouble, it is their habit of standing " off centre."

Look at the pictures of people who accomplish things. They subconsciously stand " straight." Have you ever seen even an informal snapshot of the Duchess of Windsor when she wasn't observing this rule?

So walk up to that chair, STAND DIRECTLY IN FRONT OF IT, and arch. If you are modelling professionally, you will have many occasions when your stance will be oblique and not directly in front. Don't practise this now, however, because it is a poor habit to form for social or professional contacts.

FOCUS YOUR FEET

ARCH WITH THE FOOT IN THE DIRECTION IN WHICH YOU ARE GOING. If you are going to the right, arch with the right foot. If you are going to the left, manage your feet so that you arch with the left foot.

Suppose you start to the right. Walk up to your first customer, arch with your right foot, so that when she has seen your garments, you may step out on the same foot and be on your way to your next customer, where you repeat the procedure.

This is another phase of what the model calls " thinking on your feet." You gauge your body in action as you drive your car. You will see that it requires concentration !

Should you walk up to a customer, progressing always to the right, and make a mistake, arching with the *left foot*, then what do you do ? You can't go back and start over again. No, you hide your error. You arch with the left foot as you started to, and then you casually shift your weight off your right leg to your left, so that you can arch again with the right foot and are in position to be merrily on your way once more. Thus you have learned to SHIFT THE BODY WEIGHT OR SHIFT THE ARCH.

When a woman has worked on just this much of her movement training, the difference in her body mechanism is apparent. She looks more certain of herself. I've had women up to eighty years of age work on this because of the " sureness " which it gives them.

You will find that you favour one foot or the other for making your arch. That is all right unless you are planning to do professional work. We all favour one foot just as we favour one hand.

So far so good. Now you have an attractive and efficient pause position. However, if you were going to try to stand " arched " for half an hour before an audience, you would be definitely uncomfortable, even if you changed from one foot to the other.

Your base of support is too narrow to support your body. You have too much of your body weight on one leg. You are top-heavy. Also, you look theatrical and affected. Therefore, your next move is to master the stance that will flatter your legs.

You have pictures here of every type of leg. (See Figure 29.) Which is most like yours ? Get an uninterrupted view of your legs from the hips down. You may have what you consider a " combination " leg. If they're thin and bow, or heavy and bow, practise the stance for bowed legs. A bow in your thighs usually indicates lack of muscle development and weight distribution rather than faulty bone structure.

You'll find a couple of good exercises for this in Lesson 7. *Concentrate first on a stance that will show your legs to advantage from the knees down.* Master this first. Then get going on your thighs.

So in case your legs are thin below the knees and fat above them, you'll perfect a stance for thin legs first. Then begin your exercise programme for distribution.

STANCE FOR NORMAL LEGS

First, let's consider the normal stance position for the normal leg. Virginia Mayo, Helen Hayes, Gertrude Lawrence, Joan Crawford, Marlene · Dietrich, Mary Martin, Claudette Colbert, Gene Tierney, all use this stance. (See Photograph 7). Watch them. Statistics do not prove that this type of leg is more common than the others. *So I say, if your legs are straight, be thankful for them and get busy glamorizing them !* Here is

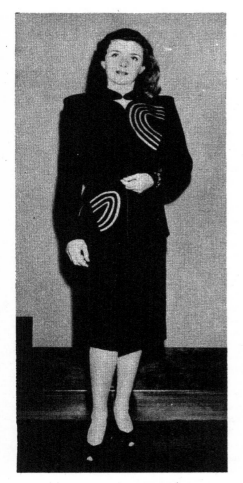

Photograph 7 Here Lenore Aubert demonstrates a natural stance for normal legs.

how you do it :

1. The feet should not be farther apart than six inches.

2. One foot should be pushed back a few inches farther than the other, so that the toe of the back foot is one or two inches behind the heel of the front foot. The back leg will carry a little more body weight than the front one. But don't settle so much on your back leg that you push your hips out of line !

3. The heel of the back foot turns slightly in toward the centre of the body. For comparison put this foot back straight and then put it back at this suggested slight slant. See how much more flattering the second position is ?

4. Both knees are *slightly* bent—never held rigid.

5. The knee of the front foot should cover the inside line of the back knee, *so bend it a lot.* The model calls this the " knee flip " and her knee may fall one or two inches over the back one, depending upon her legs. The best-looking legs need the least bend. This is a beautifying trick that every actress learns. Watch, however, that the foot of the front leg from the ankle down is held firmly. Don't let the ankle or arch drop.

Go to a mirror and see what a vast improvement this makes in the appearance of your legs. Practise it until you can go into it smoothly without calling anyone's attention to your foot-work.

STANCE FOR BOW LEGS

Of all the lessons I present, I suppose I get the biggest thrill out of the session when I show those whose legs fall into this group how to stand so that no one can tell they are bow.

Any woman with bow legs can, by handling them wisely, give the illusion of having normal legs. My own students fool me every day with this stance. I forget which ones use it. I can't tell and I defy ANYONE to tell !

Remember we said that if your legs do not meet at the ankles, calves or knees, they are considered " bow " to some extent, depending upon the distance between the calf, ankle and knee of one leg and those of the other leg.

The principle for correcting the line of the bow leg is like that involved in comparing any two objects. Suppose you have two vases. If one has a crack and you place it too near the perfect one, you will call attention to the flaw. Where you have some distance between them, the defect may never be apparent.

It is the same with bow-legs. Never, *never* place them in an identical position side by side, toes pointing straight ahead in parenthesis fashion ( ). One leg alone, without another for comparison, looks perfectly normal. Often, each individual leg is beautiful *alone*. Its flaw isn't obvious until the other leg pops up beside it for emphasis ! Here's how you disguise bow-legs :

1. Front foot faces due front. (See Figure 31.)

2. Turn the toe of your back foot to the side, so that your back foot forms almost a right angle with the front foot. As the back foot turns to the side, the body wants to turn with it. So adjust your back foot enough to ensure your body is directly facing the front.

3. Put most of the weight of the body on the back foot.

4. Have both knees bent quite a bit.

5. BEND THE FRONT KNEE ENOUGH SO THAT IT COVERS SOME OF THE BACK LEG. It is these two techniques which hide the crooked arch.

6. Do not let the heel of the back shoe show from the front. (See Figure 31.) Push the whole front leg over enough to hide this back heel.

Now look at yourself. It's so magical that it's difficult to believe. After you've practised your corrective stance for a week, you can slip into it very easily and inconspicuously. It's like money in the bank.

STANCE FOR HEAVY LEGS

Sometimes heavy legs are found on slender bodies. They need not be too great a handicap. Many successful women have " piano legs ", yet few people have ever noticed it because they handle them well and dress so as not to emphasize them. And remember, there are thousands of men in the world who like good substantial " pins " ! BUT USE THEM CAREFULLY !

If your legs are heavy, here is one sure cure for diminishing their line. Strive to create one line instead of two.

You do this by hiding the back leg. Notice the two sketches of fat legs. (See Figure 32.) Here are the rules for imitating this foot position:

1. Put front leg directly in front of back leg. (See Figure 32.)

2. Have a little more of your body weight on the back leg.

3. Keep both knees bent or " easy "—as the elbow falls, but put a lot of ease in your front

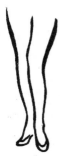

Figure 31

knee.

4. Turn toe of front leg slightly away from the centre of the body—about an inch.

5. Turn toe of back foot away from the body in the opposite direction from the front foot. For example, if the front foot turns to the left, then turn the back foot to the right. See ? This turning out also helps your balance.

6. Heels of both feet are turned in towards the centre of the body.

7. There may be three or four inches between the heel of the front foot and the toe of the back one. *This is where you get your balance.* In other words, you get your spacing between your front and back leg instead of crosswise as do those who have another type of leg.

Now look in the mirror. You've subtracted inches from your legs with this stance, haven't you ? Personally, I think this is the most difficult stance of all, and I wish I could encourage you by divulging the names of some very lovely ladies you admire who use it ALL THE TIME.

STANCE FOR THIN LEGS

The very thin legs seem to give their owners the most worry. They complain, and rightly, that there just isn't any appeal in skinny legs. Fortunately, by handling them carefully, actual inches can seemingly be added to their size.

Some of our most successful actresses, such as Irene Dunne, Constance Bennett, Joan Fontaine, Rosalind Russell, have very slender legs ; but they handle them so skilfully that their public is never aware of their proportions. Watch to see how they do it.

If your legs fall into this classification, your guiding principle at all times is this : don't separate them so much in standing or sitting that the eye is attracted to only one. Keep them close enough that they give a double line and therefore create the illusion of being twice their inches.

When you sit, you are the type who can cross her legs most gracefully ; and press the calf of your top leg against the calf of the under leg to give each more width. Your fuller-legged sister must avoid this like the plague !

When you stand, here is your most flattering stance, so practise until it's a habit :

1. Stand so that the toe joint of the back foot is even with the heel of the front foot. (See Figure 33.)

2. Have no more than six inches between feet from toe to toe.

3. Put a little more body weight on the back foot than on the front foot. But don't settle on it so much that you push your hip out of joint.

4. Back foot is placed at an angle—heel in, toe out.

5. Bend the knee of the front leg enough so that it just barely covers the inside line of the back knee.

6. The front leg covers only half an inch or less of the inside line of the back leg. Let no daylight show through the two legs from the calves up to the knee.

7. The front foot faces *straight ahead*.

So what do you get ? A double line so curved that even an expert won't know you've worried for all these years about your " skinny " legs ! AND MOVE SMOOTHLY AND RHYTHMICALLY ! Quick, jerky movements make legs seem twice as spindly as they are.

Don't forget, when you are practising your particular stance, to line up your body correctly as you learned in Lesson 3 Part A.

You must look at yourself in your entirety—not piecemeal. Because that's the way others see you. As you are from the top of your head to the tip of your toes.

Therefore, each time you assume your stance, balance your pelvis over your feet, your chest over your pelvis, and your head over your chest. These stances are the accepted glamorous ones. You can get away with the current stylised leg positions IF (see Figure 29) :

1. You have almost perfect legs.

2. You've had ballet or modern dance training (not to be confused with ball-room dancing).

3. You're wearing active sports, spectator sports, or ballet clothes.

4. You're under thirty !

That narrows it down to about 2 per cent of our girls—or possibly the models who are displaying these stances.

Do practise in your high heels. What's more ungainly than a grown woman acting as though she's wearing her first high heels ? Keep your high heels for your more exciting moments. Wear your low-heeled shoes for walking, working, general wear.

I notice that Gene Tierney is one Hollywood star who likes low heels, and the new low heels are smart. Low-heeled shoes require clothes adapted to them. Fortunately, there are beautiful low-heeled shoes made now that are as formal as high heels.

Whether you wear low or high heels will depend a lot on how you feel in either. If, no matter how flattering the low heels are, you still feel " un-dressed-up " in them, don't wear them when you're out for a new job.

On the other hand, low-heeled sandals may make you feel akin to Cleopatra. Then, they're for you !

I'd like to caution you about so-called health shoes and shoes with arch supports. If your feet hurt, go to an orthopaedic specialist. He will X-ray your feet and prescribe correct shoes for you. And you won't be out of pocket ! Because what is more costly than shoes that hurt or that you can't wear ? To say nothing of the multitude of arch supports and artificial foot gadgets that some girls fall for !

You have only one pair of feet. TAKE CARE OF THEM as thoroughly as you do your hands. You should see how dancers, actresses and models " coddle " their feet. They have to, because if their feet give out, they're finished. *You know how much older you look when your feet are*

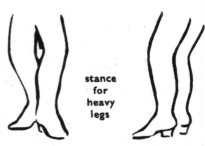

stance for heavy legs

Figure 32

82

tired or hurt. Even make-up seems to accentuate the fatigue lines at such times.

You know, too, how much more irritable you are !

Whenever I coach a new group of studio players, I am requested to give each girl a written schedule for the care of her feet. This is the one I've worked out to keep normal feet in condition—and it doesn't take a great deal of time to follow :

1. Wear flat shoes as much as you can. Stylish, glamorous flat-heeled ones.

2. Wear shoes that are wide enough and long enough. See if you can wiggle your toes around in them comfortably.

3. Have the shoe shop ease up your shoes for two days on their stretchers. Try to find someone with feet a size or so smaller than yours to " break in " your new shoes for a week.

4. If they hurt after you've worn them several times, sell them or give them away. WEARING SHOES THAT HURT YOUR FEET IS FOOLISH ECONOMY. It will catch up with you !

5. Wear hose a size larger than you think you should wear. Stretch the feet of your hose length-wise and crosswise after each laundering. Sell or give away hose that are too small for you. Foot experts will tell you that small hose cause *most* of our foot troubles.

6. Change your shoes and hose as often as you can during the day. Between changes walk around in your bare feet. Stretch your toes by opening them as wide as you can. Shake your feet. Then pull your toes under. Repeat stretching, shaking, and pulling under.

If your work is such that you must wear one pair of shoes and hose for hours at a time, then take off your shoes (hose, too) and do as much of this stretching, shaking and pulling as possible. You can do a little of this even with your shoes on—every little bit helps a lot, too. You'll find time to work them in if they seem important to you.

7. Walk around the house in your bare feet ; or if you take cold from this habit, wear woollen hose. No shoes when you exercise.

8. Scrub your feet and toes with a brush once a day, preferably while you're taking your bath. Rub them vigorously as you dry them. Use a softening lotion or oil on them, but be sure they're dry before you put on hose. Massage oil or cream into your feet as often as you have time. Minutes spent in foot massage are well

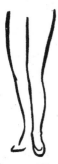

Figure 33

spent !

9. The " upside-down " position mentioned in Lesson One Part A helps your feet. Don't forget that your feet and legs fight gravity every minute they are supporting your weight. Foot elevation gives them a little chance to compensate.

10. Good posture and the posture exercises in Lesson Six Part B are extremely beneficial for your feet. So you're killing many birds here with one stone !

11. When your feet swell, burn, or you've subjected them to long hours of strain, sit on the edge of your bath and put your feet in water as hot as you can stand it for a minute or two. Then let the cold water run over them for a couple of minutes.

I've heard of alternating foot plunges in hot and cold water—but what modern home has two foot baths convenient for filling ? Hot and cold running water will serve your purpose. And you're far more likely to use it !

12. Wear "toe dividers" between your toes to correct crooked ones. Or pieces of cotton wool between your toes day and night will do the trick provided you start getting large enough hose and shoes.

13. Learn how to give yourself a professional pedicure.

14. Use a little pumice on calluses, or use the smooth side of an emery board. Soaking, oiling and massage will soon relieve this condition. Follow the directions on corn plasters for corns.

If your feet don't respond to your own treatment, consult a chiropodist for corns or calluses. These are indications of strain. Don't let the condition continue !

15. Here are a few foot exercises (see Figure 34) you should incorporate into your working day. Notice that I do not put them in the Lesson on exercising, because I feel they definitely should be part of your daily " must."

(a) Pick up your towel, wash-cloth, pieces of paper with toes.

(b) Wiggle your toes. Pretend you are playing the piano with them. Two beats with each toe.

(c) Clasp one big toe with the other and pull one towards the other. This is especially good for an enlarged toe-joint.

(d) Pull your toes.

You will recall that this schedule is for feet that seem to be normal in that they cause no pain, spasms, excessive fatigue, etc. There are, however, many feet that are past this stage. DON'T TRY HOME REMEDIES ON THEM. Go to an orthopaedic specialist, or an osteopath. He will probably have you follow a schedule similar to this, plus a few individual correctives. *If you don't get reasonable relief after following his suggestions, keep going back until you do hit on the right programme for you.*

YOU CAN'T BE GRACEFUL ON SORE FEET !

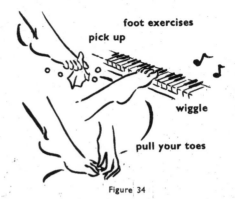

foot exercises
pick up
wiggle
pull your toes

Figure 34

Remember that many a facial wrinkle begin with an aching foot ! Indeed, so close do Atkinson's find the link between a lovely face and comfortable, healthy feet that they give pedicure and foot massage treatments in their Bond Street Salon as an important part of many of their Beauty routines.

This is a lot of leg information to digest, but isn't it fun ? And don't ever tell me you can't glamorize YOURS.

Notes:

Notes:

Self-Test Questions Based On Lesson Three

This is most important. Attractive features, shapely legs, well-groomed figure are all spoiled unless one walks and sits gracefully. Too often one meets the gauche, awkward walker with slouching shoulders, which partially ruin an otherwise very attractive woman.

After you have studied this Lesson you should be able to answer the following questions. If you have any difficulty in doing so, refer to the Lesson for further study and revision. Your answers should not be sent to the publishers of this Course.

1. How and when can you acquire good posture ?

2. Write down five benefits which you acquire from possessing good posture.

3. Write a criticism of your posture after standing in front of the mirror. Enter under two separate headings as shown :
   Good Points :   Bad Points :

4. Where to put and what to do with the hands are most people's greatest problem. Quote four points in regard to hand positions.

5. Write the words you should repeat to yourself to make sure your posture is correct and ensure your looking your best. These words should be learned by heart.

6. Study types of legs described in this Lesson; then with the aid of a long mirror find what type of legs you possess. You are fortunate if you have perfect legs. If you have not, find out exactly why they are not perfect.

7. Those who do not have perfect legs may make them appear attractive. How may this be done ?

8. How should you stand when approaching a person, socially or professionally ?

9. When practising your stance or examining yourself in front of the mirror, how must you look at yourself and why ?

10. Why is the care of the feet so important ?

If you wish to determine the progress you are making, give yourself 10 points for each question you answer correctly. If the total comes to 90 or more, it is excellent; 80 or more, good; 70 or more, fair.

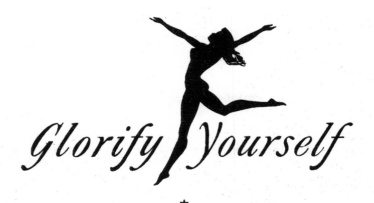

Glorify Yourself

★

A Complete and Up-to-Date Course on
Beauty and Charm by One of the
Most Famous Beauty Specialists
and Consultants in the World

Eleanore King

★

LESSON FOUR

★

STUDIO TALK •

Issued only for Students of the Eleanore King Course on Beauty. Charm and Personality.

Number Four.

Dear Student,

The chances are that to-day you will walk at least four or five miles. Without leaving your home you can cover nearly two miles in the course of ordinary light housework. If you are at business you will do rather more than this in the course of your work. Add a little for shopping or travelling, and you will soon see the miles mount up.

Since you have so much walking to do, you should learn to do it gracefully and easily. People judge you by the way you walk, and a light but assured, purposeful step will help you to make a good impression on your many public appearances.

Make no mistake. You are in the public eye when you walk into your own living-room just as much as if you were on the screen. Entering a shop is a public appearance just as much as making an entrance on the stage. You may not have thought of these occasions as public appearances but that is what they really are. And to make a success of them, you must be complete mistress of your legs and feet.

You will already have mastered the fundamentals described in Lesson Three. It is time now to apply them to walking and sitting. For sitting, too, should be a time for body composure, and should always be associated with poise. Part B of Lesson Four therefore tells you in detail what to do about sitting; about chairs; how to get into them: and what to do with your body, head, hands and feet while you are in them.

This part of the Lesson will be of special value to you if you follow a sedentary occupation. Sitting for long periods will no longer be a tedious necessity....it will be a golden opportunity for you to enhance the beauty of your body.

Yours sincerely,

Eleanore King

(over)

Page 2.

P.S. In Lesson Five we shall discuss your clothes. You will be shown a simple, ingenious method of deciding exactly what to wear and how and when to wear it.

LESSON FOUR

Part A

A Graceful Walk

I grant I never saw a goddess go;
My mistress, when she walks, treads on the ground.
—SHAKESPEARE, *Sonnets, No. CXXX*

WHY do we associate superior qualities with those who walk well? When you read the ancient Greek legends, you learned how each goddess looked—what distinguished her from other goddesses. How she walked, how she moved. In fact, her manner of walking seemed to be one of her outstanding characteristics. Supposedly, she didn't have an earthly walk. It was as though she glided with a special tread.

Poets and writers have always been inspired by a beautiful walk. Florenz Ziegfeld was so particular how his Ziegfeld Follies walked that it was almost an obsession with him.

A woman who walks beautifully is still one of the thrills of every-day life. Yet, of all the qualities which *any woman* can develop, and which pay the greatest dividends, both socially and professionally, the art of walking seems the most often neglected.

In Hollywood, where glamour abounds, you find each star taking her walking very seriously. She may insist, when you interview her, that she " just walks naturally in front of the camera." However, her practised and rehearsed movements, through intensive application, have become such an integrated part of her that you're conscious only of a lovely, composite impression when you see her. (See Photograph 8).

Not long ago I sat at the end of a very long living-room in Bel Air and watched Gene Tierney come in and greet her friends. She was very natural, but every movement was controlled —a joy to watch.

ANY WOMAN CAN LEARN

You owe it to yourself and to those around you to be just as fastidious about your walk. ANY WOMAN CAN LEARN TO WALK BEAUTIFULLY.

You can argue that you can't change your bone structure, your skin pigment, and many other qualities about yourself that you don't like ; but you can learn to be graceful, and you can learn to master this art as you go about your daily work.

Your walk tells a great deal about you. First of all, it tells how you regard yourself in relation to others. Your walk reveals timidity, shyness, aggressiveness, even carelessness.

Into my newspaper headquarters each day pour hundreds of letters from men. They don't like women's crazy hats, they don't like painted nails, and they don't like slacks, to mention a few of their pet " grouses." *But I have yet to receive a letter, or a comment, from a man who does not want the leading lady in his life to walk well.* Men instinctively seem to watch women's movements. It's a masculine characteristic.

If you ask them what they like in a woman, you won't get a comment on walking as such. They may be expressing their dislike in expressions such as, " She's slovenly," " She's sloppy."

If you try to analyse these comments, you'll realize their impression is formed to a great extent by how the woman carries herself. It's probably the same as the familiar one of " walking like a queen."

Basically, a man wants to be proud of his woman, and he wants her to be proud of herself. One of her most tangible means of expressing her pride in herself is her walk. For too many years it was almost impossible to find specific instructions on how to acquire a beautiful walk.

I hope the steps presented here are so simple that you can't help incorporating them.

Let's pretend for this Lesson that you have signed a contract at one of the studios because of your beauty and talent. You are being groomed for your first picture, which starts in about six weeks. The powers that be have decided that you must improve your walk. Here, then, is your walking lesson, step by step.

Since every part of your body must co-ordinate with every other part of your body when you walk, there is a vast amount of information to assimilate.

Do the best you can alone, for a few weeks. Then, if you aren't in a vicinity where there is a good coach, ask a sympathetic friend to help you. We can never see ourselves as others see us. Even the coaches have to enlist the assistance of another coach for criticism. You may concentrate a whole week on overcoming one bad walking habit, with total indifference to the rest of your body. Be patient! Don't expect perfection immediately, but I will make you a promise. One of these fine days, someone will say to you, " You know, Irene, you get lovelier all the time." That's your cue to say, " Oh, thank you. You're so encouraging," and be mum about your practising.

Practise your walking lesson in your bare feet, your stockinged feet, your low-heeled shoes and your high heels. Since many of your most glamorous moments will be spent in your high heels, it is essential that you learn to walk in them as though you live in them.

I think, though, that you will feel what is taking place in your foot movement more, if you practise some of the time in your bare feet and stockinged feet.

You may even interest five or six girls in

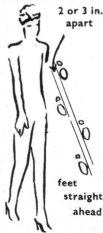

2 or 3 in.
apart

feet
straight
ahead

Figure 35

practising this walking lesson. I often think, in my own classes, that the student gets as much assistance from other students as she does from me. This is particularly true, I believe, because walking represents an over-all picture of everything you are or want to be.

RULES TO FOLLOW

Here are the rules in your walking lesson :

1. *Line up your body in correct posture, as you learned in Lesson Three Part A.*

Your body weight carried just in front of your ankle-bone ;

Your feet straight ahead ;

Your knees relaxed.

Now, tuck your buttocks under you ; carry your chest high ; feel that your shoulders are broad and relaxed ; your head high and balanced evenly.

2. *Walk in two straight lines about two inches apart.* There are many schools of thought on placing the feet. Some authorities say, " Walk in a single line."

I believe that the average woman will feel more comfortable and look more natural if she adheres to the rule of one or two inches between her feet.

Of course, the size of her knees and thighs will have something to do with the position of her feet. A slender woman can glide along almost on one line without seeming theatrical ; whereas a heavy woman will have to have a broader base for stability.

You know how difficult it is to get your Christmas tree to stand up until you have worked out the correct base and support for it. The show-girl often walks with an exaggerated crossing over of each leg in one line. I definitely do not like to have my students strive for this effect.

Stretch a ball of twine the length of your longest room. Make two lines two inches apart, or draw two chalk lines indoors or outdoors for practice. Walk along these two chalk lines for several minutes, for several days. (See Figure 35.)

The average untrained woman is amazed how much concentration it requires to co-ordinate her steps to two straight lines. You may find that you have been zigzagging all over the pavement! Feel that you can manage these two lines quite comfortably before you attempt the next rule.

3. *Point your feet straight ahead when you walk.* (See Figure 35.) Your straight lines will

94

help you with this. See that the line divides the length of your foot equally.

Walk up and down a few times, just noticing this. The chances are that one foot, or both feet, will turn in or out. Don't let this discourage you, because with a week's practice you CAN learn to point your feet straight ahead. I have seen it happen thousands of times, even in cases where the woman was a chronic " pigeon-toe " for thirty years. You must expect, though, that the longer you have placed your feet incorrectly, the more concentrated must be your efforts for correction.

Here is the best system I know for correcting foot position : Pay no attention whatever to the rest of your body for one week.

Every time you put your foot down, look at it and see if it is toeing straight ahead. Think to yourself as you walk, " Straight, straight, my feet must be straight." When you are practising on your two lines at home, repeat this command to yourself out loud. The spoken command has power to control action. That's probably why so much attention was given in Officer Candidate Schools to voice and manner of giving commands.

So, whenever you can, control yourself with specific commands.

You may have paid good money to learn to walk with your toes pointing out. You're not alone ! *This not only adds ten years to your age, but makes you look awkward and it is a gross violation of sound body mechanics.*

If you are riding a bicycle down the street and you point the front wheel to the right, your progress is somewhat curtailed, isn't it ? Yet, this is exactly what you do when you turn your toes out and still walk straight ahead. You are also straining and enlarging the big-toe joint with every step.

If both your toes turn in and you have suffered all your life with being pigeon-toed, you really have a job ahead of you.

In your case, if you walk towards a full-length mirror you will notice that your toe turns inwards because your whole foot rotates in towards the centre of your body from the ankle joint. This inward rotation has stretched the outer muscles of your legs and feet and shrunk the inside muscles. Your job now is to equalize the inside and outside muscles.

Therefore, every chance you get, make circles with your feet, so that your toes (and, of course,

your feet) circle first away from the centre of your body and then in towards the centre of it. Relax your feet as the toes point into the centre of your body ; and tense and stretch as they go away from the centre of your body.

If you were a prospective screen star and this tendency to turn the toes inwards was discovered, you might find yourself doing approximately five hundred of these circles a day. THEN, you really would improve your pigeon-toed condition rapidly.

4. *Your whole foot seems to contact the ground at one time.* Actually, however, your heel touches the ground first. Your weight is transferred to the outside margin of your foot and thence to the ball of the foot.

Think of a three-point landing : heel ; outside of the foot ; and ball of foot. Most teachers of deportment speak of only the heel and the ball of the foot, because in high-heeled shoes you aren't conscious of the outside border of the foot.

If the transfer from the heel to the ball of your foot is too slow, you will get a clumsy, " clodhopper " movement.

Be sure that the ball of your foot does not touch the ground first. Many teachers insist that you should put the ball of the foot down first. I will grant that for eurhythmics in your bare feet, this principle may have value. But try the following experiment yourself : Put on your shoes, walk towards a full-length mirror, purposely walking on the ball of your foot first. Give your honest impression of the person you see there. She looks a little insincere, doesn't she ?

Many actresses employ this means of walking when they are impersonating a deceptive character. You have enough mannerisms to overcome without adding this one. Women in the Services were taught to walk heel first, and they were a beautiful sight to see.

In your stockinged feet, as you transfer your weight from the heel to the ball of your foot, you are conscious of a powerful forward and upward movement.

The ball of your foot is a wondrous machine, responsible for moving your body forward. When you understand how delicate this mechanism is, and what a great responsibility it has, you realize why beauty and health experts advise that " You are as young as your feet are strong."

Therefore, the few minutes you spend on

massaging and exercising them are a sound investment.

5. *Keep your knees relaxed.* Just as you have learned to stand with relaxed knees, so you will incorporate this principle into your movements.

There is a caution in this respect : if your knee is bent too much as you take a step, then, before you can take another step, you must straighten it partially. Such continued straightening will give your walk a series of upward movements, or unpleasant jerks. This jerking causes the whole body to bounce up and down, and it especially affects the bustline.

A lady walks so that her bustline remains firm and controlled. To avoid ungainly gyrations have your knee reasonably firm as your heel hits the floor. On the other hand, avoid stiff knees. You have heard of "locked" knees—tense and rigid. What you are striving for is a relaxed, firm knee movement.

6. *Clear your knees.* Have a friend listen as you walk in your stockinged feet and high heels. Is there a sound ? This may be due either to fat on your knees or to knock-knees. You learned in Part B of Lesson Three that knock-knees were often caused by "knocked" ankles. Or your knees may be fat and not knocked (You will find exercises in Lesson 7 Part B on " How to Reduce Fat Knees and Thighs." While you are correcting either your posture or your weight, however, be wary about " walking around each knee." You can learn how to clear " your knees " so as to avoid this " corduroy breeches " sound.

One student told me that her husband asked her, " What have you got down there that's making such a racket ? " Don't let your knees whistle while you walk !

7. *Measure your stride.* Usually, a shorter woman has a smaller stride than a taller one. A long stride is more trying, from the angle of grace, than a short one.

Some teachers say that your stride will be correct if it measures the length of one foot. That is, you have the length of one foot between the heel of the front foot and the toe of the back foot as you are walking. There is a danger in this principle, however, because many short women have long feet in proportion to the size of their bodies.

Here is the best test I know for ensuring that you have the correct stride :

Line yourself up in your best posture. Then,

without moving your head, glance down as you start to walk. If you can see your toes or the hem of your skirt, your stride is too long. For camera technique, we warn the model, " Keep your foot *within* the hem-line of your skirt."

You may admire the long, smooth steps of a screen star. Don't forget, however, that she has spent hours practising this technique. On the whole, remember you will be more graceful if you curtail the length of your stride.

8. *Discipline your hips* Wobbly hips often ruin an otherwise graceful walk. I think it is more difficult to cure wobbly hips than any other walking habit. They are caused chiefly by two faults : first, incorrect pelvic posture ; and second, hingeing at the hip joint.

If you discover, or already know, that you have excessive hip action, then turn to Lesson Six Part B on corrective posture, and approach your problem in a scientific manner. You can't do it by walking with your hands placed over your buttocks. This may smooth them down a little, but not much. Nor can you accomplish results by walking with a book on your head.

I have seen hula hips, whose owners could balance anything from a book to a basket of clothes on their heads and still keep their hips in motion.

Very often, hip movement is due to a lazy shifting, which means that at each step there is a definite lunge on the hip joint. Almost a step, and then a sideways hingeing takes place.

Instead of settling to one side, move forward constantly without taking time to lunge with each step. This is difficult to overcome.

If you can find someone more or less your size, someone who has a graceful carriage, place your arm around her waist and walk with her. Concentrate on her forward movements which have no wasted motion to the side ; and then contrast it with your habit of taking a step and hesitating long enough to settle at the hip joint. She goes smoothly forward, while you shift awkwardly from one side to the other.

9. *Lead with your thighs.* Since your legs are joined to your torso in front of you, your legs should precede you as you walk.

So many women think of their legs being " under " them. This idea has a tendency to push the buttocks out at the back by tipping the pelvis incorrectly. When you begin to take a step, raise your thigh slightly and think of it as preceding the body. Line yourself up against a wall with your head and shoulder, spine and buttocks touching.

Now, as you walk away, notice which part of your body moves first. Usually it is the head and shoulders. You will never have a graceful line until you learn to lead with your thigh.

There is an interesting body-mechanics angle on this rule for leading with the thigh, and it is this': you must establish a base. You are moving forward an object, which is your body. By extending your leg first you establish a base on which to support the weight of your body as it moves forward from the back leg.

There is no necessity for your postponing your walking practice until you have a perfect body line-up. You will find that correct walking principles will parallel correct posture, and that one will help the other.

One day not so long ago I walked down Hollywood Boulevard behind a woman with a magnificent carriage. Before I had walked very far I heard someone say, " How do you do, Lady Mendl ? " I realized then that it was Lady Elsie Mendl, who admits to eighty-one. Had anyone asked me her age, after watching her walk, I might have said forty or forty-five.

I realized that she was incorporating what many coaches call the " youth line." It means that as you stand or walk, you adhere to the plumb-line we talked about in a previous Lesson.

If anything, the body tilts slightly backwards from the knees to the shoulders, rather than slightly backwards from the shoulders to the buttocks. This has been called the " Hollywood Walk," and it is a little exaggerated, but if you have been hurrying around for years with your buttocks trailing your head, then this exaggerated idea may help you to succeed at least in achieving a body that looks straight up and down.

10. *Chest high.* Carry your chest high—not forward. Be sure that, as you raise it you do not push out your buttocks. This is a natural tendency, so guard against it. This will help to flatten your abdomen.

Also, of course, your best cure for a protruding abdomen is to walk with your pelvis carried correctly—or your hips tucked under you. You'll recall how quickly servicemen lost their " corporations " during six weeks' basic training.

Raise your chest muscles until they are tense, then gradually relax, but don't " drop "

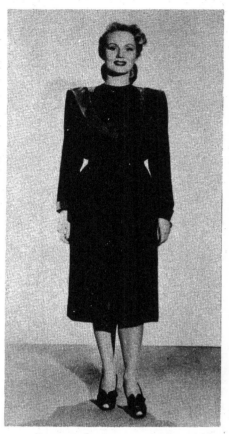

Photograph **8** For a natural walk, model your movements after those of Virginia Mayo.

your chest.

A beautiful woman must have a high, firm chest and bust line. Thus, every moment that you walk with your chest carried correctly, you are helping to improve or maintain your breasts, since they get their sole support from the pectoral muscles which are spread fanwise throughout the chest and under the arm area.

You will find that just as for correct *standing* position, the movement of your chest, shoulders, head and arms is closely related—so the same co-ordination must be maintained for walking.

11. *Swing from your rib cage.* You and I know it is impossible for you to walk from your rib cage since your legs are joined to the torso, in the

groin. Yet the leg muscles, as well as all the other muscles of your body which are used when you walk, do reach the rib cage area.

I have found that it helps my students to acquire a " long-legged " look if they have a MENTAL CONCEPTION of moving high. Many of our most famous actresses are very small : Helen Hayes, Lily Pons, Vivien Leigh, Bette Davis. Yet, as you watch them, you have a feeling of streamlines. Their stride is not necessarily long, but their legs seem to swing from their ribs. Contrast this with the women you see going along as though they were on scooters, moving only from their knee joints.

Here is a good way to get the feeling of this rib-cage movement :

As you are drying yourself after your shower or bath, support yourself by putting one hand on the wall, at arm's length. Then swing your right leg backwards and forwards ten times. Then swing your left leg. *Feel* the muscles around your ribs. This is the same muscular sensation that you should have as you swing into a walk.

Keep the feet relaxed or " soft," and bring them down lightly. Don't clump down heavily. The combination of bringing your feet down lightly, heel first, confidently, plus feeling that you are controlling your legs from the rib cage, will give a positive " lift " to others as you enter a room.

Often, before an actress says a word, you sense an exhilaration from her entrance. Her movements and walk either give you an uplift or they don't.

So it is with individuals. If you wish to impress others with optimism and radiance, you must produce it with lightness and spring in your walk. Then when you have left a room, your presence is still there.

12. *Use your shoulders for balance.* If it was important for you to have a relaxed, broad shoulder line in standing, it is even more so for walking.

When you detect any tension in your shoulders, don't forget to rotate them up towards your ears, back and down. Repeat this relaxation rotation until your shoulders feel perfectly at ease.

High, tense shoulders can ruin an otherwise graceful walk, and they make you seem so ill at ease. Be sure that your shoulders are even. Where one is lower than the other, carry your handbag or your small packages with the arm of

the low shoulder. And carry your heavy packages that have handles with the arm of your high shoulder. Also, you will want to make use of the corrective shoulder exercises in Lesson Six Part B.

13. *Your head is high.* Walk tall. Stretch up. Feel tall. Don't get the habit, however, of walking with your head always straight ahead. It's good for you to practise moving your head from side to side as you walk down the street. Move it slowly. It won't be as easy as you think, the first few times you try it, because your head is heavy, and this movement may throw you off balance somewhat.

This technique does give your carriage distinction when you enter theatres, clubs or dining-rooms.

The most important rule for you to remember about your head is to keep it in line with the rest of your body. Don't lead by a nose. For a few weeks, check the position of your head and shoulder line whenever you think about it.

Remember that you want the lobe of your ear to form a vertical line with the shoulder-bone.

There is something lovely about the carriage of a woman's head, IF SHE KEEPS HER CHIN UP. I suppose it is possible to overdo this, and look too aggresive, but I know of no such cases.

I think that Aline Kilmer in her poem, *Experience*, had a beautiful head carriage in mind when she wrote, " She walks the way primroses grow." I emphasize this habit of walking with the head held high, because it is so easy for a woman to drop her head as she starts thinking while she walks along.

Every time you walk with your head forward is adding years to your neck-line. Your neck sags in front into folds.

14. *Control your arms.* Now that you have your torso and legs working, begin to co-ordinate the arm movements with them. Usually, the last part of a student's technique to be mastered is the movement of arms and hands, and getting them to co-ordinate with the body properly.

How much should you swing your arms ? What should you do with them when moving ? If you are out for a hike, swing them as much as you wish, and really work up some circulation. But for business or social purposes, here is the rule for them. *They must be disciplined, but this must be done so casually that they seem perfectly poised.*

Measuring from front to back, the distance from the largest part of your abdomen to the largest part of your buttocks is equal to the distance your arms should swing. This gives them quite a bit of leeway, depending upon your proportions.

Women in the Services were taught to swing their arms four inches in front of the body and six inches behind it—which still isn't the wide, uncontrolled swinging so apparent among women today.

The arms hang loosely from the shoulders, elbows always held slightly bent or "easy." Forget your arms if you can. The whole arm should fit close to the body. Don't carry your elbows out.

Often you see a beautifully costumed and groomed woman who, when standing, is lovely. But when moving, she has pugilist's elbows. If wide-flung arms are your problem, here is the best cure I know :

Make sure that the inside of your elbows and wrists touch your side with every swing. Sometimes the arms hang away from the body because there is a layer of fat on the arms and on the body just under the arm sockets. In this case, these areas *will have to be reduced.*

Keep your hands down at your sides as you walk, palms turned in, as you did for your standing position. Very often one arm of a woman's body will swing back and forth, and the other will swing crosswise from one side to the other.

Keep your arms parallel ! Don't consciously swing your arms. They move, rather, because your torso moves. They help balance your body and act as levers.

When you see a line of soldiers marching, notice how little their arms move, and with what a small effort.

If you find your arm movements are out of line, then take a week to correct them. Every time you move or walk, check the position of your arms. It takes some time to discipline them but it is well worth it, for the ultimate success of your walk depends on how beautifully your arms co-ordinate with your body.

This same law applies to an actress, an athlete or a platform speaker. The arms and body must work together, to give a pleasant picture.

Sometimes when the arms are tense, they have a tendency to hang down stiff at the sides of the body, with the wrists pushing out. This betrays the fact that you are self-conscious or nervous about something. Others sense this quickly. The trick here is to have the inside of your wrist *touch* the side of your hip. (See Figure 36)

15. *Rhythm does it.* And now we come to that quality which is the difference between grace and awkwardness. RHYTHM. You can have it one month and fall out of it the next month.

NATURAL RHYTHM

What is rhythm ? It is beauty applied to everything you do. It is a beauty which others *feel* about you and cannot define.

You will notice that all through this instruction we have stressed verbal counting. That is just another way of describing rhythm. Haven't you noticed that you whistle as you walk, or that you hum a tune ? That is natural rhythm asserting itself.

As you start to walk, form the habit of saying slowly, either audibly or inaudibly, " One, two, three, four ; one, two, three, four ; one, two, three, four."

Say the words with a smooth tone. Don't count as though you were marching to a staccato beat, because such practice would defeat your purpose and make your steps jerky.

You know that our muscles have an amazing capacity for responding to the quality of the spoken word. For this reason, only nurses with soft voices are employed in wards where the

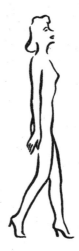

Figure 36

99

shell-shocked or the mentally afflicted are treated.

Thus, in striving for smooth motion, dictate to your body with tones soft and relaxed.

Count aloud whenever you are walking alone. Then when you are moving where there are others, *think* the count. You will catch yourself jouncing along at any old gait. Pause if you can, line yourself up, start counting again. If you can't pause, slow down and *think* your tempo. DO THIS ALWAYS AND ALWAYS AND ALWAYS, whenever you are walking. It may take you several days to analyse your walk from a rhythm standpoint.

You may have a friend who will help you to criticize yourself. If you are nervous, abrupt or jerky in your motions, then *this* is the time to practise walking· with a book on your head, because it will smooth out your motions.

On the other hand, your head may be of such a shape that you cannot balance a book on it without pushing your head out of line. In this event, the much-advertised book trick is again taboo for you.

How fast or how slow you walk depends upon your personality. Often it is devitalizing to a strong, energetic type to have to glide slowly across the room. On the whole, most teachers of deportment do recommend well-paced steps. These can be either fast or slow, but they must be even.

It is rather amusing to read that in the 1800's Lord Chesterfield recommended in his *Letters*,

" Never walk fast in the streets, which is a mark of vulgarity . . . though it may be tolerable in a tradesman."

Today the whole world likes to see a girl or woman who looks as though she knows where she is going. There is something downright unattractive about a slouching, idling gait.

To help you in acquiring an evenly paced momentum, here is one last skill :

When you are walking is an ideal time to breathe correctly. Here is a simple trick that will increase your vitality. As you count one, two, three, four, inhale for four steps. Hold your breath for four steps, and then exhale for four steps.

From now on your success will depend upon practice and application. Think of every time you walk as an additional opportunity to incorporate all these techniques.

Let me emphasize again the importance of checking and concentrating on one thing at a time. Usually, three months is required to master a beautiful walk. Think and see the ideal. Watch other women. Analyse what makes them graceful or awkward.

A cine film of yourself walking, would give you a splendid opportunity to see yourself as others see you. Study your favourite screen stars, even if you have to sit through the film twice to get your mind off the plot and on to their walking technique. How can you possibly lose on improving your walk ? You improve your health—your appearance—and you make others proud to be with you.

Notes:

LESSON FOUR

Part B

Sitting Technique

Our bodies are our gardens, to which our wills are gardeners . . .
—SHAKESPEARE, *Othello*

YOU associate poise with sitting. Sitting should mean a time for body composure. When you sit opposite a friend or a new acquaintance, you subconsciously " size him up." Then, too, the impression you make as you sit is important because so many opportunities come your way through an interview which exacts smooth, poised sitting habits.

This lesson, therefore, will concentrate on what to do about sitting ; about chairs ; how to get into them ; which ones to select ; what to do with your body, head, hands and feet while in them ; and how to get out of them.

TAKE IT EASY

One of the first rules in sitting is not to be in too great a hurry to sit down. The self-conscious woman's first impulse is to sit in the first chair

she sees, and the sooner the better. Haven't you seen a woman half-way " seated " several feet from her chair ? (See Figure 37.) You will find here shortly that those body mechanics which get you gracefully *into* a chair are different from those used in *approaching* the chair.

Haven't you heard your mother say that you can tell a man is a gentleman when he makes his coming known to you ? He may whistle, clear his throat, or call, but he will announce himself in some way.

Many a man who prides himself upon his chivalry and gentlemanly qualities will slip up on you without advance warning. A woman instinctively resents this. In the same manner, a man resents a woman who dashes through doorways. He expects a lady to pause in the doorway when the door is open ; and, of course, to knock when it is closed.

This is the most reliable background I have been able to unearth for the social law that demands that a lady pause for a second in a doorway :

She is not making an entrance : she is not

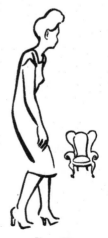

Figure 37

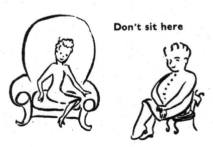

Don't sit here

Figure 38

101

being dramatic : she is exercising good taste. It works to her advantage, too. That second gives her an opportunity to get her bearings. To know where she will go, in the room, which group she will join, or, for the purpose of this lesson, where she will sit.

SELECT YOUR SPOT IN THE SUN

Learn to enter a room, seeing everything but apparently observing nothing. An actress calls this " a wide look." She will be aware of everything on the stage, but not by actually looking hard at it. As you meet your hostess and her friends, nothing in that room is as important to you as their presence. All too many women enter a room and look as though they came to see the furniture, the curtains and the furnishings. Practise never seeing the things wrong in a house, or, if you do, ignore them and make the hostess feel genuinely that it does not matter to you. If she apologizes for anything (and, of course, she shouldn't but we all do, at times) don't reply, " Oh, *that's* all right," implying that it isn't or that you DID notice. Laugh with her, say you're such a poor housekeeper you hadn't noticed, your eyesight is poor, or you're so absent-minded about domestic things, and change the subject. Be so absorbed in *her* that she forgets, also. This takes practice, but it spells the magic of real charm ! When you can come into a disorderly room, dump off some papers or magazines from a chair, and not hurt your hostess's feeling, you are developing a workable talent for radiance.

MENTALLY CHOOSE A CHAIR

As you enter the room, select a chair for

yourself, mentally. Don't wander in aimlessly and then abruptly squat on anything, regardless of how ridiculous it may make you appear.

If you are small, and there are several chairs available, find a small one or an occasional chair which will not engulf you with its proportions and on which you will not feel called upon to curl up your legs, or to sit on one leg, or both ! (See Figure 38.)

If you are a large woman, don't select some dainty, spindle-legged chair which will make you look mountainous by comparison. Always select an occasional chair in preference to one of an overstuffed variety, since you can more easily get your hips to the back of the former, thereby ensuring better sitting appearance. (See Fig. 38.)

Men are more fussy about these matters than women. Think how seldom you find men sitting in chairs which make them appear at a disadvantage. Often they stand, instead of sitting on a chair that they think will make them look ridiculous.

Of course, when you are joining a large group, there may be a scarcity of chairs ; then you'll sit on what's left and like it. Or you may prefer to wander around a bit.

I've always told my timid students to avoid sitting against the wall or in corners. It's all well and good to believe in humility, but there seem to be few males brave enough or interested enough to join you. *Besides, why go out of your way to give a first-rate picture of a wallflower ?*

Then, again, you may not be a wallflower at all, but be new to the group. Your hostess has many responsibilities without having to introduce you all round. Keep yourself available, so that it's easy to talk to you.

I read a very delightful article not long ago, urging women to " stay as shy as you are." The author pointed out that very often the shy little violet against the wall is doing a good job of having the most desirable bachelors at the party help her to overcome her timidity ! It reads well but from thousands of case histories of timid souls, I don't believe it happens this way.

The world is more apt to help those who help themselves.

If you go into an office for a business appointment, wait for an invitation to be seated. Then say simply, " Thank you."

If friends come to your home, you need not ask them to be seated—in so many words. You include that by saying, " Come in and let's have

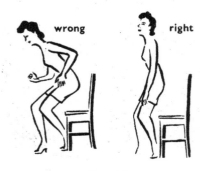

wrong   right

Figure 39

102

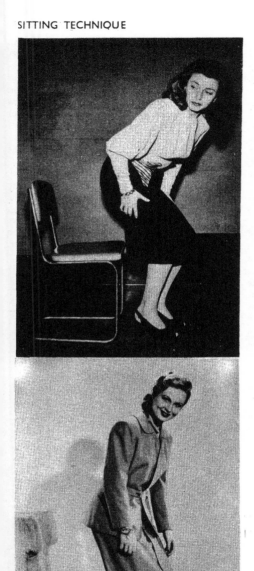

Photograph 9 The chair won't get away from you. Miss Aubert shows wrong approach.

a chat," leading the way into the room, asking if they won't take off their things, and indicating with a gesture that they should sit as you sit down yourself. Or, you might say cordially, " Do sit down," or " Come in and stay a while," or " Won't you have a cup of tea with me ?"

So You Are Ready to Sit

The time comes when you are ready to sit. Stand directly in front of the chair you have selected, and feel the chair with the back of both your knees. (See Figure 39.)

Look around at the chair casually as you start to sit. You mustn't miss it ! But do so in a casual way—not with that hurried, last-second glance indicating you're afraid the chair may have taken wings ! (See Photograph 9.)

Before you go into the actual technique of sitting, let's pause to consider here one of the most practical lessons in poise in this Course. Since you spend some part of each day sitting, use this time as an effective approach to poise.

Sit perfectly still in your chair. This sounds simple, but when you look around at your nervous, fidgety friends, you will realize how important it is to have perfect control of yourself. Just making yourself sit there quietly will have a soothing effect on your tired, jangled insides, to say nothing of its relaxing effect on the others in the room.

Here are the rules for getting into an occasional chair :

1. Assume a position of " coccyx-under-you," rounding out your back. (See Photograph 10.) Put one foot six to ten inches behind the other, and push the back foot under the chair—if it is a chair where you can do this.

2. The weight of your body is distributed between both legs.

3. Both knees relax as you bend forward through the hips, buttocks still tucked under you. (See Figure 39.)

4. Don't smooth your skirts down over your buttocks as you sit down. This does not help to keep your skirt entirely free from creases, as you hope, but it definitely DOES outline the one

Photograph 10 Try sitting gracefully as Virginia Mayo does. It isn't difficult.

part of your figure you should keep to yourself.

I never see a woman smoothing her skirts over her buttocks and reaching out with her rear as she sits, without thinking, " Well, here it is —where shall I put it ? "

5. Your hips should touch the back of an occasional chair as you sit, if you have accomplished the motion correctly.

6. Your arms fall to front and middle as you sit, so that they slide easily into your lap when you are seated. If they dangle at your sides, spread-eagle fashion, they add several inches to your width. (See Figure 38)

Don't keep your hands clasped together as you get into a chair, because that's a gesture of resignation—and it's aging ! (See Figure 38)

7. Practise getting into a chair to the rhythm of one, two, three, and keep your motions as smooth as possible. Don't settle into the chair with a last-second jerk.

You never see a leaf flutter gracefully to the ground and then—wham ! Don't spoil your unbroken line, either. Control your movements into one graceful landing. Practise this about twenty-five times with your side turned to a full-length mirror. You may be shocked at first at what you see, but after the first dozen tries you will find an astonishing improvement.

8. Control your head so that it won't flip forward. Your back is a continuous, rounded line.

A good way to practise correct sitting is to take a couple of steps away from your chair and go through the motions.

Most of the sitting action takes place in your thighs, so that every time you get in or out of a chair can be a first-rate exercise for firming, reducing and developing them.

As you lower yourself into your imaginary chair to the count of one, two, three, place your hands on your thighs and feel the reaction of the

thigh muscles. Make sure that the spine isn't doing the whole job.

Don't be surprised if you do a little " creaking." It isn't a sign of age, as commonly supposed for so many years, but one of tension. After you've practised *without* a chair for a few minutes, then go over to your chair by the mirror and see how far you've progressed.

PRINCIPLES WHICH FLATTER

Now that you're finally down, here are the principles which flatter you most, as you sit.

1. Stretch your feet out a little in front of you. This will give you a much better line than putting them straight under you on a perpendicular line with your knees. Never push your feet under a chair. (See Photograph 11) This is a negative position, and one which actresses employ when they play a subdued, timid, or eccentric character. *Keep the soles of your shoes on the floor.*

You may wish to rest your feet by having only

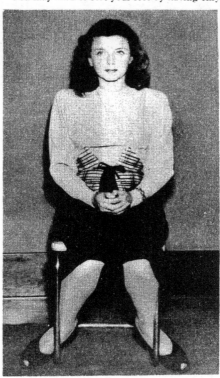

Photograph **11** Even lovely Lenore Aubert could not be attractive in this position.

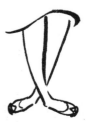

Figure 40

104

your heels touching the floor, but this is never a flattering position.

So watch that you aren't using it when you wish to make a good impression. On the whole, the things which you allow your feet to do when you are alone and off guard will be habits which they will fall into when you are with others. MAKE ALL THESE THINGS SO ROUTINE THAT YOU NEED NEVER GIVE THEM A THOUGHT, then your attention will be free to think of things apart from yourself, thereby being fascinating to those around you.

However, there are many moments during the day when you are alone or working and when you must relax.

Authorities on body mechanics assure us that by sitting correctly day in and day out we will eventually fall into these desirable habits, and will FEEL relaxed in them. But suppose you are tired to the point of exhaustion, or even ill, and you feel you *must* finish a job.

One of our greatest authorities on posture, Dr. Charles LeRoy Bowman, recommends a sitting position for such rest periods : " Recommended change for relaxation and relief, as a variation of a set position to relieve the strain of holding one position too long :

" Cross feet (not knees) at the ankle-joint. Rest the feet on the floor, holding the outer border in contact with the floor—toes straight ahead or in. " (See Figure 40)

Remember this position is for emergencies. *It is not attractive* ! You are to use it only OCCASIONALLY. If you do forget and slip into it with your best boy friend and he doesn't come back, remember I told you so !

2. This position IS flattering. Place your feet so that the toe of one foot is about level with the arch of the outer foot. Keep the front foot straight ahead, but turn the toe of the back foot slightly out.

If your legs are too short to touch the floor, then sit forward in your chair, especially when you're somewhere that your legs show.

Train your escort to put a cushion behind your back. Upon hearing this, one woman said, " But if it's your husband you'll get no cushions. You'll just have to suffer ! " When your feet don't show, sit back and be comfortable. You are the one type who may cross her feet at the ankle if this helps at least one toe to hit the floor.

3. KEEP YOUR KNEES TOGETHER ! No matter how beautifully groomed you may be nor how

much you've spent on your costume, if your knees fall apart the picture is spoiled !

It seems such an obvious point to make, yet it is painful to count the number of otherwise seemingly well-bred women who sit with their knees apart. It robs them of every inch of their femininity and allure. (See Figure 41)

4. Be sure you are sitting in the middle of your chair with your shoulders straight, your hips touching the back of the chair, and your head held straight. (See Photograph 12)

A head cocked to one side, or falling forward, plus the slump position, with the back and hips away from the back of the chair, adds about four inches to the waist-line as well as making you look down on the world AND yourself.

5. In correcting your sitting posture, don't try so hard that you overdo it. After all, you are sitting and you should be relaxed.

You have learned how to " stack up " your body parts when standing ; apply a little of this when you are sitting. The plumb-line should fall in a straight line opposite the lobe of your ear, your shoulder-bone and your hip-bone. Feel that you are balancing your chest and shoulder area over your pelvis and your head over your shoulder girdle.

You have three heavy areas to line up on your slender, broom-handled spine. Stack them thoroughly but with ease. Your weight is then divided equally between both thighs and feet.

HAND TECHNIQUE

Now that you are seated, your hands become

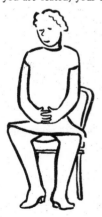

Figure 41

105

conspicuous. I wish I had a penny for every girl and woman who has written or asked me what to do about hands. They complain that their hands are too square, too short, too red, too clumsy, until you wonder if there is a woman satisfied with her hands.

So many of my high-school and college students tell me that they started to smoke because it gave them something to do with their hands.

Developing hand poise is like developing control of any other part of the body. *You learn what to do with them and then you do it.*

Whenever you are tense or nervous, your fingers are more apt to give you away than even your voice or facial expression.

You learned in Lesson Three Part A some effective hand positions to use when you are standing. In Part A of this Lesson you learned correct hand positions for walking. Almost more important than either of these are your hand positions while you are seated, because it is then that others have the most time to judge you. It works the other way, too, because it is while you are seated, especially in moments of leisure that you have maximum time to be uncomfortable about what to do with your hands.

Here are the most valuable laws I know for developing poised hands :

1. *Keep your hands still.* Keep them in your lap, on the arms of your chair, on the table or desk in front of you, but KEEP THEM STILL.

What are the mannerisms that upset you most ? We are assuming here that no well-bred woman works on cuticle, digs out her nails, or peels off her finger-nail polish in the presence of others. She knows that the first indication of a lady is that every detail of her grooming is attended to in privacy. Test yourself and see how many of these mannerisms you have :

(a) Do you tap your fingers, thereby unnerving everyone within hearing ?

. (b) Do your fingers fidget, move constantly, twitch ?

(c) Do you play with paper clips, pencils, rubber bands, matches ?

(d) Do you tear up pieces of paper into wads, or do you fold paper ?

(e) Do your hands make frequent trips to your hair, face, arms ?

If you have more than one " yes," you had better start developing constructive hand poise. You've heard even platform speakers whose

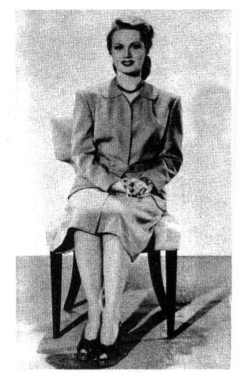

Photograph 12   Virginia Mayo illustrates how to sit gracefully with legs uncrossed.

arm movements have distracted your attention from what they were saying.

These negative mannerisms develop chiefly when you are worried, ill, depressed or tense. They rob you of poise and of the suave, charming manner which you hope is yours.

Women aren't alone in faulty hand techniques ; even men succumb. You see them stroking their cheeks and moustaches, and exploring the backs of their necks ; building temples with their fingers, cracking their knuckles, tightening their jaws, playing with their rings and watches.

No matter how nervous you feel your hands are, you can and should control them.

Recently a group of spastic young men and women asked me to contribute to their first newspaper. I was surprised when they urged me to write about hand control ; even more surprised when I received letters from them, saying how much these instructions had helped them.

If these young people, with their chronic lack of muscular co-ordination, can make progress in this respect, then you can expect virtual perfection.

2. *Don't use too many gestures.* Do not confuse nervous hand mannerisms with spontaneous gestures of expression.

Platform speakers are allowed dramatic gestures for emphasis. Some people naturally use more hand motions to express themselves than others.

I have found that it is very difficult to teach people to use gestures. Artificial gestures are seldom convincing. Where students talk with their hands, I attempt to control them to some extent, but to do so entirely would be robbing them of characteristics which enhance their individuality.

For generations, gestures and speaking with the hands were taboo for women. Men still have more freedom in this respect than women. But, after all, shoulders, arms and hands often say as much as the voice.

Many fascinating women capitalize on shrugs, waves of the hand, flips of the wrist, and vital gestures. Don't overdo them, however, and don't imitate another woman's gestures. And don't acquire them if they are foreign to you. It's better by far to have few than too many.

Just as a clever conversationalist listens as well as she speaks, so an exciting woman has long moments of utter quiet. But when she does talk her hands often help her. You think of this woman as enthusiastic, vital. Whereas you think of the woman who sits and fidgets constantly, hands and fingers never still, as irritable and irritating.

If you recognize that you do have nervous hands, then your best bet is to undergo a period of complete hand stillness.

As the weeks go by and this stillness seems more natural to you, you will experience a feeling of THE POWER OF COMPOSURE. Others will be more relaxed and at ease around you, and *this is a predominating quality in any person's charm.*

You can't create impressions of ease if you yourself are ruled by hurried, tense, irritating, confusing mannerisms.

3. Strive for length in your lap as you are seated. That means that your elbows will be close to your body but relaxed ; that your forefingers will point easily toward your knees. As a contrast, an over-weight woman who sits with her elbows extended several inches from her body, one hand stacked over the other, creates an illusion of even greater fat.

Turn your hands so that the palms face upward. Do this during your practice period. (See Figure 42.) In actual practice they will turn facing each other slightly, but do become familiar with this extended arm-and-hand line as you sit. Don't worry about your fingers looking " planted " or forced.

As you practise these positions they become very natural to you. Here's another finger trick that you notice screen stars doing between takes. *They shake their hands, even for just a second or two, because they know that if the wrist is relaxed, the fingers will assume relaxed positions.* Your fingers are neither too straight nor too curled.

See how long you can hold this simple arm or hand position. If you manage a minute the first time, you are doing very well. Practise it as you sit waiting or in the cinema or as you listen to lectures—even in church !

4. You will recall that in a previous Lesson you learned the hand position for clasping your hands in front of you while standing. You use the same finger action for this second position. Put the thumb of one hand in the palm of the other and relax your fingers.

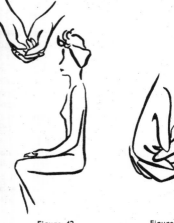

Figure 42   Figure 43

107

This position has value because it is so easily assumed, looks natural, and yet you have something to hold on to.

This is also a corrective position, because whether you consider your hands too square, too short, or too large, this shows your fingers to advantage. It acts as a camouflage agent.

5. Put one hand in the other, palms facing up, forefingers pointing toward the knees. Encircle the first and second fingers of the upper hand with the thumb and forefinger of the bottom hand. (See Figure 43) This may sound difficult but it isn't, and it is one of the most graceful hand positions I know.

Your fingers will vary slightly as you become familiar with it, so that your hands will achieve their own individuality. It's the same principle at work as when you were being taught to write. The whole class practised forming the same letters, but each person developed an individual style of writing.

6. Here is a hand position which finishing schools have presented for generations, and it is perennially popular with actresses. (See Photograph 13.) Cross your left arm to the right thigh, and join the two hands.

When you first start incorporating these hand positions they will seem forced and artificial. You will worry that others will think you are affected. They won't, though, and a week's practice will give you so much additional poise that you never will go back to your former fidgets.

SHOULD LEGS BE CROSSED ?

There was a time when it was not considered

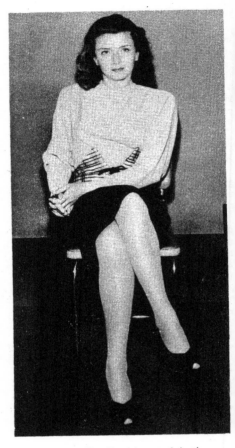

Photograph 13   Note Lenore Aubert's hands in this " off-centre " sitting position.

good form for a woman to cross her legs. Later there were specific occasions when she might and when she might not.

Today it is not considered good form to cross your legs in church, or on a public vehicle such as a bus or tram-car. It is not the best form, either, when applying for a job. Otherwise, the answer to your problem depends upon how gracefully you cross your legs, and the length of your skirt. (See Photograph 13)

You can be the sole judge of whether or not you should cross your legs. Here's how you do it. If you can cross your legs up above the knees so that the two legs fall side by side (see Figure 44), then go ahead and do it to your heart's content.

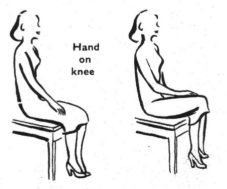

Hand on knee

Figure 44

SITTING TECHNIQUE

If, however, your knees or thighs are fat, *then don't ever cross your legs where they will be seen by others—especially when you are trying to make a good impression.*

Why present yourself at your worst ? Learn to show off your legs to the best possible advantage when you're seated. If, however, you find you can cross your legs with ease above the knees, here is your routine for making the most of it :

1. Put your hand on the knee which is about to do the crossing. For example, if your right leg is going over the left one, then the right hand stays on the right knee.

Hold your skirt down firmly with your right hand, and cross your leg to a smooth count of one, two, three. (See Figure 44.) Do not cross so fast that you look as though you had been caught short, nor go so slowly that those around you wonder if you will ever get there ! Try for in between, smooth rhythm of one, two, three. Practise it before a mirror for a minute or two.

2. Never buy a dress before you sit in front of a full-length mirror and cross your legs. Have your skirt full enough so that it makes an attractive background for your legs.

A skirt too tight and too short will ruin the lines of the loveliest legs, when you sit, and will make them look cheap.

3. Have the toe of the top leg close to the ankle of the bottom leg. Don't point the upper toe down—that's *passé* and affected—but see that it doesn't point up, either. Have it hang relaxed from the ankle.

When your legs are crossed, you have destroyed your flat lap, so hand position number 4 would look well-here, resting on the upper thigh.

There is also another hand position which is flattering when your legs are crossed : Put the fingers of one hand through those of the other, keeping your fingers linked. Now let the top thumb slide down below the little finger of the opposite hand.

Where there are arms on the chair, you may wish to put one hand in your lap and the other on the arm of the chair. Should you be much overweight, don't put both hands on the chair arms because it broadens your body.

Likewise, when you are very thin, don't have your hands stretched out too far, because you may create an illusion of scrawniness or frailty.

When you have finished reading these Lessons through once, then go back over all the pictures

here, and study the hand positions and arm lines with reference to the body.

You will soon appreciate their symmetry and begin applying them every day.

UPSY-DAISY !

The time has come to get out of that chair.

1. Before actually getting up, practise rocking forward and back in your chair. Use your hip joint for this. Remember that it is one of the most powerful, complicated joints in your body, and should do your rising jobs. Rock forward and back, smoothly, keeping your body parts lined up. (See Figure 45)

You don't want to collapse in the middle or let your head lead. Try to practise this sideways before a full-length mirror. There should be a gentle, graceful curving of your body, with the small of the back curved outward, not in.

As you rock forward, your hands fall to the front and centre, but you do not clasp them together. If your arms fall out to the sides with a flourish, you create unnecessary breadth.

Don't use your arms as though they were propellers. You don't want to put them on either arm of the chair to help to lift yourself up, either. It makes your body seem heavy and old.

2. Put one foot behind the other, or put the back foot slightly under the chair, if possible.

3. Your weight is distributed between both legs, but, just as in sitting, your thighs absorb most of the action. So in rising, you are conscious that the thighs seem to carry your weight.

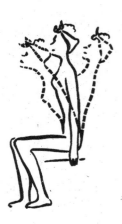

Figure 45

109

Make sure that your spine and shoulders are not doing the actual work. Get your thighs into action.

4. Make sure that your buttocks are tucked down under you, and that your back—from your hips to your head—creates a rounded silhouette.

You will notice, all through the study of body control, the importance of correct pelvic position and therefore correct buttocks position. Count a smooth, evenly paced, " One, two, three," as you stand up. You needn't rush it. You'll make just as good time by doing a rhythmical job of it.

To Sit on a Sofa

Thus far we have discussed only the technique for a straight or occasional chair. But how about sitting down on a sofa, divan, or easy-chair?

If you are five feet seven inches, or over, and slender, you may be able to negotiate these big pieces without much help. But if you're of average height or under, or overweight, then large pieces of furniture present a hazard.

Haven't you seen a woman pulling and puffing herself out of a large chair, her skirts sliding back under her ? Here are some preventatives :

1. Stand in front of the sofa. Bend your knees ; then, keeping your buttocks under you, sit on the very edge of the sofa.

2. Your hands touch the edge of the upholstery on either side of your body. (See Figure 46)

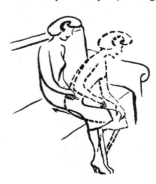

**Sit on edge . . push up
and back smoothly ! !**

Figure 46

3. Your hands and legs help to raise your body up ever so slightly and actually lift it back into the sofa.

Let me repeat : come down on the very edge, knees still bent, and then lift yourself to the back of the sofa. If you land in the middle of this deep mass, you will have to lean so that your back isn't comfortable, or use your buttocks to settle yourself into a comfortable position.

If there is a man in your family, ask him what he dislikes most about watching a woman sit on a divan. He will tell you he hates to see her " flop down," jarring everyone else on the divan. Invariably, she lands with her knees apart.

Practise your sofa-sitting technique so that you don't obviously make two decided motions—one down to the edge of the divan and the other backward. You do stop, but keep it as smooth as possible.

When you are ready to get up from the divan, use the same technique to pull yourself to the front of the divan, and then use your legs and arms to push yourself up.

Watch your skirt, that it does not cling to the sofa fabric. The lifting action helps to prevent this to a great extent. Here again you will note the wisdom of buying a fuller skirt.

Sitting on a Bench

You may find no chairs left in the room for you, but your hostess indicates a window seat, fireside bench, or hassock.

Don't feel slighted, because if you've been practising your lessons, you will really show off to better advantage when sitting without a chair-back.

Notice how many models or glamour girls are photographed without the support of a chair-back.

I'm not saying that you'll be more comfortable over any length of time, but you CAN look your most graceful. These rules apply for each height :

1. As you sit, keep your knees together.

2. Raise your chest.

3. Keep your shoulders straight and your head evenly balanced.

4. Remember your streamlined hand-and-arm positions.

5. A hassock is solid to the floor, so you will have to sit down with your feet placed side by side, bend your knees, and turn them either to the right or to the left.

SITTING TECHNIQUE

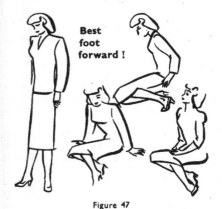

Best foot forward !

Figure 47

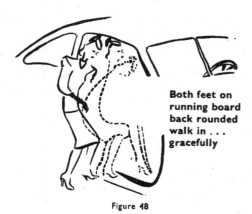

Both feet on running board back rounded walk in . . . gracefully

Figure 48

SITTING ON THE FLOOR

You may find yourself lucky to have the floor to sit on, or you may be out on the lawn, or the loggia or on the beach. Study graceful sitting positions.

It's all right for a teenage youngster to sprawl, but even she will look better in a graceful, relaxed position. Go down in segments. You've heard a lot about body-segments in these Lessons. Here's the time to make use of your knowledge. Before you start to go down, separate your feet, one a little ahead of the other, bend your knees, and sink with your thigh muscles so that your buttocks are under you. (See Figure 47.)

Then put your weight on one knee and your hands, and lower the other knee before sitting. Straighten your legs, bend them or cross them. But keep your knees relaxed and reasonably close.

Before you get up, fold your feet beside you, rise to your knees, then place one foot flat on the floor and raise your body as your other foot contacts the floor. If you will watch yourself in a mirror as you practise this for a few minutes, you will see that you are moving by segments.

GETTING IN AND OUT OF A CAR

It's heart-breaking to see beautifully groomed women sprawling and pulling and puffing out of cars.

Here's a graceful routine for getting *into* a car : Put both feet, one at a time (of course), on the running-board. Then think of walking into the car itself with your buttocks under you, your back rounded, and your head bent forward to complete the curve. (See Figure 48.)

How to get out of a car. Slide to the edge of the seat—feet facing front. Get out of the car sideways, if there is a running-board. Where you are minus a running-board, you will have to turn your body to a direct right angle to the front of the car, BUT KEEP YOUR KNEES TOGETHER.

Step down with one foot, keeping the knee areas of your legs close to each other. One knee slides against the other leg. Even if your skirt slides up over your knees, you still have a graceful line.

SITTING-DOWN WORK

You don't like to be reminded of the " typist's spread." You don't have to have a typist's spread, either !

There are thousands of women who spend the best part of their days sitting as they work, yet still have trim hips and firm abdomens. You will find, in Lesson Six Part B on corrective posture, that you can correct many posture faults when seated. You don't have the same pull against gravity which is in force wherever you stand or move.

So instead of bemoaning the fact that you must sit so much, look upon it as an opportunity actually to help the beauty of your body.

Here is a schedule that will be worth your while to copy and place in your desk. Check your sitting habits with it very quickly, once a week.

1. When you reach for the telephone, the lower drawer, or something on the floor, rock forward

with your hip joints.

Don't strain and reach with your spine. It is good for you to reach, but first get your body co-ordinated for the reaching.

2. Contract and relax your buttocks several times each hour. This will help to keep those sitting muscles firm, and prevent them from spreading.

3. Sit with your feet flat on the floor and parallel. Have your weight distributed between both thighs.

4. Don't cross your legs too much. Especially avoid wrapping one foot around the other. You will develop one leg larger than the other if you do. If you must cross your legs while you work, alternate the action.

5. Every time you sit in a chair, see if you can get the small of your back to touch the back of your chair.

If you are sitting in the same place, for several hours at a stretch, check this at least every hour. See what happens to your abdomen and chest when you do this ? When the back is flat against the back of the chair, you also simultaneously raise your chest.

6. Keep your shoulders relaxed and broad. No supervisor will resent your rotating them once every hour if she understands that in the long run this tends toward relaxation and, therefore, increased efficiency.

7. Whatever your work is, try to arrange your tools so that you are not pushing your head forward as you work. Bend forward from the hips so that the whole torso goes forward with you. Don't sit rigid and then push your head forward to see.

Wear glasses, have good lighting. If you spend your days doing copy-work, use a line-a-time or similar device to hold your copy for easiest visibility. If you are transcribing short-hand notes, use a stiff-backed notebook to serve the same purpose.

8. Even with your shoes on, you can incorporate a few foot exercises. Sit so that the outside of your feet takes the greatest weight. Raise the inside arch.

If your shoes are large enough, stretch your toes, pull them under you. When no one else is around, you can sit with your back touching the chair back, raise your feet directly in front of you, pull your toes back towards you and stretch your heels away from you.

9. Stand up one minute out of every sixty. Make those sixty seconds pay with a visible or invisible stretch. Most employers today realise the importance of increased production resulting from increased resistance to fatigue.

Well, this is the end of your sitting lesson. It's been a long one. I hope you've enjoyed it and that it will help.

Personally, when I was doing intensive studying in this field, going from one teacher to another, I felt that this lesson in sitting helped to further my poise more than any other one.

Self-Test Questions Based On Lesson Four

Having studied the Lesson on Sitting Technique, you will have realised now, if not before, the necessity to practise some exercises and conscious control when sitting; otherwise you are in danger of spoiling all your attempts towards grace and charm.

After you have studied this Lesson, you should be able to answer the following questions. If you have any difficulty in doing so, refer to the Lesson for further study and revision. Your answers should not be sent to the publishers of this Course.

1. Write down what you should repeat aloud to yourself as you practise walking on your two straight lines.

2. Quote a DO and a DON'T for knees when walking.

3. What fault in walking, above all others, often ruins an otherwise graceful walk?

4. Describe shortly how arms should be used when walking.

5. Describe a simple trick to use when walking which will increase your vitality and help you to have an even walk.

6. What is one of the first and most important rules to learn in sitting?

7. Quote here one of the most practical and useful exercises in this Lesson for acquiring poise.

8. Apart from being good taste to hesitate for a second in a doorway before entering, what advantage is gained?

9. When you are sitting, what is a good rule to remember in regard to what you should always do with your feet?

10. Quote an instance when it is not good form to cross the legs.

If you wish to determine the progress you are making, give yourself 10 points for each question you answer correctly. If the total comes to 90 or more, it is excellent; 80 or more, good; 70 or more, fair.

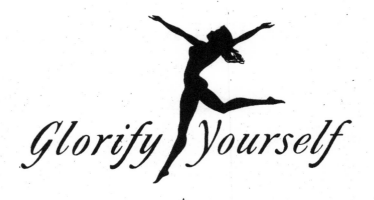

Glorify Yourself

★

A Complete and Up-to-Date Course on
Beauty and Charm by One of the
Most Famous Beauty Specialists
and Consultants in the World

Eleanore King

★

LESSON FIVE

★

Issued only for Students of the Eleanore King Course on Beauty. Charm and Personality.

Lesson Five.

Dear Student,

A wit once remarked that when a man is due to make an important public appearance he always asks himself: "What shall I say?" whilst a woman will ask: "What shall I wear?"

Certainly the question of what to wear is an important one for all women. In Lesson Five it is fully and completely answered.

First of all you learn the important RULE OF FOURTEEN. This simple rule eliminates all guess-work from the task of deciding what to wear...and what not to wear. Each article of outer wear is allotted a code number. You add up the numbers corresponding with the clothes and accessories you intend to wear; and if they total fourteen (or in some cases slightly less) you will know that your choice is a good one.

It's as simple as that! A little very easy mental arithmetic is surely a small price to pay for the knowledge of how to be well and tastefully dressed for any occasion.

The rule of fourteen is applicable to all women. When you have mastered it, you will pass on to those sections of the Lesson which deal with your individual figure type. You will also be given detailed individual guidance on what you should wear to make the best of your own special features

The dress and accessory charts included in this Lesson are fully comprehensive. There is hardly any dress problem that you cannot solve for yourself by referring to them.

I am sure you will enjoy this Lesson, since it is perhaps the most rewarding of the whole Course. By applying its principles you will benefit not only your appearance, but your pocket as well.

For good dressing is not necessarily expensive dressin Even the well-known actresses who consult me in my Hollywood Studio often have to budget carefully for their wardrobes. They have to master the rules of good dress sense. You can

(over)

do the same, and thus make sure that even on a limited dress allowance you will always have something smart to wear. Even the smallest wardrobe budget will go a surprisingly long way when it is wisely spent.

Yours sincerely,

Eleanore King

EK.5.

P.S. In our next Lesson you will learn further secrets of grace and poise, formerly available only to professional models.

LESSON FIVE

Flattering Clothes

Whosoever hath a good presence and a good fashion,
carries continual letters of recommendation.
—BACON, *Isabella of Spain*

LIFE is going along serenely enough, when suddenly you are invited to meet " the old gang." You know . . . those special friends of his you've heard so much about, but have never met before.

Even if you've been married for ever so many years, the thought of going up for inspection in the eyes of the people he likes so well is apt to become quite a mental hazard. And if you happen to be the girl he's going to marry in a month or so, the ordeal is even worse. Of course, it all starts very casually. One day he says :

" Oh, by the way. Some old friends of mine . . . you've heard me speak of Lil and Dick . . . well, they're giving a party on Saturday night and they want us to go."

You take it very easily and say, " Oh ? Good. Who's going to be there ? "

"All the old gang. No one you've met, I suppose . . . but they're grand people. In fact, the party is sort of in your honour."

" In my honour ! How'd that happen ? "

" Well, I've told Lil and Dick all about you, and they just thought it'd be nice to get together."

From there he goes on to say that the affair is going to be a buffet supper and that the girls aren't dressing. And if he's typical of most men, he doesn't know anything more about it.

There you find yourself, scheduled to meet the people who may represent your very close circle of friends in the near future.

You know it's an important occasion—and whether or not you admit it, you want to appear at your best.

If you've been very casual with him about it so far, you've scored one already. Yet, as the evening approaches, a few problems do present themselves.

First of all, in order to make the best impression possible, you want to look your best. What should you wear ?

Answer very frankly. Do you wait for occasions similar to this before buying your clothes ? Do you usually buy a dress for a dinner, a date, an interview, just BEFORE the dinner, or interview ? If you do, the chances are you are neither getting the most appearance-value for money spent nor being very well dressed.

Looking your best consistently demands an overall schedule. Twice or three times a year you decide what you *need* to buy and what you can *afford* to buy.

You shop wisely, sanely, without a deadline. I'm not saying that there are no occasions during the year when you rush out to buy a hat, an accessory, or even an occasional dress or suit. But remember, I said occasional.

In my capacity as tutor and counsellor to several motion-picture stars, I learned that even these girls must plan very carefully for their appearances. They can't afford to risk having " NOTHING TO WEAR ! "

I should like to give you the same type of advice in this Lesson that I have given these girls. If you have been shopping helter-skelter, hit-and-miss, spending more than you can afford, and still feeling insecure in what you wear, the following procedure will help you.

1. Know that you are not overdressed. *You must know when to subtract and eliminate.* To help you know that you are not overdressed there is the classic Rule of Fourteen. I first became familiar with it examining studio stills.

A still is a picture made of a star in each change of costume before it is accepted by the producer and the director. I thought perhaps this rule had originated with the studios.

I find upon consulting Grace Beardsley, one of Hollywood's outstanding costume authorities, that " according to a fashion principle written for *Lady's Book*, January, 1849, a famous Parisian couturier pronounced that no lady should own an out-door costume which comprised more than fourteen eye-arresting elements."

This means that you should be able to count no more than fourteen of everything which is visible to the eye. It wouldn't affect your under-cover articles.

Let's suppose for the particular evening that we mentioned here you decide to look pretty, smart, but not extreme. That's the way most men like you to look. You finally worm it out of your escort that the ladies are wearing short skirts. So you wear a black basic dress, with a red rose at the belt.

You want your accessories to have a festive air. Your shoes are black suède with black suède bows. Your bag is black suède with a gold initial. You wear a black cocktail hat with matching red rose.

Suppose you decide upon a gold necklace, a couple of gold bracelets, some gold earrings. You wear your engagement ring and your wrist watch. You wear below-the-elbow gloves, with gold stitching. You have a wrap and since it seems a little plain you put a jewelled clip on it.

You are miserably overdressed. And that's the first impression you will make on every one of his friends who has a remnant of taste.

You may say to me, " But I want to be dressed up. It's a party ! " Realise that the best-dressed women are often the most simply dressed.

A plain dress and hat with but one bit of jewellery are often far more outstanding than that same dress cluttered with various eye-arresting pieces. So let's start clipping.

· Remove the clip on your coat. Remove the necklace and the ear-rings. Remove the bracelets. Remove the initial on your bag.

You may argue that when you arrive at the party and take off your hat and coat, you will look rather plain in the black dress with the rose, your watch, and engagement ring. You have already paid for too dressy a hat. You bought trimmed gloves instead of plain.

Your shoes have bows which may be particularly flattering to your feet. But the combination of these three elaborate accessories makes it imperative that you slice off the jewellery. True, they may be individually beautiful, but collectively they may cause someone to ask, " Where's the kitchen sink ? "

Now let's see how this Rule of Fourteen operates, so that you will be sure about each costume you wear. A one-piece dress is one count. Buttons would be two. A suit is two. Its buttons would be one. The basic frame of a hat is one. A feather would add a count ; so

would a veil.

Each different colour adds a count to a hat. If you like fancy hats, you may as well make up your mind to stick to very simple suits and dresses. Two ear-rings count one. A pair of stockings is one.

Plain shoes are one. Bows or trimmings count one. A set of bracelets on one arm count one. The combination of engagement and wedding rings is one. A scarf is one. A bag is one unless it has contrasting colour or trimming. This goes for gloves, too.

Some items like sequins, fringe, metallic cloth, and highly beaded materials count five in themselves and require very little trimming.

RULE OF FOURTEEN FOR DRESSING

Let's see how you'd count your black dress:

Item	Count
Black basic dress	1
Red rose at belt	1
Stockings	1
Shoes	1
Bows on shoes	1
Bag	1
Gold initial	1
Hat with two colours	2
Gold necklace	1
Two gold bracelets	1
Gold ear-rings	1
Engagement ring (or engagement ring and wedding ring)	1
Wrist watch	1
Gloves	1
Gold stitching	1
Wrap	1
Clip on wrap	1
TOTAL COUNT	18

You must eliminate at least four counts.

In this case, you must omit the necklace, two bracelets, clip on wrap, and earrings—since you can't very well take bows off shoes, colours off hat, stitching off gloves, without considerable expense.

You may wish to slice off rose on dress and keep your bracelets OR necklace OR ear-rings. (But the flower has more sex appeal !)

I have found that more slender types of women with rather subdued colouring can get by with more points than women who are over-weight, " curvaceous," voluptuous, or with dazzling red, or golden, or black hair. The Chinese sign for disharmony shows two women under one roof. That's a pretty good law to apply to yourself with respect to wearing too many elaborate accessories.

If you are a definite type of aggressive colouring, keep the count even under the fourteen.

Some of our best-dressed women can be classified under a twelve count year after year.

After you've juggled with this law for a bit, you will become adept in varying your accessories and fall under the fourteen count almost automatically. You may as well make up your mind to admit this one fact. *Women of taste seldom accept overdressed women.* There are few snobbish rules that the average democratic woman adheres to ; she will, however, make an exception where taste in dressing is concerned, since she feels it is within the reach of all.

Whether you are dissatisfied with everything you own and want to start out fresh—or whether you feel there are some clothes you own that are becoming to you and yet you would like to have a guide-post for going ahead with your new purchases, your clothes philosophy should incorporate somewhat the following procedure :

1. At least twice a year write down every stitch of clothing you own. Segregate your list into dresses, suits, sports clothes, afternoon dresses, evening clothes, coats, underwear, and accessories, adding individual headings to fit your needs. Decide which of these things you are going to give away.

They may be clothes that are uncomfortable, those in which you never have a good time, or clothes that you haven't worn for some time. *There's no use letting them clutter up your wardrobe and absorb your attention.* Of those remaining, check alterations.

If you aren't clever with this yourself, do take them to a dressmaker in whom you have faith. Let her check the shoulder-pads, the belts, the waist-lines, hip-lines, and hem-lines. They may need new collars, yokes, or freshening touches. Have them all ready to wear and in first-class condition. Fit your clothes with your " good girdle " and brassiere.

Every woman or girl, no matter how thin, should wear a girdle. Our finest designers insist that their slimmest models must wear girdles.

Wear a pantie girdle if you are slender ; a pantie girdle with an open crotch if you are heavier ; or a girdle with boning if you are definitely overweight.

On the whole, your figure will look more youthful and you will protect your breasts from sagging by wearing a brassiere and girdle—and not a one-piece foundation garment. I grant there may be exceptions to this.

2. Make a list of all the places you've been to, the last year. Have an approximate totalling of where you've spent the most hours.

For example, if you are taking care of a family, most of your hours are spent around the house.

Do you have appropriate working clothes ? Have you ever thought how a man on even the most reduced budget will always have a pair of cords or overalls for his heavy work ?

On the other hand, don't you know women who spend quite a bit on their clothes annually, who do keep house, and yet who try to do a good job in broken-down evening slippers and soiled afternoon dresses ? Haven't you known teachers who are so well-groomed and beautifully dressed on Sunday that you don't recognize them ? They teach all the week in one or two drab, commonplace dresses !

The underlying principle is : allow money for clothes for your working hours.

3. From this list of places where you have spent most of your time, write down your ideal list of what you would wear if money and time were no deterring factors.

For example, for around the house you might say : three pairs of slacks of varying weights, so that there is always a fresh pressed pair when the other two are at the cleaners ; nine blouses and skirts ; two wool jackets ; two washable housecoats ; one hostess dress ; two pairs of low-heeled comfortable shoes ; a dozen pairs of socks ; four pairs of panties and four brassieres ; two cotton house dresses.

With a list like this you would feel that you could look presentable most of the time and yet have quick changes available for emergencies or drop-in callers.

4. Now list what you could afford to buy of this general list. How you distribute your money in buying your clothes will depend upon your activities, your figure, and—your purse !

There should, however, be a sensible general rule. You're not spending wisely if you own two elaborate evening dresses that you wear once a month, and only one suit to wear to work.

You should think of your clothes in the complete costume sense : to take care of your round-the-clock activities and to show you off well from top to toe.

· The best-dressed women I know do not necessarily spend the most money. So often people think that motion-picture stars pay vast sums for their clothes. It's true that the most famous ones do. But there are hundreds of capable actresses who dress beautifully economically.

Now remember, these girls are making top appearances and are competing with stars who spend fortunes on how they look. They don't have many of each type of dress, but they will have at least one of each type which is presentable at all times.

Don't forget, too, that these girls have almost perfect figures, so that on them a medium-priced garment looks much more expensive. Many of the best-dressed women I know, who have good jobs, or whose husbands have, don't squander money on clothes.

5. Study the methods that clever dressers use in assembling a wardrobe. Ask women whose costumes you admire. They'll be flattered to help you.

Magazines often run articles with such information.

6. Improve your shopping technique. Try to look your best when you go shopping. Be courteous and charming with the shop assistants. Have a pretty good idea what you want, but be willing to see their suggestions. *Avoid bargains with which you have nothing to wear.*

Bring along parts of your wardrobe to help the salesladies make suggestions for the completed costume. GO ALONE. No girl friend and no husband !

The study of clothes and how to assemble costumes is a very definite skill. It can be developed by any woman who is willing to learn. Those students who make the least progress in developing clothes sense are those who either refuse to study the basic lines involved, or who consider themselves authorities and are not open to new suggestions.

You've probably heard so much about building a basic wardrobe that the very expression bores you. Nevertheless, every well-dressed woman has a thorough knowledge of how to put her clothes together to the greatest advantage. Even where there is an unlimited amount of money to draw from, there is still the question of assembling clothes that will travel easily and lightly.

The time element for shopping is an important factor in the lives of busy women, regardless of how much they can spend. *The answer lies in buying basic clothes.*

How can you designate a garment that's basic ? As you look at a dress, suit or coat on a rack in a store, ask yourself these questions : can I wear it on three different types of occasions? If it's a dress—would I be equally comfortable in it at the football match, dancing, and the office ? You may be able to buy only one basic costume for each season, but you should be aiming at somewhat the following ideal for a period of seasons :

1. A basic dress.

2. A basic coat.

3. , Two sets of accessories, one more formal than the other.

4. A basic suit.

5. Two sets of accessories for the suit.

With a wearable, flattering wardrobe like this you can consider yourself a well-dressed woman. Most fashion authorities recommend that you buy your basic wardrobe in this order.

· Therefore, if you feel that everything you own is a hodge-podge and you can buy only one new garment, you will decide on a basic dress. On the other hand, you may be at your best in suits and go for a basic suit first.

Just as you must stick to basic lines, so you must stick to basic colours ; namely, black, brown, navy, grey and beige. And any one of these colours is as essentially basic as any one of the others. Some authorities add for sixth and seventh place, wine and deep green.

Let's suppose that you buy a black basic dress and a black basic coat. If you are ultra-conservative, you might also buy a black basic suit. Or your suit might be grey or beige, so that you could wear it with your basic coat and the accessories you bought for the dress and coat.

Even if you were to add another basic dress, it, too, might be grey or beige. Up to now, you will take out your flair for colour in your accessories. *After you own a couple of basic dresses, a basic coat and a basic suit, then you are entitled to a colour splurge.* It may be a coloured suit, a coloured coat, or a coloured dress.

How can you spot a basic dress ? It will, as we

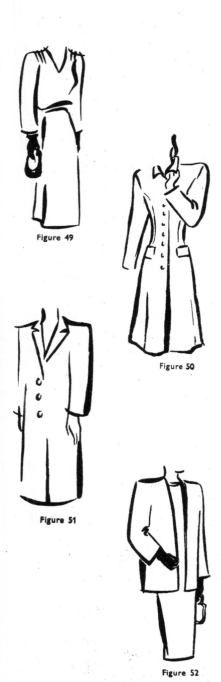

Figure 49

Figure 50

Figure 51

Figure 52

said, be of a basic colour ; it will be plain or the trimming will be such that you can change it easily. It will have a good clear neckline of its own which is not dependent upon trimming, probably either a round or a "V" neckline.

It will have fullness in the bodice, bracelet or full-length sleeves, a narrow belt of the same material as the dress, a full enough and long enough skirt, and very good shoulders. (See Figure 49.) It will be of a jersey or a sheer wool so that you can wear it practically the year round.

You can wear it to work with a smart hat, suède or leather handbag and shoes, gloves, and piqué accents.

Notice how often our glamorous stars wear just such a " little dress " in their pictures. You could wear the same dress dancing, with a hat of feathers, silk-net, or flowers, or no hat at all, longer gloves, more elaborate jewellery or flowers. You could even use the same bag and shoes for both occasions. With a quick shift to a plain hat, leather shoes and bag, you could even wear it at a football match.

I know many women discard suède shoes and bags, because they get so dusty and shiny ; but suède shoes are the most flattering you can wear.

How about a basic coat with a nipped-in waistline, flared skirt.?(See Figure 50.)Its close runner-up and my first preference for a basic coat is the standard strictly boxcut. (See Figure 51.) This coat will take you anywhere. Have an extra wool lining you can snap into your basic coat.

With one full-length coat, it's wise to invest in an additional topper or a short box-coat which ends at the largest part of your buttocks. (See Figure 52.) This can be worn with anything from slacks to a formal.

Suppose your Chesterfield is black and your topper is black, too. Or you might decide to have your topper in a colour. Don't overlook the basic value of such shades as yellow, green or purple, because you can combine them with almost any other colour. With two such coats, I think a fur coat is an admirable addition if it can be afforded.

The Basic Suit

Many women live in suits. They have all types and colours. They own few dresses. These are the women who look exceptionally well in suits, who have small hips and good legs.

The following women probably should not

wear suits at all : those who are badly over-weight ; those whose buttocks measure four inches more than their bust ; and women whose bust-line is four inches larger than their buttocks. Their proportions can be camouflaged better in a dress and coat ensemble. Be very careful in buying your first basic suit. It may be of a man-tailored variety with lapels suitable to the size of your shoulders and general height, (see Figure 53) or it may be the rounded neck and shoulder line. (See Figure 54.)

It should be simple enough so that you can wear either a blouse, sweater, or something more elaborate with it. You should be able to wear it in the country with a sweater, in town with a blouse, and to a cocktail party with a lace frill.

Some authorities warn you that a black basic suit can very quickly make you look over-dressed ; but if you are careful in your com-binations, there is no reason why you should have difficulty.

Frankly, I think that a girl starting from scratch is wise to get her coat, suit and dress in one of the basic shades, whether black, navy, brown, grey, beige, green or wine.

Then I would recommend that if these first three items were black, her next suit be grey and the next dress beige. If they were navy, the suit could still be grey and the dress beige.

If they were brown, the suit might be beige

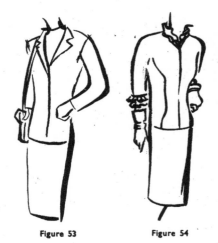

Figure 53   Figure 54

and the dress any one of the handsome colours between beige and brown. She could wear these clothes for years and they would furnish a background for a never-ending combination of accessories and colours. She would appear to have many clothes and she would be smartly dressed.

A suit or coat should look in first class con-dition for three years, and be very wearable for five ; a dress for three years ; hats for two years ; shoes and handbags indefinitely.

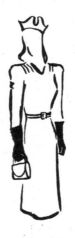
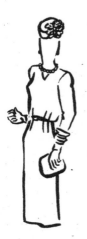
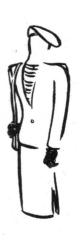
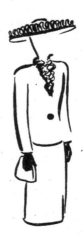

Figure 55   Figure 56   Figure 57   Figure 58

Accessory Chart

Sport Wear	Hat	Shoes	Gloves	Bag
Town Wear	Hat	Shoes	Gloves	Bag
Dressy Basic	Hat	Shoes	Gloves	Bag
Street Wear	Hat	Shoes	Gloves	Bag

ACCESSORIES

You could follow the above advice to the letter and still look miserably dressed if your accessories were wrong.

Almost anyone today can select practical, workable dresses and suits, but selecting accessories is more difficult. They indicate your taste. Let's work out an accessory chart here for the above basic wardrobe, with the hope that these selections will help you with all of your accessory problems.

KNOW THE LAWS OF PROPORTION

Are you sure you know the basic laws for proportion ? There *may* be a very small percentage of women who can buy wisely by depending on their innate taste.

I have found that most of the women that I thought were doing this turned out, after all, to be students of the laws of proportion. Before you can hope to be confident of your judgment, so that you won't have a wardrobe full of clothes you can't wear, you must study the general laws of proportion, just as an engineer must know his basic mechanics. The first proportions of the body that you should understand are these :

1. The largest part of the bust should equal the largest part of the hips and the waist should be ten inches smaller than either. That means that with a 36-inch bust, ideally the largest part of your buttocks would measure 36 inches, and

BASIC DRESS

	Dressing Down (See Figure 55.)	Dressing Up (See Figure 56.)
HAT	Felt or straw.	Flowers, feathers, veils, net or no hat ; flowers or ornaments in hair.
GLOVES	Suede, cotton.	Silk, suede, three-quarter or below-elbow length in black, white, or coloured.
HANDBAG	Suede, leather, plastic.	Suede, satin, corded, broadcloth, plastic.
JEWELLERY	Gold, silver bracelets, ear-rings, necklaces, costume clip, watch.	Rhinestones, coloured stones, pearls crystals, beads, watch.
SHOES	Suede, leather, patent.	Suede, corded, faille.
EXTRA TRIMMINGS	Cotton flounces or collar-and-cuff sets, coloured belt of suede or reptile.	Flowers, corsages, jewelled belt.

BASIC COAT

Accessories worn with the coat are determined by the dress or suit.

A BASIC SUIT

	Dressing Down (See Figure 57.)	Dressing Up (See Figure 58.)
HAT	Sports hat of any kind; or no hat.	Felt, straw, fabric, feathered or flowered hat.
BLOUSE	Cotton shirt or sports shirt ; sweater ; or shirt *and* sweater.	Lingerie blouse, novelty garments in satin, brocade.
GLOVES	Leather, doeskin, chamois, string.	Suede.
HANDBAG	Leather, straw or plastic.	Suede, dressy leather. plastic.
JEWELLERY AND TRIMMINGS	Mexican silver, silver, brass, gold, copper; leather or novelty lapel pieces, watch, boutonniere; definitely limited.	Watch, gold, silver, rhinestones, coloured stones, lapel clip, boutonnière, corsage, flowers.
SHOES	Calf, novelty leather or fabrics, patent.	Suede, patent, leather.

your waist would be 26 inches.

However, this is an ideal measurement. Few women actually measure up to this standard. A figure may vary an inch or two and still be considered good. It depends upon where the proportion is out. You're better off having your bust two inches larger than the largest part of your hips than the other way around. You also have a strange looking figure, if your bust and buttocks are—say, 36 inches, but your waist and abdomen are 31 inches. An eight-inch taper from the bust to the waist is considered good, or standard.

From a dressing standpoint, I would say that if you are more than three inches out of proportion, you have to be very careful about your clothes selections. And don't let any salesgirl change your mind. There are exceptions to rules but these body proportions are steadfast.

2. Now, let's see how the body should be proportioned vertically. From your head to your toes the body should be divided into four equal parts : (See Figure 59.)

(a) From the top of your head to your bust-line.

(b) From the bust-line to the hips.

(c) From the hips to the knees.

(d) From the knees to the floor.

You may also wish to look at the measurement chart later on in the Course.

Get out your tape measure and measure yourself.

You may be surprised to find, for example, that you are the shortest from your bust to your hips. Should your measurement show you that your waist and abdomen are also a little large in proportion to your other measurements, then what do you deduce ? Since you are the *shortest* in the very area where you are the *widest*, you are going to have to be very careful about the lines for your midriff. You will put nothing there to add further pounds.

Here are some other general laws of proportion :

1. An unbroken line looks longer. Therefore, contrasting colours, two-piece costumes, yokes, belts, or any horizontal lines create breadth. (See Figure 60.)

2. The taller you look, the more slender you look. Since most women are overweight or have large hips, they will dress for height.

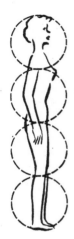

Figure 59

3. Dramatize your good points. If you have a nice flat stomach, what's the good of disguising it in a dirndl skirt !

4. Don't dramatize a weak point by calling attention to a good one.

The woman who weighs 2 stones more than she did ten years ago may still be waddling around in spindly, elaborate shoes. She will tell you rather pathetically that her pretty feet are all that's left of what she used to be. And so she emphasizes them. Others see only the lack of proportion, and her body looks even more top-heavy because of her extreme shoes.

A more stable, sensible heel with a shoe that looks as large as possible would help to proportion her and make her much more attractive.

5. Camouflage your poor lines. For example, if your waist is large, exaggerate your shoulders. Wear fullness through your blouse. Wear flared skirts.

From a proportion standpoint the larger shoulder-line and hem-line will throw your waist-line into weakness. (See Figure 60.) *Don't take the attitude that there's nothing that can be done about what's wrong with you.* Designers have laws for every possible figure defect.

6. You look larger in light colours. Light shoes and light gloves, even, make your feet and hands look larger.

7. Materials with lustre add pounds also. This goes for sequins, satin, brocades, and metallic fabrics.

8. A heavy fabric also adds weight. A tweed suit adds at least ten pounds. Unless you live in the country, you can select fabrics that will be more practical and flattering than tweed. It's too bulky and warm for most of the year, too.

9. Clinging and transparent fabrics are form-revealing. Leave the knitted materials, jumpers, chiffons and laces to those with perfect figures.

10. Learn to get a head-on view of yourself from the front, sides and back. Even if you are just going to the corner for a few groceries in a cotton dress, each detail of your appearance should look as though it were selected with reference to every other detail.

It isn't a question of money as much as it is lack of co-ordination—taking time to plan for and wear each detail of your costume with every other detail.

11. Modify your accessories to your size. Tall, overweight or large-busted women should wear large accessories.

Small women should wear accessories scaled to size. Since accessories refer to almost everything except the costume, this rule applies to shoes, gloves, handbags, jewellery, hats, cor-

a broken line

looks shorter

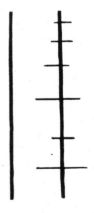

Figure 60

sages, flowers or any other trimming.

Now, let's see how far you've gone on your clothes jaunt :

1. You know how not to be overdressed.

2. You know how to go about organizing your clothes.

3. You know how to start building for a well-rounded wardrobe.

4. You understand how to select and combine your accessories so that they will be not only flattering to you but appropriate to the occasion.

5. You have an understanding of the basic body proportions and general laws of design.

Next, let's talk about specific laws of proportion as they apply to your particular figure type. You may have figured them out already yourself.

WHICH TYPE ARE YOU ?

Designers divide women into the following types :

Tall	(See Figure 61.)
Short	(See Figure 62.)
Fat	(See Figure 63.)
Angular	(See Figure 64.)
Top-heavy	(See Figure 65.)
Hip-heavy	(See Figure 66.)

You're considered short if you're under five feet two. Your height is considered normal if you're between five feet two and five feet six. And you're considered tall if you are over five feet six. These measurements represent your height without shoes.

In my classes, I dress every woman who is overweight or whose hips are out of proportion for height. As I said before, the taller she looks, the more slender she looks. I'd like to say also that the studio designer does not consider you tall until you are five feet eight in your stockinged feet.

Esther Williams, who is five feet seven in her stockinged feet, never looks too tall ; and you don't find the designers cutting her best lines with low or flat hats, either. True, a tall woman shouldn't go out of her way to wear twelve-inch vertical feathers ; but flat, turned down hats do saw her off too suddenly and give her the " droops."

128

In addition to the right clothes, a tall girl's best insurance for morale building is a tall escort or husband. For some reason, short men often are attracted to tall women.

One statuesque student of mine who is just under six feet told me that she became quick in recognizing the look in a man's eyes which said, " My, but you will have nice tall sons."

Combine these suggestions for dressing your figure with all the material in other Lessons on reducing, developing and handling it.

For example, if you have a thin neck, you won't decide what to wear on it and call it a day. You'll also find out how to develop it, how to hold it for correct posture and poise, and how to make it up correctly.

THE TALL WOMAN (See Figure 61.)

	Right	*Wrong*
HATS	Big-brimmed ; wide-crowned. Balance your body lines with wide enough hat lines when wearing smaller hats.	Hats with too much height. Hats with high, pointed crowns. Hats with too definite turned-down brims. Tiny, babyish shapes.

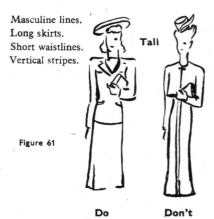

Figure 61

DRESSES AND SUITS· Suits of contrasting colour, bright, wide belts and two and three colour combinations.
Suits of every kind except bolero. Stress anything which is horizontal, padded shoulders, yokes, set-in waistlines, crosswise stripes, bands around your skirt hem.
Suits with long jackets. Break up leg lengths by trimming on skirts, such as ruffles, tunics, skirt pockets, pleats.
Skirts on the short side, depending on shape and size of legs.
Clothes that lengthen the waistline, minimizing a too long-legged look.
Large print dresses, plaids.
Dresses or blouses with neck interest.
Skirts with pleats shirred fullness or flares.
Wrist-length or bracelet, rather than cap sleeves.

Wrong:
Bolero-type jackets.
Waist-length jackets
Masculine lines.
Long skirts.
Short waistlines.
Vertical stripes.

Do   Don't

SHOES Wear high heels as much as you can. Smart low-heeled shoes.

Shoes that make feet look large.

HANDBAG Good-sized.

Small, or masculine accessories.

THE SHORT WOMAN (See Figure .62.)

	Right	*Wrong*
HATS	Small, with an upswept line.	Large-brimmed.
DRESSES AND SUITS	Long, one-colour, unbroken lines. Bolero-type suit.	Horizontal lines. Exaggerated shoulder padding.

THE SHORT WOMAN (*Continued*)

	Right	*Wrong*
DRESSES AND SUITS	Narrow belts the same colour as dress. Skirts an inch or two longer than prevailing length. Higher than normal waistline. Any vertical trimmings, such as buttons from neck to hem. Trimming about the waist.	Suits with hip or three-quarter jackets which cut you in half. Trimming, tunics, ruffles, or peplums on skirts. Fuller-than-average skirts. Shorter-than-average skirts. Large print dresses.
SHOES	High heels whenever possible.	Toeless shoes. Strapped sandals.

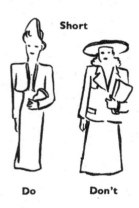

Short

Do   **Don't**

Figure 62

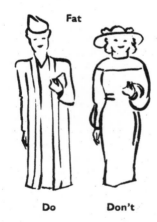

Fat

Do   **Don't**

Figure 63

THE HEAVY WOMAN (See Figure 63.)

	Right	*Wrong*
HATS	Those which stress height. Substantial brims. Sufficient feeling of width to balance hips.	Tiny, silly hats.
DRESSES AND SUITS	Colours like black, brown, navy, grey, soldier blue, deep greens and wine, blurred pastels to conceal extra pounds. Dull rayons, and sheer wools. Very narrow belt of same colour as dress. Hem-line equal in width to the hip and shoulder line. Shoulder pads to balance hips. Skirts with slight flare and longer than prevailing mode.	Intense colours. Satins, taffetas, sequins, padded or starched materials, heavy wool, corduroy. Coloured or wide belts. Short narrow skirts. Flounces, pockets, or skirt trimming.

Angular

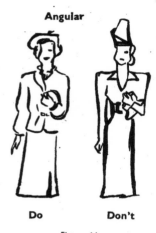

| Do | Don't |

Figure 64

Top heavy

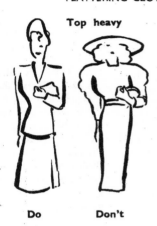

| Do | Don't |

Figure 65

THE HEAVY WOMAN (*Continued*)

| *Right* | *Wrong* |

DRESSES
AND SUITS — Suits (if you must have one) in plain colour with narrow pin stripe.
Buy clothes one size too large and have them fitted.
"V" or oval necks.
Three-quarter or full-length sleeves.

SHOES — Shoes with comfortable heel.
Wrong: Spindly high heels, ghillies. Pointed toes. Straps, Heelless shoes.

HANDBAG — Medium or large.
Wrong: Small.

JEWELLERY — Small.
Wrong: Hanging, cascading strands of beads, " quaint " or gaudy trinkets.

GLOVES — Plain gloves.
Inside seams.
Wrong: Trimmed gloves.
Outside-sewed seams.

THE ANGULAR WOMAN (See Figure 64.)

| *Right* | *Wrong* |

HATS — Hat line irregular.
Bring colour to your face with your hat.
Wrong: Stiff, straight sailors.
Hats with points or downward lines.

DRESSES
AND SUITS — Clothes with rounded lapels, jackets, collars, etc.
Clothes that fit well at the waist, hips, and wrists.
Sequins; fabrics with body, such as piqué, starched cottons, seersuckers, taffeta, heavy wools, velvets, satins, tweed.
Wrong: Garments with sharp, pointed lines.
Clothes that hang on you.
Clinging fabrics, such as chiffons, silk jerseys, flimsy crêpes.
Vertical lines.
Fussy or " old " lines for softness.
Masculine lines.

THE ANGULAR WOMAN (*Continued*)

	Right	*Wrong*
	Plenty of fullness and softness around your neck. Add ruchings, ruffles, starched piqué trimmings, flowers. Three times more amount of shirring in your blouse than average figure. Pleated, full skirts. Trimming on skirts, pockets ; draping. Clothes stressing horizontal line. Contrasting colours.	
SHOES	Rounded toes. Break foot length with bows or cut-out sandals. High heels. Smart low heels.	Pointed shoes. Old or dated-looking shoes.
HANDBAG	Medium sized, with soft lines.	Small. Points.
JEWELLERY	Bracelets—many and wide. Heavy necklaces. Strands of beads. Chokers, novelty jewellery.	If hands are thin, rings. Cascading strands of beads ; heirloom pieces.

THE TOP-HEAVY WOMAN (See Figure 65.)

	Right	*Wrong*
HATS	High, medium-sized, to avoid pin-headed look. Irregular brims or brims with transitional lines.	Large brimmed. Turned-down brims. Small or silly.
DRESSES AND SUITS	Darker-coloured, light-weight materials for top of your costume. Lighter-coloured skirts of heavy material. Longer-than-average, full or flared skirts. No extra padding in shoulders. Narrow lapels. Softened waist-lines. Trimming and bulk in skirts. Deep, substantial hem-line.	Plenty of fullness above waist. Heavy, light-coloured materials for jacket or blouse. Well-padded shoulders. Too much design on blouses and bodices. Straight, short skirts.
HANDBAG	Medium-sized, conservative shape.	Small or large. Ultra-modern shape.
JEWELLERY	Medium-sized rings ; wrist watch.	Prominent clips, lapel pins, brooches, necklaces, ear-rings or bracelets.

THE HIP-HEAVY WOMAN (See Figure 66.)

	Right	*Wrong*
HATS	High, good-sized hats, that balance hip-line.	Small or tightly-fitted hats. Turned-down brims.

DRESSES AND SUITS	Shoulders slightly padded to balance hip-line.	Straight skirts.

DRESSES
AND SUITS

Shoulders slightly padded to balance hip-line.
Lighter-coloured materials for top of your costume.
Darker-coloured skirts.
Heavy materials for jacket or blouse, such as tweed, padded fabrics, wool jersey, starched cottons, etc.
Skirts of sheer wools and silk crêpe.
Plenty of fullness above waist.
Yokes with plenty of shirring for blouses and dresses.
Fullness across back.
Full skirts.
Bolero and cardigan line, if short.
Set-in yoke waistline with narrow belt.
Wide lapels.
" V " neck.

Straight skirts.
Diagonal pleats.
Short skirts.
Narrow lapels.
Narrow shoulders.
Bright blouses.
Trimming on skirts, pockets, ruffles.

hip heavy

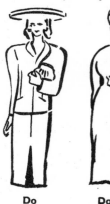

Do   **Don't**

Figure 66

HANDBAG   If tall, large.   Small, silly shapes.
           If short, medium-sized.

JEWELLERY Eye-arresting chokers, earrings, bracelets,   No jewellery or small pieces.
           rings, clips, lapel pins.

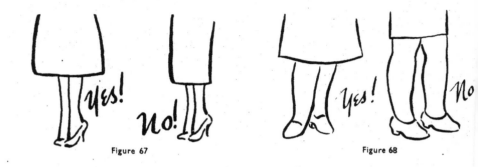

Figure 67   Figure 68

Solving Figure Problems

For These Problems:	*Do's*	*Don'ts*
THIN LEGS (See Figure 67.)	Shiny, light-coloured hose. Full or pleated skirts. Skirts as short as prevailing style allows. See shoes for angular figure.	Dark, so-called "camouflage colours Pencil-slim straight, long skirts.
FAT LEGS (See Figure 68.)	Dull, subdued-colour base. Flared skirts, longer than the prevailing mode. Plain shoes. Stable heel.	Light-coloured base. Short, tight, straight skirts. Strapped shoes.
FAT ARMS (See Figure 69.)	Armholes that are full. Three-quarter or full-length sleeves. Loose sleeves and cuffs. Medium-sized rings.	Coloured or starched cuffs. Tight or short sleeves. Bracelets.
THIN ARMS (See Figure 70.)	Cover them with full-length sleeves. Large, full sleeves of tulle or net for evening. Bracelets, rings, galore.	Tight armholes or sleeves. Dresses without sleeves. Three-quarter length sleeves, cap sleeves.

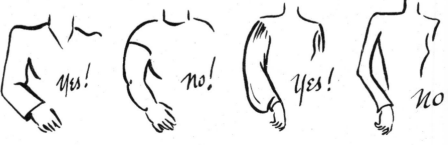

Figure 69   Figure 70

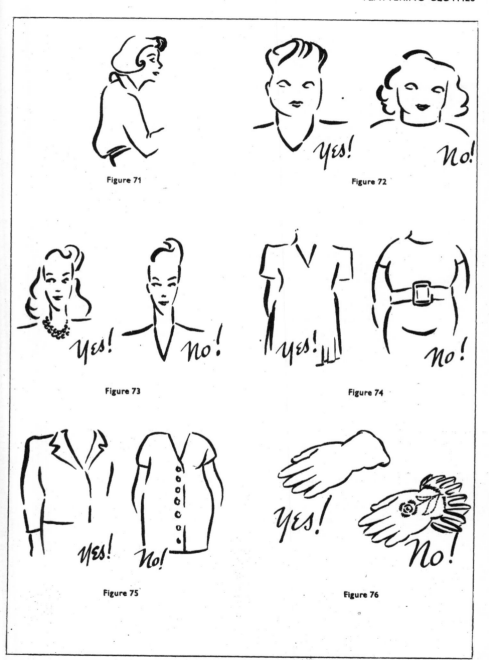

Figure 71

Figure 72

Figure 73

Figure 74

Figure 75

Figure 76

SOLVING FIGURE PROBLEMS (*Continued*)

For These Problems:	*Do's*	*Don'ts*
STOOPED SHOULDERS (See Figure 71)	Large collars that hide dowager's hump or forward curve. Necklines and blouses that distribute fullness and emphasize front and back. Hair full in back.	Collarless dresses or blouses. Long necklaces. Large lapels, front emphasis.
FAT OR SHORT NECK (See Figure 72)	Soft hairline with roll or upswept hair-do. "V" neckline. Furless coat collars. Flat furs. High hats, turned-up brims.	Heavy necklaces. Chokers. Large knot or chignon. Coats with heavy collars. Down-turned brims or wide brims.
LONG OR THIN NECK (See Figure 73)	" Lots of hair " look. (See Lesson Nine on hair). Wide shoulders and lapels. Heavy necklaces and chokers. High round necklines. Neckline fullness. Ruffles, ruching, starched bows. Chiffon and taffeta scarfs.	Collarless coats, suits, dresses. "V" necklines, and oval. Poor-fitting neck-lines. Drooping jewellery or bows. Upswept hair style. " Shingled " hair-line.
A LARGE ABDOMEN (See Figure 74)	Build up interest above waist. Stress diagonal lines below waist. Side closings. Flared skirt or skirt with pleats. Narrow belt of same material as dress.	Tight fit across abdomen. Wide belts of contrasting colour. Buttons up centre of body. Tight, short, narrow skirt. Skirt trimming.
A LARGE WAIST (See Figure 75)	Small belts on dresses of same material as dress. Colours that are conservative. Shoulders padded and hem-line fullness to make waist-line smaller in proportion. Large lapels ; above waist trimming and fullness.	Bright colours. Beltless dresses. Wide, large belts of contrasting colour. Narrow shoulders. Tight, straight skirts.
UNATTRACTIVE HANDS (See Figure 76)	Gloves that are conservative, with inside stitching. Subdued nail varnish. See Lesson Eight on graceful hand technique and make-up.	Heavy rings and bracelets. Heavy, outside-stitching gloves.

Self - Test Questions Based On Lesson Five

Many attractive women, often with good figures, spoil the whole effect by overdressing. Good clothes can be thus spoiled. The woman with a small wardrobe or dress allowance can yet be well dressed. This is a lesson of vital importance to every woman.

After you have studied this Lesson, you should be able to answer the following questions. If you have any difficulty in doing so, refer to the Lesson for further study and revision. Your answers should not be sent to the publishers of this Course.

1. What is the rule by which you may judge the correctness of your dress for any occasion? How does this work?

2. Have you applied this rule to your own dress? If so, with what result?

3. What is the advice given in this Lesson regarding the wearing of girdles and brassieres?

4. Examine yourself in regard to your working clothes. Most of your time, especially if you are a housewife, is spent at your work. Do you make yourself as smart as possible for this, in accordance with the nature of your work?

5. What do you mean by a basic garment?

6. What are the basic colours?

7. What types of women should not wear suits?

8. What is the general rule to follow in choosing your wardrobe, having regard to your own particular figure?

9. How long should your clothes last if you treat them kindly and with care?

10. Have you found the type of figure in the Lesson as nearly resembling your own as possible?

Be sure to check on your clothes for any faults.

If you wish to determine the progress you are making, give yourself 10 points for each question you answer correctly. If the total comes to 90 or more, it is excellent; 80 or more, good; 70 or more, fair.

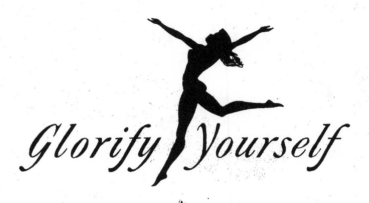

Glorify Yourself

★

A Complete and Up-to-Date Course on
Beauty and Charm by One of the
Most Famous Beauty Specialists
and Consultants in the World

Eleanore King

★

LESSON SIX

★

STUDIO TALK •

Issued only for Students
of the Eleanore King
Course on Beauty. Charm
and Personality.

Number Six.

Dear Student,

Every woman a model! That's the title of •
Lesson Six Part A. And it embodies an ideal; for to-day's
leading models set a universally recognised standard for
grace, poise and deportment.

Your own career may be home-making or business;
but you should still practise the special modelling
techniques described in this part of the Lesson, since
they are a wonderful short cut to correct body line-up.

Modelling methods also help you to make the most
of your clothes. Even the simplest dress can gain glamour
from being properly displayed. Many of the movements used
in modelling can and should be used every day in social
and business life. Whenever you turn in a doorway you
should always use the beautiful movement described on
page 9; whenever you have to approach someone and then
walk away again, you should always, instinctively use the
social pivot which is fully described on the same page.

In Part B of this Lesson we consider posture and
relaxation. You will remember the importance of
relaxation was stressed in our very first Lesson. I hope
you have been regularly practising the simple exercises I
prescribed then. Lesson Six also contains more advanced
techniques, and I trust that you will practise them
carefully. They are wonderfully soothing, and are among
the most valuable aids to beauty and charm.

Lesson Six marks the half-way point in the Course.
If you have done nothing more than read through the Lessons
and Studio Talks up to this point, you belong to that 10%
of women who realise that you are the only one who can
change yourself. If you have practised the techniques,
routines and exercises you will by now be seeing the results
for yourself. You will already be a more confident, assured
personality: your natural charm and grace will be more
fittingly revealed.

(over)

But I hope that you have gained even more than this! The cultivation of your own personal beauty is only a part of a wider, deeper philosophy of life. I shall be more than happy if I have succeeded not only in helping you to radiate charm, but to adopt a more vital, dynamic approach to life as a whole.

Go forward, now, to Lesson Six. And above all, continue to GLORIFY YOURSELF.

With continued good wishes.

Yours sincerely,

Eleanor King

LESSON · SIX

Part A

Every Woman A Model

We are, in truth, more than half of what we are by imitation. The great point is, to choose good models and to study them with care.
—LORD CHESTERFIELD, *Letters*, 18 *Jan.*, 1750.

THROUGHOUT this whole Course, you have been learning tricks, short cuts and techniques that every woman in the public eye practises—whether her career is modelling, homemaking, acting or business. There are still a few more to absorb before you join the ranks of the poised and charming. First of all, stair technique.

UPS AND DOWNS

What kind of a picture do you make as you go up and down stairs ? Or are you one of those women who complain, " By the time I go up and down stairs thirty times a day, I'm a nervous wreck ! "

Let's say that the average homemaker goes up and down stairs three or four times every hour in an average ten-hour day. These steps can be a challenge and an exercise for firming, developing or reducing her thighs and legs. And her thighs and legs cannot operate correctly unless she *is* holding her body in good alignment.

Therefore, at the same time as she is firming and reducing her buttocks, even if she makes one hundred trips during an average day, the correct stair technique will mean less wear and tear on her body and nerves—not to mention how much better she will look !

How many times have you heard, " You can always tell a lady by the way she ' takes her stairs ' " ? And it's true you do form a subconscious impression of a woman as you watch her moving on stairs. Notice how often you see an actress, especially in the films, going up or down stairs. Those wise directors know that if a woman can do them well she can't be placed in a more attractive background.

In the long run of *Life with Father*, much of the light, gracious impression which Dorothy

Stickney (who, incidentally, was my first inspiring voice and drama coach) made as *Vinnie* depended upon her floating up and down stairs dozens of times. As the stormy Katherina in *Taming of the·Shrew*, Lynn Fontanne seemed to have no stairs beneath her at all as she swept up and down in a rage ! Lily Pons' *Lucia* is twice as effective because of the stairway exits and entrances allowing her floating trains full sweep.

Of the skills you have learned in these Lessons, stair work is the most simple. Your success at it depends upon a few basic techniques and your willingness to employ them each time you are confronted with stairs.

UP, UP, UP !

Before you start up a stairway, pause at the bottom, bend your knees quite a bit, and tuck your buttocks under you. (See Figure 77.) Full instructions for controlling the buttocks are found in Lesson Three Part A. Put your whole foot on the stair if you wish. (See Figure 77A.) It is just as good form as placing only the ball of the foot there. (See Figure 77C.) The whole foot on the step ensures that you keep your back straight and your hips controlled, for no dress on earth can hide protruding buttocks and wobbly hips as you ascend.

Say to yourself, " Up, up, up, up."And here's the trick : never unbend your knees much! Then you will go up smoothly with never a jerk. Incidentally, you ensure a controlled bust-line by maintaining stable knee action on stairs.

I used to think that men collected at the bottom of stairs in hotels and clubs because they were hopeful of seeing a few well-turned legs and knees.

Since watching hundreds of full-busted, over-

143

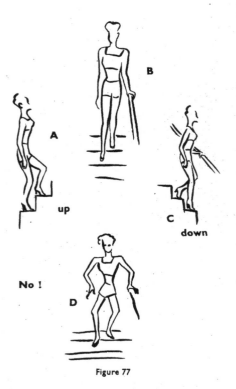

Figure 77

Put a book or posture board on your head to help. Say aloud " Up, up, up, up, up," in an even smooth voice. It is perfectly good form, also, to place one hand on the railing and to look down at the steps. Don't appear to be peering down, though.

You will notice that your thighs do the work with this method. Keep your feet in two lines as you ascend, about two inches apart. (See Figure 77). It's all well and good for our showgirls to come downstairs crossing one foot over in front of the other, but it is too " stagey " and affected for practical use.

Down, Down, Down !

Before you come downstairs, pause, get your buttocks under you, line up your body correctly, bend your knees, and go down, again *keeping your knees bent*. You will learn by practice how much to bend your knees and still ensure an unbroken line. (See Figure 77B.) You're actually controlling an up-and-down motion with your knees and thighs. You will have a tendency at first to move up and down stairs too fast, but that is all right.

After you have mastered the feeling of the bent knees, then you can relax and take the stairs more slowly.

developed women bounce down stairs, I'm beginning to think their interest might well be focussed on the over-action of the bustline ! A lady must have a controlled bust-line.

The average person bends her knee when she steps up. As she places her weight on this foot in order to go up *another* stair, she straightens the knee. Then she takes another step, again adjusting the knee for the next step. This knee adjusting on each step causes the body to bounce, so that there is a series of jerky up-and-down lines.

If these women could see themselves only once, they would be cured for life ! Keep your knees bent and relaxed and never unbend them. To get the feel of it, walk around the room with your knees bent " Seven Dwarfs " fashion for a few times. Then without unbending them, start up the stairs and keep them bent until you reach the top.

As you descend, say " Down, down, down, down," on each stair. Say it aloud, if you can and to yourself when others are around. Let your knees rotate inward a little, to ensure that there is no space between them. (See Figure 77C.)

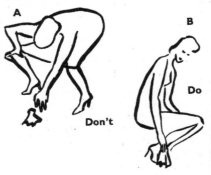

Figure 78

If you will consciously apply these principles for several weeks every time you find yourself on stairs, you will have adopted a joy-instilling habit which is yours to keep for the rest of your life. Here, then, is a lesson which takes you ten minutes to learn, two weeks to master, and adds grace for the rest of your life *if* you remember to do it each time.

Don't Trip on It

Women often complain about feeling nervous on stairs, in long skirts. Here's your cure. Bend over, slip the folds of your dress in your fingers at about the knee-line, straighten your body, and bring the skirt up with you. It doesn't matter if you bring it halfway up your legs in front.

A long skirt picked up even to the knees won't be unflattering. Don't scoop up your skirt to the side, causing it to wrinkle unnaturally and your rear to become too prominent. Many very long skirts, or trains, have a little hem-line tape to slip around your fingers to help you pick them up on stairs.

Know that you never look more feminine than you do coming down a stairway, so make the most of it.

Pick It Up Gracefully

How do you look when you pick up your handkerchief or a piece of paper from the floor ? Do you bend over, with your knees straight, your rear out ? (See Figure 78 A.) You couldn't possibly look more unattractive. See how much better you look this way : as you stoop, bend both knees in one direction.

Don't squat, with knees apart, unless you're wearing shorts or slacks. Round your back and go down with your knees bent, your thighs taking the action. (See Figure 78 B.) Come up the same way.

How to Pick Up Heavy Objects

Maybe you have to pick up a heavy box. Get close to the box. Bend your knees. Balance your torso over your thighs. Put your hands and arms under the box. As you lift it, feel that the strongest part of your body is carrying the

greatest part of the load. That is, your thighs and pelvic region. (See Figure 79 A.) Don't expect your arms and upper back to carry the load. (See Figure 79 B.)

Even if you have to move a heavy piece of furniture, manage to have the pelvic area or strongest part of your body do the work. When you lift a heavy object overhead, raise it first to your waist-line and then keep it close to your body as you raise it overhead. (See Figure 79 A.) Don't extend your arms in front of you and then strain your back trying to reach a high shelf. Stay close.

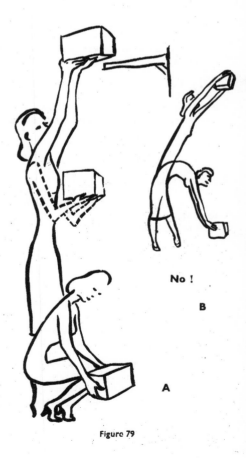

No !

B

A

Figure 79

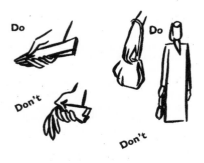

Figure 80

HOW TO MODEL HATS

In modelling a hat, lower your head to the front, then slowly raise it. Use either a slow military or social pivot and as you turn to the side drop your head, first slightly to the side, then to the back

Start taking the hat off from the back of the head and bring it forward to the front. If you take off the front part first, then you show the lining. Have your arm movements well timed for this.

HOW TO CARRY YOUR GLOVES

When carrying or showing gloves, have them palm to palm and finger to finger, as they are when new, and then put your thumb down on the fingers. (See Figure 80.)

If you hold gloves by the top or clasp them around the part intended for the wrist, they hang limp and stringy. If you're modelling, you can hold your gloves with both hands to call attention to them as you pause. Or imitate the model with this glove trick to control your hands when you're nervous and gloved. In daily life, *wear* gloves instead of carrying them. When you wish to remove them, pull each finger a little at the tip. Don't roll them off by pulling at the top so that you turn them inside out. Form the habit of placing them palm to palm and putting them in your bag.

A well-bred person puts her accessories or belongings in one spot, so that they do not clutter up a table, divan, or whole room.

HOW TO CARRY YOUR HANDBAG

Handle your bags with your fingers only—not your whole hand. Put your bag either under your arm, or if it has a handle, slip your wrist through it. (See Figure 80.) When modelling a bag carry it as though it's yours. When you clasp a bag by the handle and carry it down at your side, you add five years to your appearance. (See Figure 80.)

TIPS FOR MODELLING OR WEARING COATS

When modelling a coat, remember that you are presenting line. Be sure the coat fits you at the shoulder seams. Then it will hang correctly. Adjust it only at the shoulder line and keep your hands from fidgeting, pulling, patting, and smoothing the garment. This same advice holds good for wearing coats. To show the lining, hold the garment between thumb and forefinger of one hand, and with the other, hold back the coat so that the customer may see the lining. (See Figure 81A.) This is a simple trick but it preserves the line as you show the lining. If you pull the two flaps back you ruin the line.

Another tip is to slip one hand or both hands in your pockets, so that only the thumb is visible. (See Figure 81B.) Sometime during your showing, push back the front of the coat and put your hand on your hip. You may slant your fingers either up or down for this hip gesture. (See Figure 81C.) The fingers pointing downward

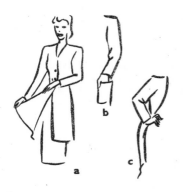

Figure 81

146

with the inside of the wrist on the hip-line, is an appropriate hand pose on more formal and elaborate clothes. The fingers pointing up with the inside of the wrist on the hip-line is a hand position more appropriate for sports wear.

How to carry a coat. Haven't you seen women practically ruining beautiful coats by carrying them carelessly? They stamp themselves also as negligent.

Here's how a model is told to carry her coat, and a well-bred woman uses the same technique : fold it so that the shoulders are even and put it casually over your arm. It's such a simple principle but it makes a world of difference in the complete impression you give to others.

HOW TO PIVOT

Since every woman is turning constantly, I insist that every one of my students master at least five pivots. They help to develop balance, co-ordination and poise more quickly than any other method I know. Of course, every model must master a series of pivots. Different coaches present different pivots by different names. As you know, a pivot is a turn.

The first pivot you will work on is essentially a balance pivot. The poorer your balance, the harder you should work on it. Or should I say that difficulty with this pivot is an indication that you have poor balance ? Here it is called the Military or Ziegfeld Pivot.

MILITARY OR ZIEGFELD PIVOT

The first pivot, then, which you will work on

is one whose chief aim is to develop balance. Haven't you ever felt your ankles were wobbly ? Many women who lack poise do not realise it may be caused by lack of balance.

Spend several hours practising this one pivot, so that you will be sure of your ankle strength and general co-ordination before you go on to any of the others. It is called the " Military Pivot " because it is copied from the soldier's " about turn " command.

Here is how it's done : Put your right foot into the arch position. (See Figure 82.) Now cross it behind the left foot, so that the toes of both feet face the front with weight equally distributed between both feet. Do this several times, counting : right foot in arch, cross back, so that both toes point front, with weight equally divided. Now put your weight on the balls of your feet and turn your body towards the foot which crossed back, or back foot, and pivot. (See Figure 82.)

You are now facing in the opposite direction and you have made a half circle. Try it again : right foot in arch, cross back, weight on toes, and pivot.

After turning halfway around, bring your back, or left foot, forward into the arch position. This time arch with your left foot. Left foot crosses behind the right foot, weight on your toes, and PIVOT. (See Figure 82.)

Practise it over and over until it is smooth and lovely to watch. In a real-life situation you could use this only for practising balance.

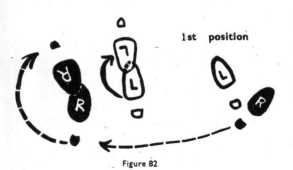

Figure 82

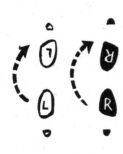

Figure 83

147

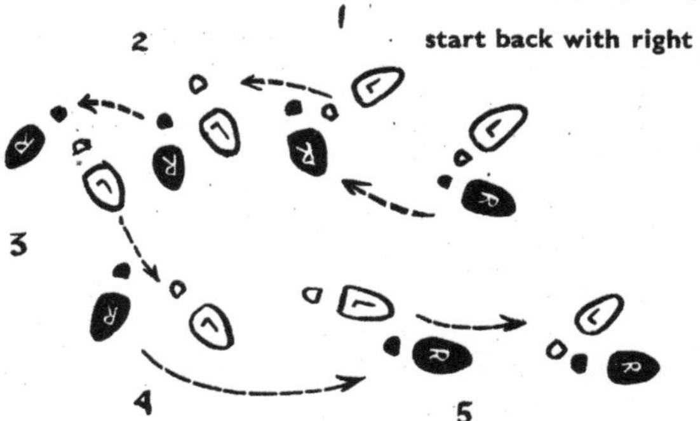

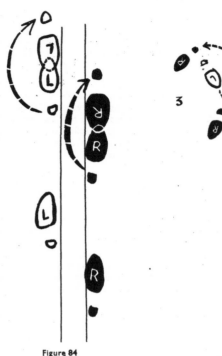

start back with right

Figure 85

Figure 84

off the floor, and turn your feet and body so that your two toes are now facing where your heels were when you started. (See Figure 83). This turning will hereafter be referred to as " shifting."

So here is your practice exercise as an approach to the walking pivot : toes both straight ahead, one foot ahead of the other, put your weight on balls of feet and shift. Then shift back. The balls of your feet never leave the floor. Keep shifting until you can do it with ease.

2. Toes both straight ahead, feet in arch position. Step out with foot in arch position. Count one, two, three, four, and stop. Don't move feet or take them off the floor. SHIFT. (See Figure 84).

Now, step out with the front foot (the foot which is front since you've shifted). If you learn just this one thing in this whole Course the chances are you will handle your body better than 60 per cent. of our women. Do it again. Step out one, two, three, four, shift. You will have to pause a second to get your balance after shifting. Then walk again.

However, a model will often use this if she is showing floor-reaching, frilly clothes. Or she may use it to model a bouffant evening dress, in which case she turns very slowly to the count of five.

This slower pivot is often called the Ziegfeld Pivot, because Ziegfeld used it so often on the stage to dramatise his beautiful chorus girls. You have achieved a movement of beauty when you can execute this pivot slowly and smoothly.

WALKING PIVOT

This pivot is the most fun of all, and the one you will use dozens of times each day. It's simply an efficient, graceful way of turning. Also you will recognise it as the one you see models use more than any other. Here is your technique for it step by step.

1. Put one foot in front of the other. Now shift your weight to the balls of your feet, heels

Practise this for about ten minutes by the clock until you are positive of it. Then take six steps, shift, step out with the front foot and return six steps. Gradually add one more step through six, seven, eight, nine and ten, until you can go to the end of your room, shift, or turn, start out with the front foot and walk down the length of the room again.

You see why it is called " walking pivot "?

148

You never really cease moving, although there is a slight pause after each pivot. The shift itself can be slow or fast. You'll have occasions for both, depending on the time element.

Now, suppose you are practising this pivot only for modelling purposes. Walk to each chair in your practice room, shift and walk away. What have you accomplished? You know how to model the back of your garment. Thus far the customer has seen only the front or side of your dress. You may have to count as you walk towards your imaginary customer : one, two, three, four, SHIFT, and one, two, etc., away to the next one. Or if your customer seems interested and asks you a question, you return again for her inspection and pause long enough to answer her question graciously. The more you practise with your imaginary audience the better you'll perform for an honest-to-goodness one.

How to Turn in a Doorway

One of the most beautiful movements which any woman executes is her turn in a doorway. The technique for ensuring a smooth exit is the same whether you're using it in your home or as a professional model. Walk to the door, turn back towards those in the room, then turn towards the door again, and walk through it.

More specifically, here's how : Walk to the door. Don't walk through it or pause a foot away from it. *Pause exactly at the door, or in the doorway.* Do your walking pivot, which turns you facing the room again, arch, and pause a minute. Pivot again (half turn) so that you are once more facing the door and go out.

Keep your eyes and head turned as long as possible towards your customers or towards the group you are leaving. This technique for turning gracefully in a doorway requires only a little practice, and it's well worth the time you spend on it.

I repeat that even if you know you will never model a single garment during your lifetime, practise this for the ease it will give you in homes, offices, stores and in gatherings of all sorts. You are constantly turning. And men have a way

of watching you as YOU MOVE. It's their deep-rooted sense of rhythm.

Social Pivot

If you do not intend to put this foot-work to professional use, you may not use the military pivot for anything but balance practice. *The social or detail pivot, on the other hand, can be used to advantage dozens of times each day wherever you are.*

Follow the diagrams carefully. In this pivot your aim is to turn your body half-way round as smoothly as possible. However, you walk around instead of pivoting on the balls of your feet as in the other pivots. Here's how you do it : Right foot in arch, stand directly in front of a chair, step back slightly with right foot (but do not cross back as you did in the military pivot).

Now turn the whole left foot two or three inches to the right. Now pick up the right foot and take a little step of perhaps two inches to the right with it. Then take another step with the left foot, and one more with the right foot to ensure turning your body half way around.

Thus far you have taken five steps and your body is turned around so that your back is to the chair or customer. Bring your back foot (in this case the left one) forward into an arch as you pause. (See Figure 85) Keep your head turned in the chair's direction as long as you can. Your head lingers.

As you practise the social pivot, count : arch, cross back, one ; turn left foot, two ; turn right foot, three ; turn left foot, four ; turn right foot, five ; and bring your left foot forward into an arch. You have just taken a little walk and have covered perhaps two feet in distance. The social pivot is the forerunner of the other more difficult ones, so be sure you master it. Get so that you can count : arch, turn one, turn two, turn three, turn four, turn five and arch.

Then pivot back to the chair or customer again, showing the front of your costume to her. (See Figure 86)

When you have practised this for about ten minutes—and don't rush it—then start putting the hand motions in with it. As you start turning back with your right foot, pick up your left hand to about your waist. (See Figure 86).

Then, as you count three, bring your right hand to the waist-line into the hand position you learned in an earlier Lesson.

Let me repeat this : To be well co-ordinated in all movements you use the opposite hand and foot at the same time. You do *not* use your right hand, for example, with your right foot. If you are starting out with your right foot, you pick up or use first the *left* hand. If you are using the left foot, you pick up the right hand.

CO-ORDINATION PRACTICE

To get this timing, practise the following exercises : Your hands at your waist with palms. facing up. Begin walking with your right foot. As you step out with the right foot, drop the left hand. Then after you take three or four steps, drop the right hand to your side.

Now, let's go back and put this hand timing in with the social pivot. Into your arch with your right foot and as you cross back with your right foot, pick up with your left hand. (See Figure 86). Left foot turns two, right foot turns three (as you pick up your right hand), left foot turns four, turns five, and into your arch with your right foot, as both hands assume position at waist.

This is one of the most difficult things to accomplish in this whole Course, so take it slowly. Concentrate on your feet at first. When you are sure you have them disciplined, then get the hands working.

If you get the co-ordination going smoothly between your hands and feet in this pivot, you need not worry about their co-ordination in anything else you ever undertake. It's a lot of fun once you have it and you have a right to feel pretty superior about perfecting it. Also I've never known a girl or woman who perfected this co-ordination and who ever had to worry about clumsy hand motions again !

If you are modelling, you would use this pivot to show a dress with beautiful detail. Hence its name. The turn is slow and casual enough to display whatever the designer intended the customer to like.

Those of you studying this material for poise training will use this pivot dozens of times daily. It's slower and more casual than the crisp walking pivot. You will use it as you are saying good-bye to a friend or hostess. How many times have you found yourself stepping back awkwardly bumping into someone or something, apologising stupidly, and retracting in haste and confusion to hide your embarrassment ?

Do you rush your introductions and good-byes because you are ill at ease doing them ? Here is your cure. Turn to an imaginary friend and without saying a word, go through the pantomime of saying good-bye, shaking hands, using the social pivot as you leave. Then pretend you have forgotten one last word, and use the social pivot to face your friend again, say what you wish, and social pivot away once more.

There are more detailed instructions in later Lessons on meeting people and leaving them. Here we are concentrating solely on foot-work to make it smooth and inconspicuous. Spend fifteen minutes on just this technique. Practise this pivot in front of every chair in your living room. " Sell " a dress to each chair. Show your customer the front of it, then the back, and then the front again.

FLOATING PIVOT

Your next turn, the floating pivot, is based on the footwork of the social pivot. It is beautiful and the one which your model uses when she is displaying lovely, full-skirted evening dresses. It is her most " showy " dramatic pivot.

If you want it for your everyday non-professional life, you will use it in your home when you are serving, passing cigarettes, or emptying ash-trays : or when leaving papers on the boss's desk in your office.

Chiefly, this large pivot teaches you not to be afraid of space. You learn to gauge your body into space just as you learn to judge distances

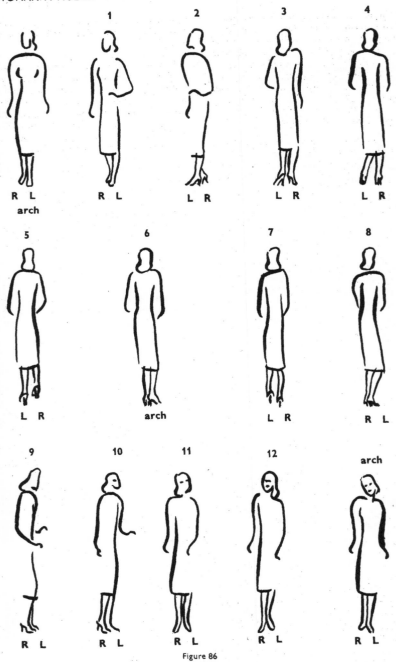

Figure 86

151

in your car as you drive. Think of it as an advanced co-ordination drill. Even if you never use it except when you practise, you have made an investment in gracefulness. You use the same motions as you did for the social pivot except that your steps are a little larger. For this you may use as much space as you wish—half a room if you have to. Counting one, two, three, four, five, arch, to waltz time ; but *don't dance*. Get some abandon in your movements.

Let's work at it now. Stand in front of a chair. Right foot into an arch, (see Figure 87) , turn one, with your right foot ; turn two, with your left foot ; turn three, with your right foot ; turn four, with your left foot.

By this time your body is turned halfway round with your back to the chair, and you step five forward, then into the arch, which makes six. Practise this until you can do it smoothly, covering quite a bit of space, and then not so much space, for you want to be able to gauge spaces. Your counting goes, arch, turn one, turn two, turn three, four, five, arch. *Keep your head turned towards the chair until you are at least halfway round.*

When you are positive you have the footwork, then add the hand motions to it. They represent the same co-ordination as you used in the social pivot, except that your hand movements are slower.

As you step back with your right foot, you raise your left hand. On the count four, raise your right hand, bringing both hands into position at the waist. Now as you go back with your left foot, drop your right hand. As you turn on the count of three or four, drop the left hand until, as you come to count five, your hands are both at your sides in their original position.

When you have completed your five arch count, you are just halfway round. In other words, if you start out showing the customer the front, you end up showing her the back at the termination of the count. Some women try to turn all the way round and make quite an ungainly picture. Never try to complete a circle as you turn.

FORWARD PIVOT

Last, but not least, we come to the forward pivot. Again, if you are not contemplating a modelling career, think of this pivot as you did the floating pivot—as a drill in co-ordination and gracefulness.

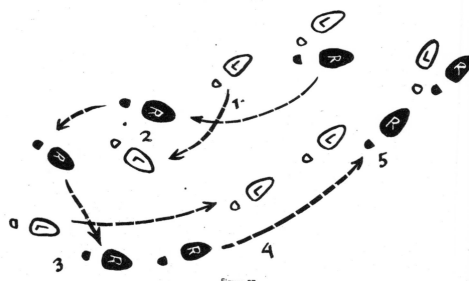

Figure 87

This is the only pivot in which you go forward at first. Stand squarely in front of a chair. Arch with your right foot, and step forward with that foot. Your aim is to show the customer, or chair, the front of your garment, and then instead of stepping back to show her the back of it, you step forward to do so. That is a most flattering movement and many models use it almost exclusively, because it shows how a skirt falls with the wearer's movements.

Go into your arch with your right foot, step forward and turn to the right, your right shoulder leading out.

As you step forward count one ; then, turn two with your left foot (still turning to the right); turn three with your right foot ; turn four with your left foot (your body is now completely turned around and your back to the buyer); and you take one more step to straighten out your movements to the count of five, and arch with your left foot. (See Figure 88). So your count as you go forward is like this : Turn one, turn two, turn three, turn four, five, and arch. Keep all your steps just like a very casual walk.

There is a tendency on this pivot to dance through it, so be sure there are no affected movements as you turn—just a smooth walk around, done so casually that no one is the wiser.

You could use the same hand movements you learned for your social and floating pivots. For variety as well as for promoting hand poise, however, you might incorporate the back hand position you learned in an earlier Lesson.

Place your hand, palms out, at your belt-line in the back. Don't let your elbow stick out horizontally. Place the arm rather at an up-and-down angle, your wrist itself relaxed, fingers curled. Your elbow falls to the side of your body rather snugly. For this pivot count six while the hand is going up the back and six down. Up one, two, three, four, five, six ; down one, two, three, four, five, six.

When you are certain you can do it well, put your hand movements in with the forward pivot.

CO-ORDINATION ROUTINE

Your co-ordination routine goes like this : As you step forward with your right foot, pick your left arm up from the side and let it creep up the back for the whole count of six, and as you come back, let the arm slide down to the side to the entire count of six. It's fun. When you've polished it up a bit, look at it in the mirror.

For practice, walk up to within six or seven

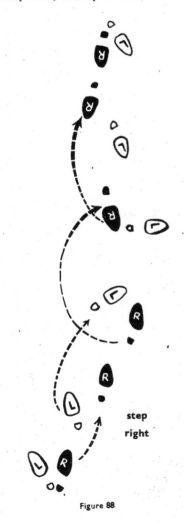

step right

Figure 88

153

feet of each chair in your living-room and begin your forward pivot. As you turn, going towards the customer, you will pick up your hands to your front waist-line.

This ensures an unbroken back-line for the customer. As you step away from her, to show her the front of the gown once more, you may incorporate the hand to the back waist-line, exposing a clear front line this time.

In addition to knowing these pivots, a model must put them together so that she can show any garment, from a bathing suit to an evening dress, or just accessories, or lingerie, or whatever it is her employer is selling.

In order to do this, she puts her routine together much as a dancer builds individual steps into a dance. Just as different coaches have different names for the various pivots, so, too, routines vary. A wise model will stud, as many as possible. Each organisation or employer has a different version : some insist that you use *no pivots whatever.*

Our idea here is to offer the fundamental routines to be mastered. If your body co-ordinates itself naturally into definite trained patterns, you can adjust yourself to new routines in only a few minutes.

FOR MODELS ONLY

Watch your tempo. Listen to the speech of a popular announcer or platform performer. Notice that his appeal lies in changing the tempo of his speech, which is never too monotonous— he varies it : fast, loud, slow, or moderate tempo. In just this manner, an outstanding model will vary her steps, moving slowly, speeding up, or slowing down on the pivots. She also wishes to avoid monotony. For short skirts the tempo is usually faster, especially for tailored costumes. For cocktail and evening fashions, the timing is slower and more languid. For sports costumes, the model may use the same footwork but be definitely out-of-doors in her freshness and vigour.

We shall consider here three routines, all of which are interchangeable : (1) short-skirt routine, (2) detail routine, and (3) long-skirt routine.

SHORT-SKIRT ROUTINE

Suppose you are modelling a tailored suit : walk up to your customer, arch, as you hesitate a moment, take three steps back so that the customer can see your garment better. Come forward again three steps into the walking pivot. Then to the next customer. Let me repeat this routine :

1. Walk up to your customer and arch for a second or long enough to answer questions.

2. Take three steps backward, facing her always, arch, and pause for a second.

3. Come forward again three steps into the walking pivot and as you turn this time, you are on your way to the next customer. Don't forget to let your head linger as you turn away.

This routine is lots of fun because you can adapt it to music of varied tempos. Try doing it over and over as you hum the chorus of "A Pretty Girl is Like a Melody." Practise to music whenever possible.

Your customer has now had ample opportunity to see your garment closely—also at a little distance, and to see how the skirt falls during movement. Keep in mind that you are working to show the garment to the best possible advantage. Your walk and turns must be so beautifully executed that no attention is centred on them. At least, this is the theory the model works on, but undoubtedly in every sale there is the factor that the buyer believes she will look as lovely in the costume as the model does when she shows it.

DETAIL ROUTINE

Suppose your employer is showing a garment whose appeal depends upon its detail. Perhaps it's that basic dress in a basic colour—the type women buy year after year and yet the manufacturer has made it up-to-date with a new cut and detail. You want to show off the workmanship. Your modelling, then, will be much slower and more deliberate. Here are your rules for a detail routine :

1. Walk up to your customer and arch as you hesitate a second.

2. Do your social pivot and arch.

3. Walk away four steps and arch (your back to your customer).

4. Do the social pivot, bringing you face to the front again.·

5. Using the walking pivot, go on to the next buyer, or if this customer shows interest, come forward again and display the costume.

Notice you have twice turned your body very slowly, the first time close to her, and the second time a few feet away. As you have taken these slow pivots, she has had plenty of time to see all the fine handwork on the garment.

LONG-SKIRT ROUTINE

Now, suppose you are wearing a housecoat, or a dinner dress, or a formal evening dress. Your long skirt makes it possible for you to take larger steps. You want to show off the fullness and cut of the skirt as you move and turn. Here's your routine :

1. Pause several yards from the buyer and as you come towards her, do the forward pivot, bringing your hands up your back waist-line as you will recall having practised in your Forward Pivot Lesson.

2. You come out of your forward pivot about an arm's length away from your customer, with your back to the customer, thus allowing her to see the back. Arch, pause, and then make another forward pivot, coming out of it to show her the *front* of your garment. Arch, pause, then quarter pivot out of your arch and on your way again.

ON A RAMP

If you are on a runway, or if you have plenty of space, then go into your floating pivot, for it is the most showy and beautiful pivot to watch. Walk six or eight steps, then use your floating pivot again, or your walking pivot. Especially be careful to vary your tempo on a ramp.

Here are some pitfalls to avoid in modelling :

1. Never look affected in your movements, gestures or expression.

2. Concentrate on your garment or the customer—or on something away from you as a personality.

3. Keep your arms and hands close to you—and keep them, oh, so casual.

4. If you make a mistake in what you think you should do, learn early in your practising to hide it. No one will ever know the difference.

5. Walk as though you *own* your costume.

6. Adapt your showing to your supervisor's suggestions.

7. Avoid poses. *Don't act like a model* ! Be yourself. Glorify yourself !

Notes:

LESSON SIX

Part B

Posture And Relaxation

Since the body is the pipe through which we tap all the succours and virtues of the material world, it is certain that a sound body must be at the root of any excellence in manners and actions.

—EMERSON, *Lectures and Biographical Studies*

THE fastest way to streamline your body is through posture. By that I mean that one bright morning you are taught how to " hold what you have."

If you are an alert student, you will look better proportioned by lunch time. You haven't lost a pound or an inch, but you are carrying yourself so much better that you GIVE THE ILLUSION of vitality and control associated with what we mean by liquid grace. You learned earlier on in the Course how to line yourself up correctly, and in a previous Lesson you learned how to walk gracefully. You are probably looking 75 per cent better already. There are, however, certain corrective posture exercises that will help you to diminish a double chin, sway-back, stooped shoulders, knock-knees, or dropped arches.

You have already read the techniques you can apply to correct these as you go about your daily schedule. There are, in this Lesson, exercises that you will actually have to find time to do. Even if you have always been proud of your posture, these routines will ensure that you maintain it. They will not only help you to distribute your weight advantageously, but they will develop a flexibility associated with youth.

Among your own acquaintances, you may know two women of approximately the same age and size. One you definitely classify as middle-aged. The other is flexible. You never associate age with her at all. IF YOU TAKE ONLY THREE MINUTES A DAY FOR ACTIVE EXERCISES, THESE POSTURE ROUTINES SHOULD BE YOUR FIRST " MUST."

RHYTHMIC APPROACH

Think of these posture routines as rhythmics— something that you do which is controlled, yet relaxed, because one of the great benefits you derive from these rhythmics is an ability to relax.

You are training each set of muscles to fall into the harmonious positions that Nature originally intended.

Through the years, women have done many exercises which were not intended for the female figure—exercises that built muscle over fat and often developed tense bodies. These posture rhythms are different. They're easy after you get the hang of them ; they're soothing and you'll like them. Lie down on a mat or rug and tune in a little music on your radio. As you know, music has great therapeutic value, so let the combination of the music and the rhythmics refresh you.

The complete group has been designed by posture authorities to help any part of your body that is out of line, whether that part is your head, neck, chest, shoulders, abdomen, buttocks, legs or feet. YOU MUST DO THE WHOLE CYCLE EVEN IF ONLY ONE SMALL PART OF YOU NEEDS ATTENTION.

RHYTHMIC ONE. Here is your first posture lesson, which is as effective for men as it is for women. Lie on your back. Bend your knees so that your feet almost touch your buttocks. Keep your feet flat, your knees together or slightly apart. No tension anywhere.

This position hereafter will be referred to as the "hook position," which it is called in all corrective physical education classes.

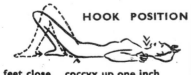

HOOK POSITION

feet close   coccyx up one inch

Figure 89

156

Close your eyes and imagine that you are picking up the end of your spine about ONE HALF-INCH or ONE INCH from the floor. Most of your back should touch the floor, except the very end of your spine, or your coccyx. Pick it up. Hold it up there a second. Then relax by lowering coccyx to floor. (See Figure 89). Repeat several times.

You may feel some muscular reaction at first but don't worry about it. You're working unused muscles. Close your eyes again, and pick up the lower part of your spine. Hold it up there for as long as you can, and relax again. Each time try to hold it to one more count until you can reach ten.

RHYTHMIC TWO. Assume "hook position" (bend your knees, get your feet as close to your buttocks as you can, toes and heels touching). Close your eyes. Keeping your tail-bone up, feel that you are sinking down, down into the earth with your back. Imagine that you are lying out on the lawn—green and soft—and that you are sinking into the cool grass. Push each part of your back down just as though you were a growing thing rooted to the earth.

This is the beginning of all rhythmic work. Push your back in until even the very smallest part of it (or the hollow part) is pushing into the floor. Be sure you keep your coccyx up. As soon as it falls into the floor the real corrective part of the exercise has ceased.

You may get your back down to the floor faster in this manner : Place your hands lightly over your abdomen. Pinch the gluteal muscles of your buttocks together, and push your abdomen down until it seems flatter.

This approach is not as technical as the preceding one, but I have noticed that many of my

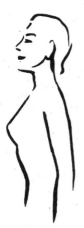

Figure 91

students get faster results this way. Whichever method you use, you are striving for every part of your spine to touch the ground, and as soon as you have accomplished that, you will find that your stomach is flat, or has actually caved in. (See Figure 90).

Try to lie in this position near a mirror and see how your stomach has disappeared. This just shows you what you can accomplish in an upright position if you are standing properly.

Here, then, are the commands which you give yourself as you lie down, saying them aloud in a soft, relaxed voice : " Coccyx up, tuck, sink down all along my back." Keep the coccyx up and the back pressing down, tucking constantly. Count as you do it, each time trying to hold it one count longer. Repeat ten times, or until you do it with comparative ease.

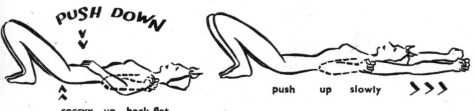

PUSH DOWN

coccyx up back flat

Figure 90

push up slowly

Figure 92

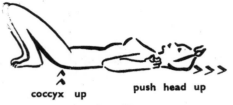

coccyx up   **push head up**

Figure 93

If you are young and your body is flexible, you will react faster than an older person who hasn't exercised for years.

Chest line-up. (See Figure 91.) Now, you are ready to think of the chest region. The chest is so important that we speak of it as the " heart of magnetism." It should be firm and high. A woman may have overdeveloped breasts and still have a " caved-in " chest.

In too many women the line from the shoulder to the spot where the breast begins to enlarge is a sad, sunken area which designers try to disguise with pockets, fullness, shirrings, gathers, etc. Even if your breasts have sagged or if you are flat-chested, you can develop the actual chest expansion with exercise and correct posture. In a later Lesson you will find some additional methods for developing breasts. You know, too, that correct chest alignment influences good head, shoulder and arm alignment.

RHYTHMIC THREE. This rhythmic is designed to help you (a) carry your chest high without effort and without pulling the whole rib cage forward or pushing the buttocks out; (b) increase your chest span. And strangely enough, if you are already full-busted, this phase of the posture work will help you firm and tighten over-developed tissue.

Lie on the floor in the " hook position," and imagine you are lying on a soft green lawn. Close your eyes and push your whole spine down into the earth. Gradually slide your arms up over your head, keeping all of the arms touching the ground as you do so. (See Figure 92.) Push your arms out straight, slowly and smoothly, an inch at a time. Start pushing your arms up only a few inches at first. Then work up to ten inches, or until the arms are straightened out directly over your head, counting slowly.

Here again, the minute the coccyx falls down or the back pulls up away from the floor, you must begin over again. *This is the imperative part of this whole field of corrective rhythmics.* Practise this twelve times daily, for several days until you can do it with comparative ease.

When you can straighten your arms and still have your whole spine touching the floor, you don't have to worry about the position of your buttocks. You're all set.

Head line-up. Next, let's get the head lined up. A previous Lesson had complete rules for head control and posture. In this Lesson you are out to get rid of a double chin, dowager's hump, or increase the length of your neck.

Don't laugh when I say that you can lengthen your neck with corrective posture exercises. It is not unusual at all for a student to measure three-quarters of an inch more after six weeks of these posture rhythmics. I don't know, but I maintain that most of the three-quarters of an inch develops in the neckline. People generally carry their heads improperly.

Now, you may be a tall girl, to whom the thought of another three-quarters of an inch is poison. Here is assurance for you. You don't ACTUALLY grow three-quarters of an inch. Let's

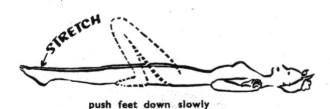

push feet down slowly

Figure 94

158

say you straighten that much, and if there is one thing the tall girl must learn, it's this : *she cannot stoop to conquer.*

Many a tall girl tries to make herself smaller by crouching and stooping. You succeed only in looking pathetic. I recall a tall student who told me that she was dancing with a man shorter than herself. She had mastered a knee crouch which made her total height a couple of inches less. She had been getting by with it for months, so she was very much surprised one evening when her partner said, " Be your size, Agnes, I can take it ! "

Remember, too, that *good head posture will do more for a youthful, beautiful neck than any other one thing you do.* It will help you retain a youthful neck, or assist you in recapturing one which is already pushed out of line.

RHYTHMIC FOUR. Assume " hook position," coccyx up, your whole back touching the floor, your shoulders relaxed. Now push your head up away from your shoulders. Feel that you are pushing up on top of your head. Push up hard. Stretch. (See Figure 93.)

As you stretch your neck up, also push your neck down until the back of it touches the floor. This may be the last part of your body to get lined up. That is so because you have carried your head wrong for so many years. You may never get your neck to touch, but keep trying. Your commands, now accumulating, go like this : Flat on your back, " hook position." Tail-bone up. Tuck hard. Push your back into the earth. Rotate your shoulders into position. Push up to the top of your head and press your neck down.

RHYTHMIC FIVE. Now for some leg action with your correct body line-up. At first, as you

combine your leg action with the rest of your body, you don't realise that you are actually laying the foundation for walking upright correctly. Haven't you heard a woman say, " I look all right when I'm standing still, but the minute I start to walk, out she pops " ? She hasn't learned to co-ordinate leg action with corrective pelvic position.

Lying down is an easy way to master this trick, because your muscles are not fighting the pull of gravity.

Assume " hook position " as you command : " Tail-bone up, back flat, shoulders flat, broad, arms bent, elbows close to sides." Slowly push your feet down two or three inches to the count of two. Then three. Then four and work up to ten, or until you have almost straightened out your knees. Put most of the weight of your feet on the outside foot structure, and as you straighten your knees, only your heels will be touching. Stretch those heels, too. (See Figure 94.)

After the third count, it is permissible to let the coccyx drop and adjust itself, but *don't* let the back pull up more than an inch from the floor. When it does, begin all over again. Practise this three times daily for another two days.

RHYTHMIC SIX. You are now ready for your final posture test. Assume " hook position," close your eyes. End of spine up. Sink down through the back, shoulders flat and broad, arms bent, elbows close to your sides. This time you use your arms *and* legs. Push your arms up until they are straight and your legs down until they're straight. Straighten simultaneously and count first twenty, then thirty, then fifty.

Count ten while you keep your arms and legs

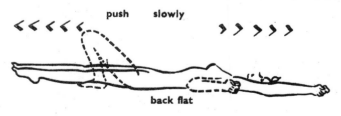

push   slowly

back flat

Figure 95

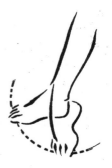

Figure 96

may feel that you make no headway whatever, but bit by bit you will strengthen the arch.

RHYTHMIC EIGHT. This is an exercise to help further to correct the pronation. It is so effective that I even recommend it for those who have normal feet.

Walk around the room and pretend that you are scraping little mounds of sand with your feet. Of course it's perfect if you can practise it in the sand.

Here's how it goes : Step forward with your right foot, weight on the outside border, toes relaxed, and rotate the forward foot in towards the centre of your body until it forms almost a right angle. (See **Figure 96**).

stretched out full length with all of your back touching. When you can do this, you are indeed a fortunate individual, for you are mastering perfect carriage and control over each different section of your body.

Now step forward, placing the heel of the left foot in front of the toe of the right foot, AND THIS TIME rotate the left foot (which is now forward) in towards the centre of the body until IT forms almost a right angle. Repeat movement with right foot, and continue twelve times with alternate feet. You keep your heel stationary and rotate your foot inward with a half-circle movement. Your body-weight falls on the forward rotating foot. Count, " step, scrape, step, scrape." This exercise may seem a little difficult at first, but I would like to urge you to perfect it, since I know any number of stars who

SINCE THE BEST DEFINITION WE CAN FIND FOR POISE IS CONTROL, YOU ARE WELL ON YOUR ROAD TO THAT COVETED QUALITY. (See Figure 95)

You will be so intent upon your spinal alignment as you do these Rhythmics that you may at first overlook the benefit you are giving your feet and legs. Each time you do Rhythmics One to Nine, you are strengthening and correcting whatever foot and leg problems you may have acquired as a result of faulty posture. You are also stretching the heel and knee ligaments, which have a tendency to shrink through wearing high heels.

Foot correctives. In a previous Lesson you found a schedule for taking care of reasonably normal feet. These Rhythmics here are designed particularly for pronated ankles, which means that you carry too much of your body-weight to the inside borders of your feet. You may speak of it as fallen arches or flat feet. Pronated ankles are not only harmful to your health, but also make your feet so unattractive.

RHYTHMIC SEVEN. Stand with as much of your spine touching the wall as you can manage. Your feet four inches away. Your knees should be relaxed but not bent. Put your weight to the outside borders of your feet. Keep your toes flat and raise the inside border of your feet. You

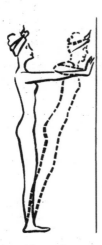

Figure 97

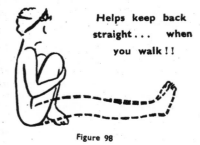

Helps keep back straight ... when you walk ! !

Figure 98

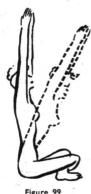

Figure 99

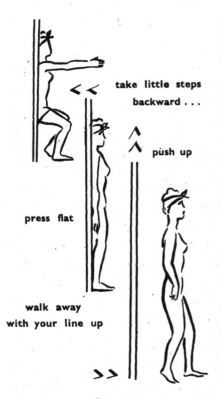

take little steps backward . . .

push up

press flat

walk away with your line up

Figure 100

claim that it has strengthened their feet for their long hours before the camera.

RHYTHMIC NINE. Here is another exercise for stretching your heel and knee ligaments. This is most important if you feel stiff and " rooted " to the ground as you walk.

Stand facing the wall, arms extended, palms touching wall, hands about twelve inches apart. Be sure that the heels remain firmly planted together, toes straight ahead, and the body in correct posture. You allow the body to sway towards the wall until the nose touches the wall, feet remaining on floor. (See Figure 97.). Do not allow abdominal muscles to relax, and keep your back straight. Continue this exercise fifteen times.

You will notice definite stiffness after the first few times, but with continued exercising you will have a much more flexible walk. More spring through the ankles, so you'll feel and sound lighter-footed.

Knock-knees. If you are troubled with knock-knees, the chances are it's caused by pronated feet. By practising Rhythmics One to Nine, you will be correcting your knock-knees, too. Of course, what you consider knock-knees may be excessive fat on your knees, and in that event you may want to do the exercises found in the Course for reducing knees.

As I said before, you may be weeks achieving this or you may learn it in only a few hours or a few days, depending upon how well you are lined up to begin with. *But the encouraging thing about this rhythmic approach is 'that if each day you correct your posture deviations the merest fraction of an inch, in thirty days you have an accomplishment to be proud of.* And will others be proud of you !

SITTING RHYTHMICS

When you have worked with the above rhythmics for a week, or as long as you need to perfect Rhythmics One to Six, then you are ready to start some sitting correctives.

You will recall that I stressed the importance of correcting serious postural problems lying down, because this position avoids the gravity pull. The same principle is at work in correcting your chest, shoulder and head posture problems in a sitting position.

Your progress, therefore, will be to get as much control as you can over each segment of your body in a recumbent position. Then you strengthen that control with sitting correctives, and finally you are ready to put your new control to a standing, then walking test.

RHYTHMIC TEN. Sit against a flat surface in a cross-legged fashion. By this time, every part of your spine should touch the wall. On the other hand, your body may fall into its old sway-backed habits the minute you sit up.

Here are some cure-alls ; as you sit with your back as flat against the wall as you can get it, raise your knees up to your chin—or as close to your chin as you can get them—and clasp your hands around your legs. This usually flattens out that back curve. Now slowly straighten your legs in front of you, keeping your back against the wall as you do so. As you straighten your legs, pull your abdominal muscles in. (See Figure 98).

RHYTHMIC ELEVEN. Sit against a flat surface in cross-legged fashion. Raise arms over your head, palms facing each other, and bend body forward. Round your back and as you straighten it against the wall see if you can't make each vertebra of your spine touch.

If you still can't get the small of the back to touch, then you either need more practice in Rhythmics One to Six, or you should consult an orthopaedic specialist about your postural deviation. Frankly, the average sway-back can

be corrected with six weeks' conscientious application and practice of these principles. You can be your own judge.

If your back is just as far away from the floor or wall after six weeks of these Rhythmics, then it's a doctor for you. If you have made, for example, a correction of an inch in thirty days, that's pretty good progress. All you need is more practice. (See Figure 99.)

RHYTHMIC TWELVE. Sit against a flat surface, cross-legged fashion. Bend your arms, elbows close to your sides. Slowly raise your arms over your head until they are straight. All parts of your arms should touch the wall during the whole exercise.

The benefit of this exercise derives from keeping *every part of your spine touching the wall as you stretch your arms.* The first time you try you may be able to raise your arms only a couple of inches before the spine pops away from the wall. That's all right. Then start over again. Personally, this is the most difficult exercise that I have ever done. But it is excellent for improving your chest, bust-line, neck, and shoulder-line.

STANDING RHYTHMICS

RHYTHMIC THIRTEEN. You have now earned your standing medals. Go over to a wall. Get your head, shoulders, buttocks and heels touching. Is your back flat against the wall? Or is there still some space between the small of your back and the wall? There should be no more than one inch. Should you have more space than this, you need more practice on the Rhythmics from One to Nine.

Also, try this : Stand with your back to the wall. Your feet six to eight inches from the wall, fourteen inches apart, knees bent. Now push torso back to the wall. Slowly walk back to the wall, straightening your knees and taking tiny steps. Do this until your spine is flat against the wall as you stand with knees normally relaxed. After you've done this about six times, let's see how well you retain this correct line-up as you walk. (See Figure 100.)

With all this talk about your back flat against the floor and the wall, you may get the idea you are SUPPOSED to have a flat back. *You should have a normal curve of your spine.*

Your purpose in trying to get the small of your back near the wall and floor is to control abdominal and back muscles, plus the pelvic muscles, so that as you make your daily rounds you will not have MORE THAN what is considered a normal curve.

WALKING RHYTHMICS

RHYTHMIC FOURTEEN. Repeat Rhythmic Thirteen. When you have finished straightening your knees, and your back is against the wall, stand perfectly still. Keep your feet in the exact position where they are. Raise your right foot slightly AND your right thigh, and step forward. Take four steps, turn round, and walk back to the wall.

Are you still lined up as well as you were before you started walking ? I think you probably will be. Next time take ten steps and go back and check yourself : then twenty.

If you are more than a stone overweight, you may have to wait until you have reduced a little before you can achieve perfection in these Rhythmics, but don't wait until you are the size you want to be before going ahead with the ones in this Lesson.

Your posture exercises must accompany your reducing exercises and your diet. They will keep you from becoming flabby and will make you FEEL and LOOK so much better while you are regaining your desired shape. Combine this corrective walking technique with your previous walking Lesson.

Notes:

Self - Test Questions Based On Lesson Six

Another essential Lesson studied, for going up and downstairs, walking correctly and general poise are matters sadly neglected today. They should be part of every woman's education.

After you have studied this Lesson, you should be able to answer the following questions. If you have any difficulty in doing so, refer to the Lesson for further study and revision. Your answers should not be sent to the publishers of this Course.

1. What trick can one use to prevent bouncing and jerkiness when ascending stairs ?

2. Describe a good exercise to practise to get the feel of the correct posture for walking upstairs.

3. What should be the position of your feet as you ascend the stairs ?

4. State shortly the main points to remember when coming downstairs.

5. How should you bend down to pick up anything from the ground ?

6. Have you practised any of the pivots which you feel may be useful to you in your social life or your work ?

7. What is the minimum time you should allow per day for actual exercises ?

8. What is one of the greater benefits derived from practising rhythmics ?

9. Describe shortly a rhythmic exercise by means of which you can appear three quarters of an inch taller.

10. Describe an exercise which will help to cure stiffness when you walk and increase spring and light-footedness.

If you wish to determine the progress you are making, give yourself 10 points for each question you answer correctly. If the total comes to 90 or more, it is excellent; 80 or more, good; 70 or more, fair.

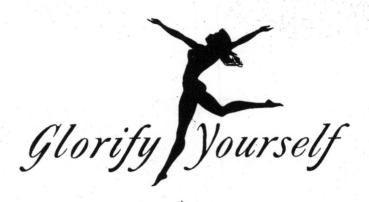

Glorify Yourself

★

A Complete and Up-to-Date Course on
Beauty and Charm by One of the
Most Famous Beauty Specialists
and Consultants in the World

Eleanore King

★

LESSON SEVEN

★

STUDIO TALK •

Issued only for Students
of the Eleanore King
Course on Beauty. Charm
and Personality.

Number Seven.

Dear Student,

We begin the second half of our Course on Charm
and Beauty by considering the most vital of all beauty
aids - perfect health!

Health and beauty go hand in hand. And so I have
devoted Lesson Seven to some practical, easy-to-follow
diet and exercise schedules.

By means of the special Chart included in this
Lesson you can select the diets and exercises most suitable
to your particular figure requirements. An individual
progress chart will help you to keep a permanent record of
the improvement in your face, figure and general health
which will certainly come about if the correct procedures
are conscientiously and intelligently followed.

And remember - nothing is more truly attractive
than the radiant glow of perfect health.

You will need just a little determination to stick
to your diet. There is, of course, no question of putting
you on a starvation menu. The chances are that after a
few days you will stick to your diet from choice, having
rediscovered that simple and natural foods can be highly
appetising as well.

As for the exercises, your best motto is: "Little
and often". It is not violent, but <u>regular</u> exercise that
is the secret of the modern, streamlined figure. The clear
directions and numerous diagrams in Part B of this Lesson
will show you how to keep yourself in perfect trim from
top to toe.

Yours sincerely,

Eleanore King

EK.7.

P.S. In our next Lesson you will learn the secrets of good
conversation. This is a topic of vital importance, since
the truly attractive woman radiates charm not only by the
way she looks but by the way she talks.

LESSON SEVEN

Part A

Dieting For Size

For as one star another far exceeds,
So souls in heaven are placed by their deeds.
—ROBERT GREENE, *A Maiden's Dream.*

IS there a woman who isn't interested in her size ? So many skills involved in being your loveliest can be read about and applied without much effort. But reducing or putting on weight is another matter.

You'll want to know how your weight, measurements and proportions compare with the average. Study the Weight and Measurement Chart here, and then measure yourself. Even if your weight is exactly as the average indicates, remember that you are working with the AVERAGE weight.

The weights and measurements in this Chart have been compiled from records of my students who are actresses, models and others whose professional work demands they keep extra slim and shapely. In addition, they diet entirely under my supervision, and with the approval of a doctor.

The normal average woman must in no wise undertake drastic slimming without first consulting a doctor. Simple methods such as refraining from sweets, chocolates, pastries and generally cutting down on starchy foods such as potatoes and bread, are what any woman can tackle for herself. Nourishment can be secured by taking more of the slimming foods, such as fruit and raw vegetables. Also exercise of a not too strenuous type, such as is recommended in Part **B** of this Lesson and also in Lesson Eleven, as well as walking, can be taken without other advice.

Again, I must stress that the student must not attempt *drastically* to reduce her weight in order to conform to the weights and measurements given in the Chart without medical advice —a few pounds—yes, but not a stone or more.

MEASURE YOURSELF

Record your weight and measurements, without clothes, in the Personal Measurement Chart here. A model is measured, dressed, minus her coat. You may wish to weigh yourself every day, but once a week is often enough to use your tape measure ! Be sure you measure in the same spot each time, because even a half-inch variation might make considerable difference No use fooling yourself ! Make two copies of your measurements and keep the information to yourself ! Here is how the experts measure you :

Height, without shoes.
Chest, under armpits.
Bust, largest part.
Waist—waist-line should be level with elbows, but measure so many inches from the floor.
Abdomen, over navel.
Upper hips, level with tip of hip-bone.
Lower hips, largest part of buttocks.
Thigh, largest part ; measure from floor.
Knee, over knee-cap.
Calf, largest part.
Ankle, above ankle-bone.
Wrist, below wrist-bone.
Arm, measure halfway between shoulder and elbow.
Neck, level with bottom of chin.

You will recall that in the Lesson on clothes selection, I mentioned that the ideal body from top to bottom is divided into four equal parts. In other words, the following areas should measure the same : from the top of the head to the bust, from the bust to the top of the hip-bone, from the hip to the knee, and from the knee to the floor. Nothing much can be done to change these proportions. Correct choice of clothing is the only hope. But there are some measurements we can change, and you read about these also in the clothing Lesson.

DIETING FOR SIZE

In the ideal figure, the largest part of the bust is supposed to equal the largest part of the hips, and the waist should be ten inches smaller than either. If your bust is 35, then your hips should be 35 and your waist should be 25. A variation of two inches one way or the other still gives you a nice figure.

Get busy, though, if the tape-measure shows much more than that. THE TIME TO TRIM OFF INCHES AND REDUCE WEIGHT IS WITH THE FIRST EXTRA INCH AND THE FIRST SPARE POUND ! That's the advantage of knowing exactly where you are out of proportion.

So many of my students have a conviction that they are too heavy in spots, but they haven't known exactly how they varied from the ideal.

After you have measured and analysed your figure, your proportion problems will fall into one of these five classifications :

Group One : You are almost all right. Your weight may be a pound or two over the average and your measurements an inch or two over the ideal.

Group Two : You need to lose about ten

PERSONAL MEASUREMENT CHART

Before studying this Chart in relation to your own measurements, read again the first column on previous page.

Height	Age	Weight	Neck	Bust	Waist	Wrist	Abdomen	Hips	Thigh	Calf	Ankle	Arm
5' 0"	15–35	7 st. 2 lbs.	11¾	31½	23⅜	5⅜	28	31½	18⅞	11¼	7¼	9¾
	35–60	7 st. 6 lbs.	11⅞	31¾	24	5½	28¼	32¼	19¼	11⅞	7¾	9⅞
5' 1"	15–35	7 st. 7 lbs.	11⅞	32¼	23¾	5¼	28¼	32	19	12	7¼	9¼
	35–60	7 st. 11 lbs.	12	32⅜	24¼	5⅜	28¾	32¼	19¼	12¼	7½	9¾
5' 2"	15–35	7 st. 12 lbs.	12⅛	32¼	23¾	5¼	28¼	32¼	19½	12¼	7¼	9¼
	35–60	8 st. 2 lbs.	12¼	32¾	24¼	5⅜	28⅞	32¾	19½	12½	7½	9⅞
5' 3"	15–35	8 st. 3 lbs.	12¼	32¼	24	5⅜	29	33	19½	12¼	7⅝	9¼
	35–60	8 st. 7 lbs.	12⅜	33	24⅞	5½	29½	33¾	19¾	12½	7½	10
5' 4"	15–35	8 st. 8 lbs.	12¾	33½	24½	5½	29½	33¾	19⅞	12⅞	7¼	10
	35–60	8 st. 12 lbs.	12½	33¾	25	5⅞	29¾	34¼	20¼	12⅞	7⅞	10¼
5' 5"	15–35	8 st. 13 lbs.	12⅝	33¾	24¼	5½	29½	34¼	20½	12¼	7⅞	10¼
	35–60	9 st. 3 lbs.	12¾	34	25½	6	30	35½	20½	12⅞	8	10¼
5' 6"	15–35	9 st. 4 lbs.	12¾	34½	25½	6	30	35½	20¼	12⅞	8	10½
	35–60	9 st. 8 lbs.	12⅞	34¾	25⅞	6¼	30⅞	35¾	20⅞	13	8¼	10½
5' 7"	15–35	9 st. 9 lbs.	12¾	35	26	6¼	31..	36	20½	12¾	8¼	10¾
	35–60	9 st. 13 lbs.	13	35½	26½	6¼	31¾	36¼	21	13¼	8¼	11
5' 8"	15–35	10 st. 0 lbs.	13½	36	27	6¼	32	37	21¼	13½	8¼	10⅞
	35–60	10 st. 4 lbs.	13¼	36½	27½	6½	32¾	37½	21¼	13¼	8⅝	11¼
5' 9"	15–35	10 st. 5 lbs.	13½	36½	27½	6½	33	37½	21¾	13½	8⅝	11¼
	35–60	10 st. 9 lbs.	13¾	37	27½	6½	33¾	37¾	22¼	13¾	8¼	11½
5' 10"	15–35	10 st. 10 lbs.	13⅞	37½	27¾	6¼	33½	37½	22¼	13⅞	8½	11¼
	35–60	11 st. 0 lbs.	14¼	38	29	6½	34¼	38½	22¾	14¼	9	11¾

These measurements and weights are for the modern " streamlined " actress or model figure. For heavier-than-average bone structure allow about seven pounds more and an inch for torso measurements. For very small bone structure, deduct five to ten pounds. For a well-proportioned figure, the bust and hip measurements should be about the same and the waist-line about ten inches less. Within an inch or two—either way—is good.

pounds and in spots you are three to five inches over the ideal measurements.

Group Three : You are more than fifteen pounds overweight and exceed the ideal measurements considerably.

Group Four : You are more than ten pounds UNDERWEIGHT.

Group Five : You are an overweight teen-ager and your measurements don't conform at all ! Let's consider each group separately, but first of all, let's abide by these Diet Don'ts.

IF SHE CAN, SO CAN I !

Because other women's achievements are inspiring, I am repeating here some of the letters received from those who have reduced successfully :

" Now that my lower extremities are under control, due to some wonderful exercises and diet, I can hardly believe the tape-measure when it reads 35½ inches around the hips. Before my intensive work, it was 39 inches."

" There are many reasons for the self-confidence which is new to me. One is that I have—by following the exercises you prescribed for me and my doctor's tips on diet—completely re-vamped my figure. It is really amazing to find how much more poise you have when you know that you are just what the doctor ordered in size and shape. These are my improved measurements :—

	12 *Weeks Ago*	*Today*
Height	5′ 5¾″	5′ 6″
Weight	9st. 10lbs.	8st 13lbs
Neck	12¾″	12½″
Bust	37″	35½″
Waist	26½″	25″
Abdomen	34″	30″
Hips	37½″	35½″
Thigh	22″	20″
Calf	12¼″	12½″
Ankle	8″	7″
Arm	11″	10¼″

" Two years ago I had an appendix removed and six months later I began to gain weight. I was around 9st. 9 lbs. at the time of the operation. I gained until I reached 11st. 8 lbs: By that time I was desperate !

" I am 55 years of age, 5′ 4¾″ tall. The 28th of October I started on your reducing schedule. I ate everything I usually ate, except that the doctor said I could cut my food down to 1,000 calories a day; I didn't eat potatoes, white bread, pastries or chocolates. I bought bread that was low in calories, 49 to a slice. By the 10th of December I was down to 9st. 13 lbs."

DIET DON'TS

1. DON'T diet without consulting your doctor first. DON'T fall for fad diets. They are dangerous and are seldom effective.

2. DON'T skip meals and then overeat at dinner-time.

3. DON'T skip breakfast.

4. DON'T eliminate the so-called protective foods.

5. DON'T take overdoses of vitamins.

6. DON'T take the attitude that if a little will reduce, less will be better.

7. DON'T insist on being ten pounds slimmer when you honestly feel better and have more energy with ten additional pounds.

8. DON'T consider certain foods reducing, such as lemon juice and grapefruit.

9. DON'T forget to add the calories of the liquor you drink daily.

10. DON'T confuse dehydration with fat reduction.

11. DON'T drink more than one glass of water with your meals, but *water is not fattening*. You should drink eight glasses daily.

12. DON'T expect to be hungry, weak or irritable on a well-balanced reducing diet.

13. DON'T take any form of medication without your doctor's recommendation. If you could see the nervous, broken women in my classes, many of them now with faulty vision and uncontrolled nerves—the products of self-administered, so-called " reducing " medicines —you'd beware !

14. DON'T expect massage alone to reduce you.

15. DON'T believe that weight can be rubbed or steamed off.

16. DON'T TALK ABOUT YOUR DIET unless others are genuinely interested ! Especially don't talk about your diet to men !

A well-balanced reducing schedule will include

three activities : (1) diet, (2) exercise, (3) massage. Of the three, diet will most effectively rid you of extra fat.

Exercise is essential, because it gives your muscles tone and redistributes weight correctly. In this way, you reduce those areas where you most need to do so.

However, exercise *alone* will not reduce any amount of weight. You might get rid of, say, five or ten pounds through exercise, but, if you're more than 1 st. 11 lbs. overweight, you can't depend upon callisthenics. Combine exercise with diet and you effect the best results, plus attractive weight distribution.

Massage is not essential in your reducing schedule, but it helps to stimulate circulation and prevent flabbiness. By increasing the muscle tone, it shortens the muscles and improves the measurements.

I would like to add a word of caution about steam cabinets and vapour baths. As yet, statistics do not prove that these devices are valuable. Many women think they are reducing when they are actually being dehydrated. If they stay on a diet also, fat reduction takes place. But don't confuse losing a pound or two in a steam cabinet with loss of fat. And don't stop drinking water just because you think that liquids bloat or fatten you. *You still need eight glasses of water a day.*

Group One : So you need to take off an inch or two here and add an inch or two somewhere else ? You may even be five or ten pounds underweight and still have a waist-line or abdominal measurement that's out. Or you may be a few pounds under the average and a few pounds over it within the space of a few days. I think even the finest figures should adhere to the following schedule :

1. Do active callisthenics fifteen minutes a day, concentrating on those areas that need help most. Include formal posture rhythmics here.

2. Walk thirty minutes a day. Walk quick. Wear low heels. Take long strides.

3. Drink one pint of skim-milk daily and take your tea and coffee plain. Take no fried foods or gravy. Eat no more than three slices of bread

daily. Cut down on desserts and sweets.

4. Be conscious of correct posture at all times.

Isn't this simple ? It's a basic health-plan, actually. If you can augment it with sun-baths, longer walks, active sports, so much the better for your figure and your stamina.

Group Two : Since most authorities on reducing caution against losing more than 1½ or two pounds per week, you can lose approximately eight pounds in one month safely. And you will lose a lot of the extra inches with it. Here's the type of schedule that my students in this category find effective :

1. Do active callisthenics thirty minutes a day, concentrating on those areas that need help most. Include formal posture rhythmics here.

2. Walk at least thirty minutes daily. Every ten or fifteen minutes extra is still better. Walk fast. Wear low heels. Take long strides. Breathe deeply.

3. Be conscious of correct posture at all times.

4. The following diet gives you an idea of your daily eating habits :

REDUCING DIET

Before breakfast : Juice of one lemon in hot water.

Breakfast

1 large glass orange juice.
2 to 4 pieces of Ryvita or 1 slice of toast with ¼ pat butter. Add 1 teaspoon of honey if you crave something sweet.
2 eggs, boiled or poached ; or 2 eggs scrambled in top of double saucepan with tablespoon of milk.
No cream or sugar in beverage.
Fresh fruit if desired.

Mid-morning

Fresh fruit, glass fruit or vegetable juice, hot beverage.

Lunch

1 bowl vegetable or clear soup.
½ slice bread, or white crackers with ¾ pat butter.
Large salad with as little dressing as you can manage, ½ cup cottage cheese.
1 glass skim-milk.
No cream or sugar in beverage.
Broiled lean meat and fresh fruit dessert, if desired.

Mid-afternoon

Fresh fruit, skim-milk, fruit or vegetable juice, hot beverage.

Dinner

Large salad.
Soup if desired.
6 ounces of meat or meat substitute, broiled, boiled, baked, or roasted.
2 servings vegetables. One baked potato every other day.
½ slice of bread with ¼ pat butter.
No cream or sugar in beverage.
Fruit dessert.

Before Bed

Cocoa made with skim-milk, tomato juice, grapefruit juice.
You might ask your doctor about taking a food supplement in the form of vitamins.

ALL-OR-NOTHING DIETS

There are some women who cannot be consistent in their diet. They would rather deprive themselves of several foods some of the time and be able to eat almost as they wish the rest of the time.

A group of such women worked out a diet with a dietician. These women live in the country, where they entertain a great deal at week-ends. They wanted to join in the social rounds on Fridays, Saturdays and Sundays, with few food limitations. So they live the year round, Mondays, Tuesdays, Wednesdays and Thursdays, on this 4-day diet :

4-DAY DIET

(will take off seven pounds)

Breakfasts

• (all the same)

Glass of orange juice. Cup of black coffee or tea.
Use one quarter grain saccharine, if sweetening necessary.

Lunch—First Day

1 broiled lamb chop, 2 sliced tomatoes.

Dinner—First Day

1 broiled steak, 2 sliced tomatoes, 1 grapefruit, and coffee or tea.

Lunch—Second Day

1 lamb chop, 2 sliced tomatoes.

Dinner—Second Day

1 broiled lamb chop, 1 hard-boiled egg, 1 large helping of spinach.

Lunch—Third Day

1 lamb chop, 2 tomatoes, glass orange juice.

Dinner—Third Day

2 scrambled eggs, 2 tomatoes, fruit jelly.

Lunch—Fourth Day

Small broiled steak, 2 tomatoes, orange juice.

Dinner—Fourth Day

1 broiled lamb chop, 2 tomatoes, coffee and glass orange juice.

EAT EVERYTHING LISTED. IT'S THE COMBINATION THAT REDUCES.

ON-AGAIN, OFF-AGAIN DIET

Here is another diet that you may like, but talk with your doctor about it *first*. Interestingly enough, many men I know have lost great quantities of weight on this one.

The theory is that the body takes sufficient nourishment in twenty-four hours to last it for forty-eight hours. Therefore on Sundays you eat as you normally do, but Monday you live on only three glasses of milk. Don't even go near the table when your family is eating. When you're the cook, you can't very well go on this diet !

Tuesday, you eat everything you would normally, but Wednesday you're back on three glasses of milk again.

Every other day you eat what you normally would, assuming you won't gorge yourself. And every other day you drink only three glasses of milk. Of course, you can always drink water.

Group Three : You really have to get busy ! Plan your menus so that you have the correct food available. You may feel you have a long road ahead, but my students easily lose between seven and ten pounds a month. Your doctor will know whether or not you need medication. He will also tell you that less than 5 per cent of our overweight people are glandular cases. True, some families seem to have larger structures than others. *More often, however, it's their eating habits and not their inheritance which causes the weight !*

Here's a sensible basic schedule to help you plan your new figure and happiness :

1. Three exercise periods of twenty minutes

each. Do posture, reducing and relaxation routines.

2. Walk at least forty-five minutes daily. An hour is better. Wear low heels. Walk fast. Breathe deeply, and follow combination breathing and walking exercise explained previously.

3. If possible, have two massages weekly.

4. Practise good posture constantly.

5. All active sports, such as riding, swimming or golfing are helpful. Avoid playing badminton or cycling until after you're the size you wish to be, because these activities have a tendency to build fat over muscle.

6. Follow faithfully the diet your doctor gives you. It may be somewhat similar to the suggested menus for Group Two and Group Five, from which so many of my students who have more than ten pounds to lose seem to get such good results.

Looking over these diets, reducing isn't such a formidable task, now is it? You'll find that after you lose the first ten pounds, you'll have more energy. You won't be so tired. Remember, no one is perfect. Just because you weaken and accept food not on your diet, it doesn't mean that you can't mend your ways and start the next morning with even more resolution to be the size you want to be!

Group Four : So you want more pounds, and especially, more curves! I have found this to be true of you girls who *think* you are too thin. *Often you're not!*

Your heavier friends give you an inferiority complex about your size. They say, " You don't eat enough to keep a bird alive!" Or, " You're so THIN!" " You're nothing but skin and bones." Worst of all is that kind soul who calls you " that skinny devil." They mean these remarks as compliments, usually. *But you don't get that idea!* You may be ten or fifteen pounds underweight and still be healthy and energetic. You may be small-boned. Many of our most successful women are of this type. Look at the list of them : Helen Hayes, Lily Pons, Joan Fontaine, Olivia de Havilland, Lana Turner, Vivien Leigh. Their daily schedule would annihilate many six-foot men.

You probably burn up your calorie intake before it can form storage fat. Here is a schedule from which many, many thin girls have gained pounds and inches :

1. Do ten to fifteen minutes of special callisthenics. *You do need exercise!* You'll do many formal posture routines too!

2. Walk thirty minutes daily. If you are habitually tired and move without energy, then increase your rate of movement. Increase it for a week regardless of how you feel. Force yourself to do this. If you are the nervous, quick-moving type, then walk more slowly and with rhythm. Move rhythmically all day and slow down your gestures.

3. Be conscious of good posture all day.

4. Get as much sleep as you need to feel your best, even it it's ten hours a night. Or maybe you need stimulation and NOT rest.

5. Rest BEFORE you get tired, if possible. Learn to relax on a table at the office or on the floor of the rest-room. Better still if you can rest with your feet eighteen inches higher than your head. Thin folk seem to rest and relax best when completely stretched out.

6. Check up on your eating habits. Don't think that the way for you to gain weight is to gorge yourself with rich pastries, gravies, sweets. Usually this form of eating simply wrecks your complexion and causes digestive disorders. Check your eating habits with the following food habits :

EAT DAILY

1. Cereals—with cream and sugar.

Oatmeal	Grapenuts
Shredded Wheat	Wheat germ
Macaroni	Rice

2. Vegetables—

One Serving	*Two Servings*
Potato	Lettuce
Beans	Beetroot
Peas	Cauliflower
Carrots	Celery
Spinach	Cabbage
	Brussels sprouts

3. Milk—at least 1 pint.

4. Three servings fruit ; one large glass fruit juice before bed.

5. Soup creamed.

6. Meat—5 ounces ; cheese dishes.

7. Eggs—1.

8. Beverages ; Milk, buttermilk, egg-nogs, hot malted milks.

9. Desserts : Cream puddings, cake, ice cream.

Here are some suggested menus for gaining weight :

Breakfast—First Day

Fruit.
Oatmeal with cream and sugar.
2 scrambled eggs.
3 slices bacon.
Toast—1 slice.
2 tbs. marmalade.
Cocoa.

Lunch—First Day

Creamed soup.
Macaroni and cheese.
Carrots.
Lettuce salad—French dressing.
1 slice bread—spread with butter.
1 cup milk—hot or cold.
Pudding.

Dinner—First Day

Cream soup.
1 serving (5 oz.) meat.
1 potato—preferably baked.
Escalloped tomatoes with mayonnaise.
1 slice bread—buttered—1 pat.
Choice of dessert (custard, ice cream, cake, pie).
Coffee.
1 cup warm milk before going to bed.

Breakfast—Second Day

Fruit.
Wheat germ cereal with cream and sugar.
1 poached egg on 1 slice toast.
3 slices bacon.
2 tbs. jelly marmalade or jam.
Coffee.

Lunch—Second Day

4 oz. cottage cheese—1 slice pineapple.
2 peanut-butter sandwiches.
Hot cocoa.

Dinner—Second Day

Hot soup.
1 serving (5 oz.) meat, fish or fowl.
Baked potato with glazed pineapple.
Beetroot.
1 slice bread—1 pat butter.
Dessert—cheese and crackers.
Coffee.
1 cup warm milk before going to bed.

You may even lose weight and inches with this schedule for a few weeks, *but stay with it !* Your

system may be sluggish and toxic and react slowly. You'll soon be the envy of all your friends.

Group Five : There was a time when if a girl from eleven to sixteen worried about being overweight her parents and friends dismissed it, saying, " That's just adolescent fat, dear. You'll outgrow it—be a LITTLE girl as long as you can ! " If these same parents and friends could hear the suffering and inferiority complexes their complacent attitudes provoked ! Children are cruelly frank. Also, they like to tease. If you've ever been called " Fatty " by your childhood friends, you'll know what I mean.

We're wiser in handling overweight teen-agers these days. Your first " must " is this : YOU MUST BE UNDER A DOCTOR'S CARE IF YOU ARE GOING TO REDUCE. He will recommend how much exercising and dieting you can do. You may be interested, also, in this sensible diet which appeared in a recent issue of *The Ladies' Home Journal* :

FOOD FOR ROMANCE

Breakfast

½ grapefruit (may be varied once or twice weekly with 1 cup strawberries, ½ cantaloup, or 2 medium peaches).
½ cup whole-grain cereal, hot or cold.
2 tablespoons wheat germ. Milk.

Mid-morning

Milk or fruit.

Luncheon

(Note that one hot and one cold dish are included. Bread and milk allowance, see above, makes good supplement.)

No. 1.

Hot consomme or hot tomato juice, liberally sprinkled with parsley.
Mixed green salad with 1 hard-cooked egg, lettuce, cottage cheese, pepper, no dressing.
(Salads can be lavish mixtures : Endive, chicory, cucumbers, radishes, spring onions and raw cabbage are all good. And of watercress ! The dark-green salads and leafy vegetables are especially beauty-making.)

On Alternate Days—No. 2.

Large tomato juice with juice of ½ lemon.
Or ¼ grapefruit.
2 eggs, boiled or poached ; or lean meat.

4 *P.M.*
Milk or fruit.

Dinner

Lean meat, fish or poultry, average serving.
Once a week, liver.
Baked or boiled potato, medium size. Eat skin.
Vegetable : Large serving from list below.
Green salad, 1 tablespoon French dressing.
Celery and carrot sticks. Eat celery tops !
Fruit, raw or cooked with minimum of sweetening.

Approved Vegetable List

Asparagus   Chicory
Artichokes   Cucumbers

Beans   Kale
Beets   Leeks
Broccoli   Lettuce
Brussels sprouts   Spinach
Cabbage   Tomatoes, fresh oi
Carrots   tinned
Cauliflower   Turnips
Celery   Turnip tops.

Remember that dieting is no mystery. It's common sense and mathematics. Don't be too discouraged if you fail the first time. Learning to reduce and to control your weight is like learning to budget your finances. You may become confused and depressed, but you win only by TRYING AGAIN.

PERSONAL PROGRESS CHART

Make A Note Every Week Of Your Weight And Measurements

	Weight	Neck	Bust	Waist	Wrist	Abdomen	Hips	Thigh	Calf	Ankle	Arm
Present Weight and Measurements											
1st Week											
2nd "											
3rd "											
4th "											
5th "											
6th "											
Weight and Measurements After 3 Months											
After 6 Months											

LESSON SEVEN

Part B

Exercising For Size

Our acts our angels are, or good or ill,
Our fatal shadows that walk by us still.

—JOHN FLETCHER, *The Honest Man's Fortune*

BY this time, you may be saying that since so much work and exercise are required to reduce even one pound of fat, then why bother? You'll diet. That's enough.

Suppose you are almost the correct weight, but still your hips are too large, or your bust is too small. *Your hope is exercise.* Even the very thin girl, and the girl who is almost perfect, must exercise. If she doesn't, the muscles become flabby and soon sag or stretch. Stretched muscles add bulk and that spells extra inches, which look as bad as extra weight.

Here's the general analysis of the minimum of exercise you should get:

1. With almost correct weight and measurements, do five minutes daily of callisthenics for the whole body and another ten minutes for those areas that need it most.

2. With an underweight condition, do ten minutes of general twists, stretches, and posture rhythmics.

3. With more than ten pounds to lose, try to exercise thirty minutes daily. Break your period into two fifteen-minute sessions at first.

GET AS MUCH ACTIVE EXERCISE OUT OF DOORS AS POSSIBLE !

Before you start exercising, list those exercises

you need—or mark them in the Lesson. You'll, need the illustrations for the first few times you go through them. Then copy them on one sheet and have it handy for quick reference when you're down on the floor with the window open ! It takes several weeks to remember them all.

Since so many of the women who come to me want to add or subtract curves quickly, I'll give you here the most effective exercises I know for each part of the body. I don't believe in confusing you with too many, since the average woman's greatest problem in doing exercises is that SHE DOESN'T KNOW ANY TO DO ! So we'll keep them few, simple, but good.

1. *How to streamline your face.* Be happy that your face is full, because it will always seem softer and younger. However, if it isn't just a case of being pleasingly curved, then take heart in the knowledge that as you reduce generally, your face also becomes streamlined. The exercises for lips, tongue and jaw in Lesson One and the neck exercises given in this Lesson will also help.

2. *Streamlining the neck.* A slim neck makes you look fifteen years younger, so watch it ! Fortunately, one of the first places you lose weight when you diet or reduce is the neck. Re-read the head and neck techniques in Lesson One.

Ninety-five per cent of a youthful neck is good

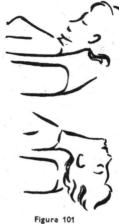

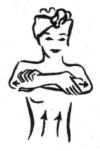

Figure 101

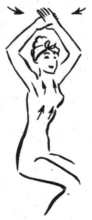

Figure 102

PUSH

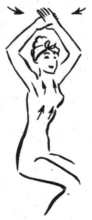

Figure 103

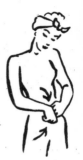

Figure 104

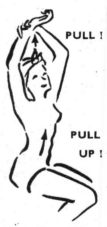

PULL !

PULL

UP !

Figure 105

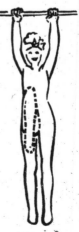

Figure 106

head posture. Since we know that good head posture means good posture generally, incorporate your posture techniques in your campaign for the loveliest, most graceful neck in town. Don't let a day go by when you neglect your neck exercises, for it's comparatively simple to do them since you can work them into your daily schedule even when you're away from home.

(a) Drop your head as far backward as possible. Open your mouth to get more stretch. Without moving the position of your head, bring your lips and teeth together. Then push the tip of your tongue up to the roof of your mouth. Rub it along the roof of your mouth, but keep your teeth together. Continue for a second or two. Open your mouth and bring your head back to position.

(b) You may wish to vary the above exercise by opening and closing your jaws twelve times. Don't overdo these chin exercises at first. Stop BEFORE your neck feels tired.

(c) Tense the muscles of your throat and slowly turn your head to the right. Try to see over your right shoulder. Slowly raise your head until your chin points at ceiling. Then lower your head until your chin reaches your shoulder—or as low as you can. Repeat motion to the left. TAKE THESE NECK EXERCISES SLOWLY AT FIRST.

(d) Here's a neck exercise that's especially relaxing. Lie on a bed on your back with only your head hanging over the side. Slowly raise your head to body level and then slowly lower your head. Repeat twice and increase to six over a period of a week. (See Figure 101.)

3. *For streamlining the bust.*

(a) I do not know of any authentic exercise for reducing the bust. As your weight decreases generally, your bust reduces also. Beware of fake bust reducing.

(b) Should you be well proportioned everywhere except in your bust, then ask your doctor about a glandular upset.

(c) *Massage will not reduce the bust.* Be cautious, too, about having any electrical or mechanical form of bust massage. I emphasise this, because I have seen many women whose bust-lines were ruined through these methods.

(d) Be sure your brassiere fits well. Remember

Right toe with left hand

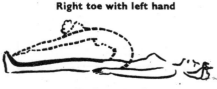

lie down slowly

Figure 108

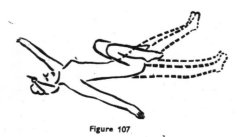

Figure 107

that the largest point of the bust should fall on a line halfway between the elbow and shoulderbone. If your breasts are pendulous, wear an uplift brassiere. Check brassiere straps after every washing because they do stretch and shrink, causing an unattractive droop in your bust-line.

(e) Where exercises will not reduce the bust, at least they will keep the breasts firm. When women reduce, there is a danger of the breasts becoming flabby. So as you diet, do exercises to keep the bust firm. If your breasts are already flabby, you can restore tone to them through exercise. How much you restore depends upon how long they have been allowed to deteriorate.

You have no bone tissue to depend upon in keeping the breasts firm. Therefore, be sure to keep the pectoral muscles, which extend fan-shaped under the breasts and arms, as firm and as well toned as possible.

(f) The posture exercises for the shoulders, neck and arms are excellent in helping to keep the breasts firm and high.

(g) Extend your arms shoulder-high in front of you. Cross your right hand so that it grasps the skin three inches below the elbow of the left arm.

Now cross your left hand so it grasps the skin three inches below the elbow of the right arm. Spread your fingers and push them into the arms. As you push your fingers into the flesh, push the hand as a unit up towards the elbow. If you do it correctly, you get a powerful pull. The breasts should rise with each tension. *Do no more than twenty-five of these daily.* (See Figure 102).

(h) Assume sitting position. Raise arms overhead. Bend elbows. Push the web of one thumb area into the web of the other. With each push the breasts rise. *Begin with ten times and increase to no more than twenty-five.* (See Figure 103.)

(i) Many women with large breasts forget that

the chest itself must be held high, or they will soon look like Miss Sagging Bosom—regardless of how firm the breasts themselves are.

Do the arm exercises given here to help keep the pectoral muscles in good condition, so that they, in turn, will do a good job of supporting the breasts. Do also the posture exercises to help the chest.

4. *For streamlining abdomen and waist-line.* You haven't any bones in your midriff, so you have to guard against bulges especially in this area.

(a) Knead skin around waist and abdomen gently until it's pink. Repeat several times daily. (See Figure 104.)

(b) Any stretching, turning or twisting activity will help your waist-line. So stretch—whether you're lying in bed, sitting down, or lying down. Put your arms up over your head, clasp the wrist of one hand with the fingers of the other hand, and pull your ribs up out of your waist-line. Pull hard. Relax. Repeat frequently during exercise period and during day. (See Figure 105.)

(c) Put an exercise bar in your home within easy overhead reach. Stretch and pull hard. Don't try to chin yourself, but after a week's stretching, you can try pulling the knee of one leg up to your chest. Then the other leg. Then both legs. After a few weeks' practice on your bar, you can combine neck exercise by letting your head fall backwards. (See Figure 106.)

(d) Lie on back, arms outstretched to sides at shoulder level. Keep shoulders and arms touching floor throughout exercise. Bend knees up to chest and slowly straighten out legs down to the right. Raise legs over chest again and slowly straighten out legs to left. Increase pace as you become familiar with exercise.

After you've exercised for a week, try raising your head off floor two inches as you straighten

Knees to nose—tips to toes

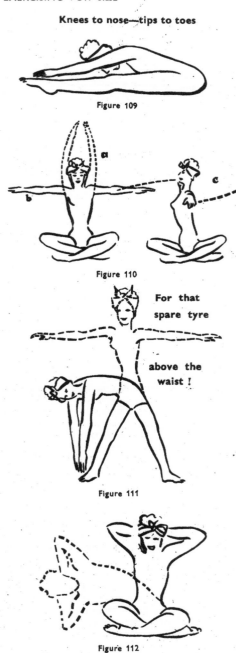

Figure 109

Figure 110

**For that
spare tyre**

**above the
waist !**

Figure 111

Figure 112

out legs. This is a splendid exercise for neck. (See Figure 107.)

(e) Lie flat on back, arms at sides. Raise arms, touching floor over your head. Keep arms extended in front of you as you come up to sitting position and then try to touch right toe with left hand. Stretch forward as far as you can and then lie down, bringing your arms overhead in original position.

Next time you sit up try to touch the left toe with the right hand. Repeat six times and increase to ten over a period of several weeks. (See Figure 108).

(f) Sit on floor with feet extended flat in front of you, feet and knees together. Try to touch your nose to your knees. Get as close as you can. Each day you'll get closer. Try also to touch your toes with your fingers. (See Figure 109.)

(g) Sit on floor with your legs crossed, tailor-fashion, in front of you. Raise arms overhead, palms facing each other twelve inches apart. Move arms until extended to sides, shoulder height. Elbows tense. Turn to right. Assume front and back position. Then arms back to sides. Up overhead. Back to sides. Turn to left, arms assuming front and back position.

It may sound complicated but it isn't, and it does involve stretching, reaching and twisting —three very important phases in getting and retaining a small waist-line (See Figure 110.)

(h) Assume standing position. Feet far apart. Bend at waist and touch floor at right with both hands. Your knees needn't be stiff or straight, but slightly flexed. (See Figure 111.)

(i) Assume sitting position, legs crossed. Put finger-tips behind ears. Bend sideways to the right at waist and touch right elbow to floor. Return to upright sitting position. Repeat exercise to the left. Begin with twelve times and increase to twenty-five over period of several weeks.

At first you may not be limber enough through your waist to touch the floor, but you'll gradually do better. If your back is touching the wall throughout this exercise, you benefit from a posture standpoint, too. (See Figure 112.)

(j) If I have time for only one exercise for the abdomen, here is the one I do : Lie on the floor, arms extended shoulder height, knees bent, feet flat close to hips. Raise your hips off the floor.

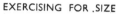

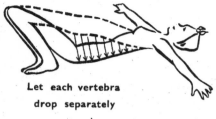

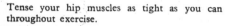

**Let each vertebra
drop separately**

Figure 113

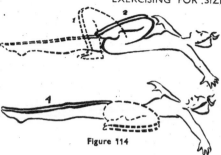

Figure 114

Tense your hip muscles as tight as you can throughout exercise.

Starting with your neck, let each vertebra slowly drop until gradually your whole spine relaxes into the floor. Start with a count of 25, then 50, with 100 your goal in a few weeks. Watch someone else do this and you'll see why it reduces and firms even distended muscles after childbirth. (See Figure 113.)

(k) *Don't forget that the posture routines outlined in the Course are part of your waist-line and abdominal exercise schedule.*

(l) Pull your waist-line up out of your hip-line whenever you think of it, all day long.

5. *Streamlining the back.* As you reduce generally, your back will reduce. Every exercise given here in a lying-down position is also good for the back, since the friction helps to break down fatty tissues. The stretching, twisting and bending exercises given for the hips, waist-line and abdomen also help to streamline the back. The posture exercises are definite aids.

In fact, *you can't have a pretty back unless you have good posture.* Swimming is especially good for the back, too.

6. *For streamlining the hips.* Most women and girls worry about their hips being too large. If you gain a few extra pounds, you're certain to put most of them on your hips. Measure your hips across the largest part of your buttocks, which is frequently referred to as the lower hip area.

Recall that we said that ideally the hips should not be more than an inch larger than the bust ? Even if there is a two-inch difference, your hips still look almost perfect. I've noticed that a tall girl can often get away with larger hips, proportionately, than a short girl.

(a) Lie on the rug at first and as you become accustomed to exercise, work on the bare floor. *Keep your arms extended shoulder height at sides and keep shoulders on floor throughout routine.* Bend knees, placing feet as close to body as possible. Roll hips to right, keeping knees bent, until all of outside of right leg and hip touch floor. Bring bent knees up over abdomen and waist-line area as you roll hips to left, again keeping knees bent, until all of outside of leg and hip reach floor. Begin with twenty-five stretches.

Work up to two hundred. Exercise at moderate

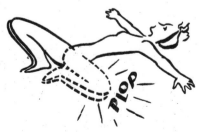

Figure 115

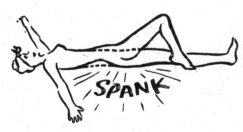

Figure 116

181

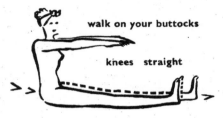

walk on your buttocks

knees straight

Figure 117

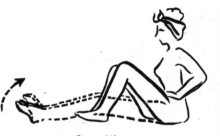

Figure 119

pace. (See **Figure 114**.)

(b) You may wish to try a little more strenuous form of the above hip-reducing exercise, but GET YOUR DOCTOR'S CONSENT FIRST. Here it is : Lie on rug at first and as you become accustomed to exercising, work on bare floor.

Keep your arms extended shoulder height at sides and keep shoulders on floor throughout routine. Bend knees, placing feet as close to body as possible. Raise hips off floor, turn to right, and spank hips and sides of thigh into floor.

Repeat turn and spank to left. Let hips and legs go plop ! *Don't put any tension in this.* Begin with fifty times and increase to two hundred over a period of several weeks. (See Figure 115.)

(c) Lie on back. Keep arms extended shoulder height at sides throughout entire

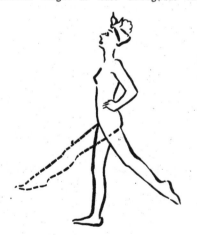

Figure 118

exercise. Bend right leg. Raise hips off floor and spank your left hip into the floor fifty times.

Find a fat spot and really go to work on it. Next bend left leg and spank right hip. This gets your upper legs and lower hip area. That spot so many women speak of as a " hip hollow."

Increase count to two hundred over a period of several weeks. Be sure you use no tension in this exercise. (See **Figure 116**.)

(d) Slap hip area briskly with fists until skin is pink. Repeat several times daily.

(e) Sit on floor in shorts, or nude, with your feet extended in front of you. Raise arms, to shoulder height and extend them directly in front. Walk around the room on your buttocks, fast. Do this a couple of times daily. (See **Figure 117**.)

(f) Stand without shoes and extend right hand to wall at shoulder level, elbow relaxed. Swing left leg as high front and back as you can ten times. Then touch wall with left hand and swing right leg for ten counts. Increase to thirty counts. This exercise not only streamlines your hips, but it also helps you achieve flexibility for a graceful walk. (See **Figure 118**.)

(g) Sit on floor with your knees bent, feet on floor. Straighten legs in front of you six times, legs clear of floor by three inches. (See Figure 119.) Breathe in as you straighten your legs, because this helps to firm the abdominal muscles too. Repeat, straightening both legs upward to the right six times. Repeat, straightening both legs upward to the left six times.

(h) REMEMBER YOUR POSTURE TUCK-UNDER ALL DAY LONG HELPS TO FIRM AND REDUCE YOUR HIPS. I don't mean they should be tensed constantly, but tucked under correctly.

7. *Streamlining your thighs.* Your legs may

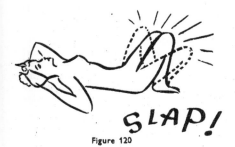

Figure 120

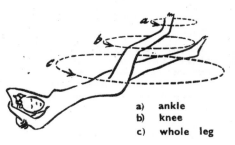

Figure 121

be too heavy above the knee and too thin below it. Do reducing exercises for the whole leg. You'll find that as your thighs lose fat, your lower legs will put on a few curves. It's that old distribution angle again. In addition to your leg exercises, do these :

(a) Lie on your back, on a bed or the floor. Bend your knees and place your feet comfortably close to your buttocks. Keep feet together, soles touching floor. Separate your knees, then bring legs together with a slap. Repeat fifty times and increase quickly to two hundred. Here's an exercise that does help to reduce thighs and it's not strenuous. (See Figure 120.)

(b) Don't forget reducing by slapping, described in routines for fat hips.

(c) Lie on floor on your right side, with your right arm folded under your head, and left hand in front of you for support. Begin with legs straight, left leg above right leg. Raise left leg as high as you can and lower six times. Roll to left and raise right leg six times. Increase count to fifty over period of several weeks. (See Figure 121).

8. *Streamlining the legs.* You CAN reduce your legs. Some of my students have even surprised me with their results. What you accomplish depends upon you.

I remember so well two girls who came to me in June and said that the following September they were going to the University. They were good friends, and they had one figure flaw in common : well-proportioned bodies, but very large legs. I showed them what to do and said there was no use taking lessons for it, since I couldn't do the actual exercising for them. By the end of August they were the proudest girls in town. Immediately, they bought suits with straight skirts, because all their lives they had had to wear flared ones to help to camouflage

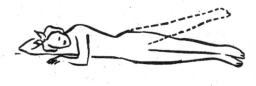

a)	ankle
b)	knee
c)	whole leg

Figure 122

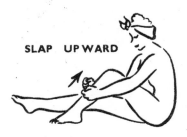

SLAP UPWARD

Figure 123

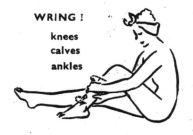

WRING !

knees
calves
ankles

Figure 124

their legs. One reduced her knees three inches, her calves almost two inches, and her ankles one and seven-eighths inches. The other girl did almost as well. *They spent three hours a day doing formal callisthenics, walking or swimming.* And they did not tell their friends what they were doing !

(a) Lie on back. Raise right leg, keeping your ankle and knee relaxed. Circle out from your ankle ten times. Let your toes describe the circles. This gets the ankle. Then describe ten outward circles from the knee. Your foot leads, getting the knee and calf. Next describe ten circles with your whole leg. *Keep knees bent slightly and leg relaxed.* Repeat, with your left leg.

Now raise both legs and circle out from both ankles ten times, both knees ten times, and then from both hips—you'll do well to make five circles the first time. Relax. You'll feel this in your abdominal muscles, too. Increase the count gradually.

Students who get sizable leg reduction do from two to four hundred circles, breaking their exercising into two and three daily periods. (See Figure 122.)

(b) Slap your legs with your fists until they are pink. Start at the ankle and slap on up the *inside* of the leg to the thigh. No downward trips, though. Start subsequent slapping from *outside* the ankle UP the leg. Then work on the other leg. (See Figure 123.)

(c) Try " wringing " your ankles, calves, and knees with your hands. Use the same hand motions as though you were wringing out a rag. (See Figure 124).

(d) If your legs are solid as well as fat, don't cycle, play tennis, or badminton until they're softened up with the above exercises.

Often it seems that strenuous sports build muscle over fat. Should your legs be soft and fat, do add sports to your daily exercising. Once your legs are the size you wish, then go in for all physical activities to help maintain them.

9. *How to streamline bow-legs.* You will recall that in a previous Lesson bow-legs were described as those which do not meet at the ankles, calves or knees. That is, the legs do not touch in any of those spots or perhaps may come together in only one of those places. You cannot change

the bone structure, but you can help to build firm, well-rounded muscles.

Suppose at that part of your calves where they should meet there is a space of two inches. Suppose you develop the inside of your calves until there is only one-half inch space between them. Then your legs won't even seem bowed. This improved muscular contour, in addition to the techniques you learned previously for handling them gracefully, makes you forget that you once worried about bow-legs !

These exercises are, therefore, designed to help to develop the muscles on the inside of the legs :

(a) Sit with your feet out flat in front of you, shoes off. With heels together, try to make your legs touch at the calves. Slowly lower your toes to the floor—stretching hard to keep calves touching the whole time.

You may never quite manage perfection, but it's this slow contracting that gradually helps to develop the inside leg curve you want. Some of my students tie a towel tightly around their calves as they do this exercise. Or you may have a friend who will try to keep your calves together with her fingers as you do this exercise. (See Figure 125.)

If you are not more than ten pounds overweight, vary the above exercises by raising your hips up off the floor, supporting your weight on your heels and hands. Again lower your toes towards the floor, trying to get the calves as close together as possible.

(b) Skip with a rope without unbending your knees as you hit the ground. Keep them bent the whole time. Begin with one minute and work up to ten. (See Figure 126.)

(c) Sit on floor, shoes off. Bend knees and touch soles of feet together. Keeping soles touching, as far as possible, slowly straighten your legs. (See Figure 127.)

10. *Streamlining the arms and shoulders.* I suppose women wouldn't be as self-conscious about heavy arms if the latter weren't so apparent. Each year more designers show short-sleeved dresses. It's a comfort to realise that arms can be reduced.

You may feel that your arms are too thin

below the elbow and too fat above it. You reason that your hands and forearms will get even more slender with exercise. That isn't the way it works. Exercise will redistribute the weight correctly on your arms.

(a) The posture routines in a recumbent position will help mould your arms into graceful lines. Also the stretching and bending exercises you do for your waist-line and abdomen help to streamline your arms.

(b) Lie on floor. Bend arms at side, so that elbows are close to sides. Raise elbows and slap them vigorously down to the floor forty times. Then bend arms, with elbows out at sides. Raise elbows and slap them vigorously down to the floor for another forty times. Increase to one hundred or two hundred over a period of several weeks. (See Figure 128.)

(c) Bring your arms up in front of you, level with your shoulders, palms facing each other. Making the wrists lead out, slowly bring the arms to the side, level with the shoulders, and back to centre again. Repeat ten times with elbows and fingers tensed ; then ten times with elbows and fingers relaxed. (See Figure 129.)

(d) Extend your arms in front of you, shoulder height, palms facing ceiling. Group the tips of the fingers of each hand around the tip of the thumb. With great tension in the fingers and elbows, slowly open the fingers to the count of twenty-five. Stretch fingers far apart. *Keep elbows tense.* Slowly close fingers to the count of twenty.

This exercise will help to firm that upper-arm flabbiness which is so unpleasant to your escort when he takes your arm to help you across the street or dance floor ! (See Figure 130.)

11. *Streamlining the hands.* Usually overweight people have fat hands. With body reduction, however, the hands soon lose that pudgy look which blocks graceful gestures. Exercising helps to keep them vital-looking, flexible and young, too. (See Figure 131.)

(a) Shake your fingers vigorously for two minutes or until they feel heavy.

(b) Stretch the fingers by pushing the finger-tips of one hand against the finger-tips of the other. After stretching, clench your fists hard. Alternate the stretching and the clenching for six.times.

(c) Extend your arms in front of you, shoulder height. Make fists of your hands and slowly move them to the right, making small circles from your wrists as you do so. Then move arms to the left, continuing circles. This helps wrist flexibility and also helps to reduce those little fat rolls at the wrist. You'll be surprised how tired your arms get with what seems to you a mild exercise !

(d) Holding the little finger of one hand with the thumb and forefinger of the other hand, make circular movements. Repeat with all fingers.

MORE PLEASE !

You want more weight, more hips, more bust— more curves ! One reason so few thin girls add weight is because they get discouraged before the end of the first month. The most successful beauty salons in the country list this as their prime reason for failure with so-called skinny girls.

One salon told me it collected a large fee for six weeks in advance from very thin people. Then for financial reasons alone, the client is more inclined to stay with her schedule until results are noticeable. So, remember, you won't show many results from exercising for a month : but when you do, will you be proud !

How to develop a thin face and neck. When I first began working with lovely Virginia Mayo, talented Samuel Goldwyn star, her face and neck were so thin she didn't photograph well. She embarked on a series of facial exercises that I recommended.

In six weeks her cheeks were considered so full that her first screen role went to another Goldwyn player ! She told me later that she had practised her facial routines an hour a day ! Few girls have her persistence. Here's what to do !

1. Blow ! Simple, isn't it ? Take a breath, keep your lips closed, and blow hard. Direct

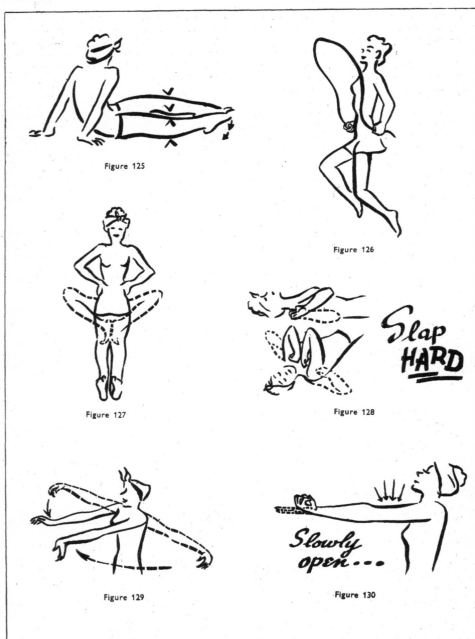

Figure 125

Figure 126

Figure 127

Slap HARD

Figure 128

Figure 129

Slowly open...

Figure 130

the breath into your upper lip, then lower lip, sides of your lips, and cheeks. You can do this standing, sitting or lying down.

It will be a little more difficult for you to catch on to the directed blowing for filling in hollows in your neck. Girls are often sensitive about having " bony " necks. Look at the models in your fashion magazines. They're thin and their bones show. It's their bone structure that's so arresting. But if you insist—take a deep breath, hold it. Direct or force the breath to the neck areas.

At first you'll think this is completely a MENTAL exercise. Continue with it a few times. Then place your fingers lightly on the areas you're trying to fill in and you will feel increased fullness where you are directing your breath. This is something you can work at as you're going about other tasks.

A recommended position for these facial routines is to lie with your feet several inches higher than your head.

2. The inverted position referred to above lends additional stimulation and circulation to the face and neck, and therefore helps to nourish it. Begin with five minutes a day and increase to an hour. Refer to the complete discussion of this position outlined in the Course.

3. The exercises given in this Lesson, for reducing necks will also help to develop them. You are re-vitalising sluggish muscles. As their tone quality is improved, the muscles react in correct weight distribution.

4. DON'T NEGLECT THE POSTURE ROUTINES. A beautifully carried head is usually supported by a graceful neck. Vivien Leigh's neck is certainly slender, but oh, so lovely, because she carries her head with such great distinction and pride.

How to develop your bust. In many of my classes, the women form inner cliques called " better bosom boosters " ! With proper exercise, they often develop the CHEST two inches.

The breast measurement may not increase, but the new high chest-line makes them seem

much better proportioned ; and they look so much better in their clothes. Here is their schedule. (A few of these exercises will help to firm the pectoral muscles, which support the breasts, but a concentrated dose will do the developing.)

1. Do posture routines, particularly those involving the upper part of the torso. Spend ten minutes a day on these alone if you have time.

2. Assume correct posture, either sitting or standing. Extend your arms at shoulder height in front of you. Cross right hand so that it grasps the skin three inches below the elbow of the left arm.

Now cross your left hand so that it grasps the skin three inches below the elbow on the right

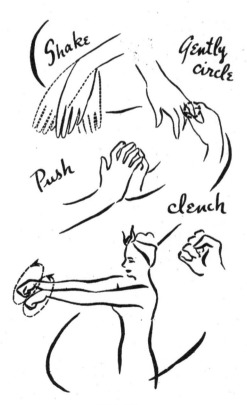

Figure 131

arm. Spread your fingers and push them into the flesh, push the hand as a unit up towards the elbow. If you do it correctly, you get a powerful pull on the pectoral muscles.

The breasts should rise with each tension. Take it easy at first for about twenty-five times, three times a day for two weeks. Then increase count gradually to three hundred.

3. Assume correct sitting posture. Raise your arms over your head. Bend elbows. Push the web of one thumb area into the web of the other. With each push, the breasts rise. Begin with twenty-five times, three times daily for two weeks, and increase count to three hundred. Keep chin back, so that you get assistance for your neck, too.

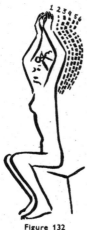

Figure 132

4. Assume correct sitting posture, arms stretched over head, palms facing. Push arms back as far as you can six times, with palms one inch apart. Then separate palms five inches and push back six times. Then about two feet and push back about six times. Rest and repeat several times throughout the day. (See Figure 132.)

5. All shoulder, arm and neck exercises will help to raise and develop your bust.

6. Badminton, tennis and swimming will help to develop your bust.

7. *Whatever you do, don't go around looking flat-chested.* Worse still, don't take the attitude that you're the only flat-chested woman in the world and grieve over it. Before I started counselling women, no one could have told me how a girl or woman will get an inferiority complex over just some such thing as this.

Ask any buyer how hard it is for her to keep a stock of brassiere padders ! Someone must be buying them, so you have plenty of company. You may look well proportioned when undressed but need help to look your best in your clothes. Take time when you're buying your brassieres. Experiment with several " cheaters " that the assistant brings you. Slip your blouse or dress on to see which one is best for you. Or make

your own "fillers." As one salesgirl laughingly told me :

> *Where God has forgotten,*
> *You can stuff with cotton !*

Don't add too much at once ! It isn't that others will notice, particularly, but you'll feel self-conscious. And sew them in, covering the inside with net or a lightweight fabric.

8. Check your chest, shoulder, and head line-up constantly. KEEP YOUR CHEST HIGH !

9. The following illuminating information on developing breasts was printed in the March 1946, *Fascination Magazine* :

" Experiments conducted by a physician, and independently, by a woman surgeon, revealed that the growth of the human mammary glands depends on oestrogenic hormones, and that the ultimate development of normal proportions is contingent on the body supply of oestrogen and what are known as ' corpus luteum ' hormones (ovarian).

" Active mammary growth can be induced by injections of 150,000 to 300,000 International Units of hormones per week. One objection to the treatment was the number of injections required over a period of many months. The

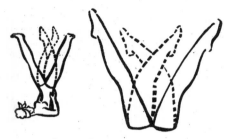

Figure 133

physician decided to use the same number of hormonal units in a permeating ointment base. While other female sexual organs were activated during treatment, the breast also took part in the change. However, the most effective treatment proved to be a combination of Progesterone and Progestin or Estradiol benzoate.

" There has been little unanimity of opinion among the medical profession of late years concerning the therapeutic effectiveness of permeable ointments in general.

" In some medical quarters it was denied that the ointment use of oestrogens could produce specific effects on the body.

" Today, hormonal ointments are sold without prescriptions, at many salons at high prices. But it must be stressed that every patient is, so to say, a law unto herself and that treatment MUST be under the direction of a reputable physician.

"Where rudimentary breast structure is present, treatment by oestrogens is of definite value. In many instances the disproportion between the physical development of the breast and the general configuration of the body is actually due to a poor distribution of breast tissue. In other words, there is adequate breast tissue but it is so unevenly distributed over a wide area that it forms a large ' pancake ' and never gives a breast-like appearance. In these cases a simple surgical procedure produces the desired effect.

" The widespread tissue is gathered and held together by different parallel layers of sutures. It is then firmly anchored on the cover of the underlying great pectoral muscle and the skin is adjusted to the reconstructed proportions."

How to develop your waist and abdomen. It seems almost a sacrilege to write this expression ! Imagine anyone wanting more of either ! But I know from experience that there are those of you who do. All I can say is that as you gain weight generally, your waist and abdomen will increase soon enough. CAUTION : Continue exercising as you gain, however, or you'll find yourself large in the waist and abdomen and thin everywhere else.

How to develop your hips. Do the exercises given in this Lesson for reducing hips, BUT DO THEM ONLY TEN TIMES. You need only a little stimulation to help to fill out curves. You must exercise your hips to some extent or they will spread all in one spot, and then you are a strange looking girl ! Do your hip-bones protrude ? Cover little cotton pads with net and with adhesive tape keep them on the spots that cause you embarrassment.

How to develop your legs. Do all leg exercises slowly and with tension. These are classified as contractile exercises.

1. Lie on back. Raise right leg, knee rigid, toe pointed. Very slowly and with tension make OUTWARD circles from ankles, toes leading. Begin with six and increase to one hundred within several weeks. If you've ever had a sprained ankle, or feel your ankles are weak, do a few inward circles, too. (By " in " I refer to the centre of the body, and by " out " I mean away from the centre of the body.)

2. Lie on back. Right knee bent, toe pointed. Make circles out from the knee. Begin with count of six and increase to twenty-five over period of several weeks.

3. Lie on back. Right knee rigid, toe pointed. Slowly and with tension make circles with whole leg from hip. Begin with six, increase to fifty over period of several weeks.

4. Repeat whole routine with left leg.

5. Repeat whole routine with both legs.

6. Skip with rope, keeping knees bent the whole time. Don't straighten them as you touch floor. Begin one minute daily and increase very

slowly, because this is strenuous exercise. If you're over forty, or much overweight, your doctor may say no to this.

7. Stand with your spine touching wall. Bend your knees as much as six inches and sink your whole spine against the wall. Then very slowly push the upper leg away from the wall. Keep your feet flat on the floor, your heels as close to the wall as you can manage. Push the thigh region forward—as far out as you can go, retaining your initial foot position. Your head and shoulders remain touching the wall also.

Count five as you bend your knees, five as your thighs go forward, and five as you straighten knees and bring all of body back against wall. Relax and repeat several times. Make sure the thigh muscles are doing the work.

8. Raise your legs in the air, and rest your whole body on head and shoulders, supporting yourself with your arms and hands on hips. Stretch legs as far apart as possible. As you close them, cross them scissors fashion. Begin with twelve and increase count to fifty over several weeks' time. This is especially good for the hollows in your thighs, too. (See Figure 133.)

How to develop thin hands. Do the same exercises as those given for fat hands in this Lesson. REMEMBER TO USE SMOOTH MOTIONS.

As I said before, all exercises were purposely put in this Lesson of the Course—not only because I thought they would be more easily referred to here, but also because I know that few women actually will exercise. If you've even read through to here, give yourself a pat on the back. You belong in that 10 per cent of women who realise that YOU are the *only one* who can change you. I know that YOU will *Glorify Yourself* ! !

Self-Test Questions Based On Lesson Seven

In these days of speed, road, rail and air travel and sedentary occupations, very many of us do not get nearly enough exercise for our health and beauty. Therefore, this Lesson is vitally important: You should get into your own daily routine whatever extra exercise you feel you need.

After you have studied this Lesson, you should be able to answer the following questions. If you have any difficulty in doing so, refer to the Lesson for further study and revision. Your answers should not be sent to the publishers of this Course.

1. Are you using the PERSONAL PROGRESS CHART at the end of Part A of this Lesson ?

2. Have you decided whether you are just right, overweight or underweight ?

3. What is a well-balanced schedule to follow if you wish to reduce ? State it shortly in three points..

4. No matter what group your figure falls into, state four points that it is advisable for any woman, other than an invalid, to follow daily in order to keep healthy and trim.

5. If you have followed any diet, however slight, or any of the routines suggested, do you feel any better or more energetic after, say, four weeks of trial ?

6. If you are thin and wish to put on weight and round off your curves, state six points you should have been following recently.

7. What is one essential to health in the way of daily exercise for any woman, no matter what her occupation ?

8. Have you picked out the exercises which you require to meet your special needs? You will know which parts of your body require reducing or improving and rounding off. Make a short list of these, then go through this Part of the Lesson, marking the Exercises you need to practise.

9. Have you made a separate sheet of these exercises for your easy, quick reference when carrying out your daily routine ?

10. For how long should you persevere with regular exercise, either for reducing or increasing weight, before you can expect any real improvement to show ?

If you wish to determine the progress you are making, give yourself 10 points for each question you answer correctly. If the total comes to 90 or more, it is excellent; 80 or more, good; 70 or more, fair.

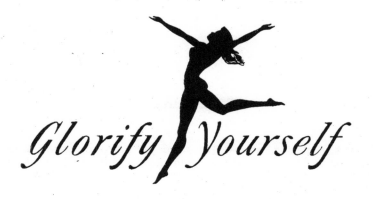

Glorify Yourself

★

A Complete and Up-to-Date Course on
Beauty and Charm by One of the
Most Famous Beauty Specialists
and Consultants in the World

Eleanore King

★

LESSON EIGHT

★

STUDIO TALK •

Issued only for Students of the Eleanore King Course on Beauty. Charm and Personality.

Number Eight.

Dear Student,

In the first seven Lessons we have covered such important matters as facial radiance, the care of the skin, correct posture and tasteful dressing. If you have conscientiously carried out all my suggestions on these subjects, you will already have increased the charm of your appearance.

But appearances are not enough. Charm depends not only on the way you look, but also on the way you talk.

And so Lesson Eight is a brief but detailed guide to good conversation.

Don't forget that the Course is designed to groom you for public appearances. In a previous Studio Talk I pointed out how you are constantly in the public eye even though you may never appear on stage or screen. Nevertheless you are learning the same techniques of beauty and charm that I teach to the world's leading actresses.

My actress pupils have to learn not only how to radiate charm before the cameras, but also how to deliver their lines effectively.

And it's just the same for you. You have a part in the great play of life; and your lines are your everyday conversation.

Conversation has been described as the great universal need of mankind. It is the bridge which you must cross to meet your fellow men and women. There is hardly any occasion when you may not be called upon to converse.

Your knowledge of conversation will help you to find more pleasure and profit in all human associations. If you will follow the simple technique described in this Lesson, you will never again feel lonely in the midst of a group of people. You will add to your poise and self-confidence. You will achieve a fuller, more dynamic expression of your personality.

(over)

Page 2.

Incidentally, this Lesson is not all my own work. I got seven hundred men to help me with it.

I asked them to tell me frankly what they most liked, and what they most disliked about the girls they met. Their answers are given on pages fourteen and seventeen.

Some of these remarks are almost brutally frank. I feel, however, that they form an invaluable guide not only to good conversation, but to feminine charm in general.

Yours sincerely,

Eleanore King

EK.8.

LESSON EIGHT

You Talked Yourself Into It

*Wise, cultivated, genial conversation
is the last flower of civilization . . .
Conversation is an account of ourselves.*
—EMERSON, *Miscellanies : Woman*

I HAVE been amazed at the number of books and courses in our libraries and schools on every phase of speech *except* conversation.

There are whole departments devoted to diction, grammar, public speaking, debate, drama ; but have you tried to find concrete material on conversation ?

Yet every day you must talk with people ; and more than in any other way, you are judged by what you say and how you say it. Because there is so much space devoted to the quality and development of your speaking voice, I shall devote most of my space here to what you're going to say.

I BELIEVE THAT YOUR ABILITY TO SAY THE RIGHT THING AT THE RIGHT TIME WILL HAVE A MORE DESIRABLE INFLUENCE ON EVERY PHASE OF YOUR LIFE THAN ANY OTHER ONE QUALITY YOU CAN POSSESS. *I also believe that you can develop outstanding conversational ability.*

You do not have to be born a clever conversationalist. You are not striving to be a great wit. It's delightful to have such people around. It's stimulating. But the average person is slightly uncomfortable, too. The source of his discomfort springs from his inability to keep pace. And therein lies the secret of all good conversation. Conversation is an exchange of feelings, thoughts, attitudes. The moment you forget this exchange idea, your conversation swerves from its natural channels and you are in danger of offending.

It is well to understand at the outset that your conversational technique depends on how well you know the other person or persons involved. If they are friends of long standing, you may violate many conversational principles and still retain their friendship.

You must have one person or two people in whom you can confide. *But where you do not know people, you must play the game, if you wish to be well-liked or even acceptable.*

Conversation is for stimulation. It is for pleasure. It is a leisure pastime. It furnishes the spice of everyday life   Just remember what O. Henry says in his *Complete Life of John Hopkins*, "Inject a few raisins of conversation into the tasteless dough of existence."

As in developing in any other skill, you learn to talk well by working at it. Some people talk all day every day, but because they are unconscious of the underlying rules of psychology, they are more apt to slide downhill conversationally than uphill.

People are divided into two groups as far as their conversation is concerned :
(1) those who talk too much and
(2) those who talk too little. Even those who talk too much are accepted and welcome if they abide by correct conversational techniques.

The most helpful advice for the great talker is to measure out his remarks. He should deliberately count how many times he says something in relation to every other individual in the group. He should not contribute a second remark until every other member in the group has expressed himself.

The first time you try this, the shock may kill you ! You find that you are contributing four or five remarks to other people's one. But if you get it down to two remarks to every other person's one, and abide by the laws, you will be making headway.

THE STRONG SILENT TYPE

The non-talker. You must begin talking to people. Don't fall back on that old one, " But I never meet anyone interesting."

The mark of an outstanding individual is his ability to draw out and create outstanding personalities with those he contacts in everyday life.

If you are going around the world, storing up your conversational technique until such time as you meet a set that you consider worthy of your efforts, don't be hurt if you overhear someone say about you, " snobbish and dull."

Basically, the person who does not talk is an

egotist—often much more so than the one who talks too much. There are two underlying reasons for not communicating with others.

First, you may feel that you are too timid. Who isn't timid ? But that's no reason for you to spend your life in patting yourself on the back, and stroking your precious timidity complex. You are spending too much time thinking about yourself !

Second, you don't talk to others because it doesn't seem worth your while. That means you're a snob. You feel superior to others. The best cure for this would be for someone to take a vote on what the people who see you every day think about you. *That might startle you into saying something.*

In all my career, working with thousands of people, I think the one most objectionable personality was a young man who had progressed very well in his own line.

He came to me for an intensive course in conversation. He said he could talk where business was concerned, but outside of working hours he was practically speechless.

There was no warmth whatsoever to his personality. The harder I worked to help him, the less progress he made. Sensing my own innate dislike of him, I tried to compensate by giving him extra help because of this. Finally, one day I had the answer to my lack of progress. I was trying to encourage him to talk with those around him, just to show a friendly, human interest.

For example, towards the girls in his office. We had spent considerable time in sample conversations. First, I would be the lift attendant, then the receptionist, then the telephone girl, or one of the secretaries.

A couple of weeks later I asked him how he was progressing in this regard. He looked at me disdainfully and said, " These girls always get the idea that I am leading them on when I try to be nice to them."

His basic trouble was that he genuinely felt himself so desirable that should he converse with any girl, regardless of her station, for a few minutes a day, he imagined she would begin to build matrimonial bridges.

Even I did not have the heart to tell him that 98 per cent. of these girls were probably feeling sorry for him and thinking, " What a dud ! "

So if you are consoling yourself with the fact that you are the strong silent type, better start talking. Take a genuine interest in those around you. (See Photograph 14). Get to know something unusual about everyone you contact all day long. You needn't be inquisitive, but show a normal interest in their lives and in them.

YOU'RE OFF !

For the remainder of this lesson, let's assume that you are invited to a new city for a month. Let's take up here the various conversational techniques that you will want to perfect or brush up.

1. How to meet people successfully.
2. How to begin a conversation, which includes introduction technique.
3. The pattern of the short conversation.
4. The long conversation.
5. Conversational Do's and Don'ts.

HOW TO MEET PEOPLE SUCCESSFULLY

But they couldn't chat together, they hadn't been introduced.
—W. S. GILBERT, *Etiquette*

One morning a telephone call came into my office from a man who wanted to employ three people by the hour to shake hands with him for as long as it took him to do a good job.

Most people assume that anything as natural as shaking hands needs no practice. Yet in my classes I have been surprised to find that at least 50 per cent. of my students not only make a very poor job of shaking hands, but frankly admit that they dislike doing so.

On the whole it seems there are very few people who shake hands without inhibitions. Yet there are others who grow up watching their parents shake hands naturally and enthusiastically and they take it in their stride.

I shall never forget a prominent hostess who said, " I never shake hands with my guests as they arrive, but I always try to manage it when they leave." Imagine doling out your handshakes ! Either make a good job of it or don't bother at all. If you know you bungle your handshaking, then start practising. It's important, because it is through your handshake that a new acquaintance forms an impression of you.

If your handshake were being filmed your coach would break down your technique into three phases.

1. What you say, and your facial expression.

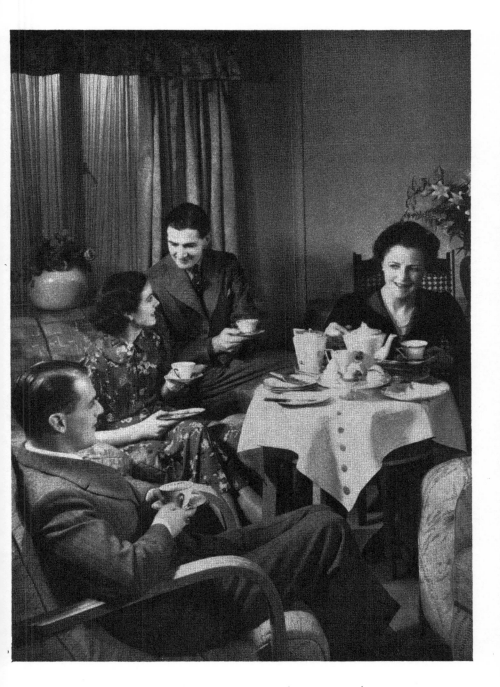

Photograph 14.—Good conversation can make you more popular

2. Your actual handclasp.

3. Your body co-ordination.

1. When you are introduced, your standard reply is " How do you do ? " Put as much friendliness and warmth as possible in your voice and try to repeat the person's name.

No matter if you meet a hundred people in one hundred minutes, you still say, " How do you do ? " Look directly into the eyes of the persons you meet. Don't look at her gold filling, the mole on her chin or the feathers on her hat.

If it's a man, don't look at his bald head. Eyes that jump from item to item on your clothing seem restless, disinterested, uncertain. Such eyes are supposed to be furtive. They're far more apt to be timid. *You'll recall in the lesson on radiant expression that I stressed the point that there's nothing about a person as important as the person.*

A snob is more interested in apparel and possessions than he is in the person. Carrying this principle a step farther, you should be able to walk into a home or office and see nothing but the person you've come to visit.

2. Theoretically, the hand should be extended, palm up. In actual practice your hand turns slightly to contact the palm of the other person. (See Figure 134.)

Your handshake is over so rapidly that it's impossible to realize how many factors go into its success. It's like a wedding, where hundreds of hours go into preparation for a beautiful twenty-minute ceremony. Here are some techniques to observe.

(a) Keep the web between your thumb and forefinger open as you extend your hand. That allows a firm clasp. What is worse than feeling hard, cold knuckles ?

(b) There should be definite pressure from the palm of the hand. Therefore, keep the palm as flat as possible.

(c) Don't dig with your fingers.

(d) Your elbow should be straightened, but your arm should form a curve.

(e) Don't hug your elbow to your side as you shake hands. This is attributed to a suspicious, miserly nature. It is also more apt to be caused by timidity.

(f) Make it obvious to the other person that you intend to shake hands. Haven't you been

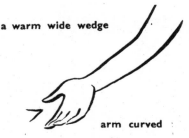

a warm wide wedge

arm curved

Figure 134

embarrassed by the person who walks up to you smilingly, without giving any indication of shaking hands, and upon being directly in front of you, darts out a hand ?

Your movement should be so spontaneous, unstudied, gracious, that the other person senses instinctively that you do intend shaking hands. When you are the hostess welcoming a guest, learn to cross a room with an extended hand.

(g) *Don't pump up and down* ! All you need do is clasp the hands with one or two pressures. If you're stuck with a hand pumper who seems to be enjoying his work, your best cue is to ignore his pumping completely.

On the other hand, if you're enjoying it, you'll flutter your eyelashes, look up at him pleadingly, down at your hands demurely, and gently try to pull your hand away. IT ALL DEPENDS.

(h) *It is always a woman's prerogative to extend her hand first.* Make it very obvious whether or not you intend doing so, because the man

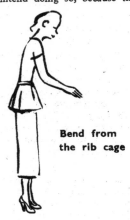

Bend from the rib cage

Figure 135

watches for an instantaneous cue from you. Should he override the rules of good form by assuming that you plan to shake hands with him, you will, of course, be gracious and cover his blunder.

Theoretically, the man waits for you to extend your hand upon all subsequent meetings. I'm happy to say that many well-bred men do not stand upon this stuffy law of formal etiquette, if they feel you are their friend.

3. *Charmed* . . . . Many women could take a lesson from the army officer's introduction technique. At Officers' Candidate School, the students are instructed to hold themselves rigid from the waist down and to bend forward no more than six inches for their bow of acknowledgment. Contrast this with the average woman's technique as she makes the rounds in the living room. She bows from her hips, so that her buttocks protrude ; stands with her feet apart, often crossing them awkwardly. Or she may be acknowledging introductions by bowing her head vigorously up and down.

A woman's technique differs somewhat from a man's : her feet assume a closed position, such as the arch which you learned in a previous Lesson. Her knees are relaxed. Her buttocks are controlled and pulled under her, and she does not move from the waist down. Her rib cage, shoulders, and head move forward about three inches. Usually a taller woman can manage more bowing forward. (See Figure 135.) Practise just this much from chair to chair in your empty living room. Keep your feet uncrossed. As you pause for your introduction, your feet assume the arch position, so you have one foot with no weight ready for action.

The underlying principle of graceful motion is TO ARCH IN THE DIRECTION IN WHICH YOU ARE GOING. If, when you are acknowledging introductions, you are moving to the right, always arch with the right foot. Should you forget and arch with the wrong foot, you can always shift your weight, change your weight and step off correctly. This takes a few moments to master, but it will ensure a poised, attractive demeanour.

There is a theatrical saying, " Your poise is as sound as your foot-work is sure." No matter how composed you feel inwardly, if you give a bulky, awkward, ungraceful appearance, you do not impress others as a poised individual. Sooner or later your awkward motions will embarrass

you, too.

Who can cover gracefully such blunders of movement as bumping into someone, backing into a chair, stumbling over a waste-basket, missing a stair ? On the other hand, if you have trained your body, your feet and your arms to act mechanically and smoothly in co-ordination, you will give the impression of poise even though inwardly you do not feel it.

HOW TO BEGIN A CONVERSATION

Meet Miss Smith. By this time, you have made the rounds, you have met everyone, and you begin your conversation. The man is always presented to the woman, a younger woman to an older woman and a single woman to a married woman.

In this day and age, unless there is a great difference in age, the only one of these observations you need follow to the letter is that you must mention the woman's name *first* when presenting a man to her. Thus you will say, " Miss Smith, may I present Mr. Jones ? " Or more simply, " Miss Smith, Mr. Jones."

Do not make a distinction in introducing two people. It is poor form, for instance, to say, " Miss Smith, I'd like you to meet my very dearest friend, Mr. Jones." It is better to mention later in the conversation what a dear friend Mr. Jones is ! You may innocently say, " Miss Smith, I want you to meet one of the most brilliant girls in this town, Miss Jones." You do not intend to imply inequality, but you have done so ; and it is considered poor form.

The person who does the introducing is socially bound to start the conversational ball rolling. The more simple and effortless this cue is, the better for all involved. Thus you say, " Miss Smith, may I present Mr. Jones ? Mr. Jones has just returned from Europe." That at least calls for an exclamation, " Oh, really ! How interesting," from Miss Smith. Even if she misses her cue and says no more than " Oh ! " then either he or the introducer can cover it up by saying " Yes, I (he) was working there for six months." And you hope by this time that Miss Smith has recovered sufficiently to say, " Did you like it there ? "

Suppose, however, this happens to you. " Miss Smith, Mr. Jones. Oh, please do pardon me, some other guests have arrived . . . " whereupon the introducer leaves you cold.

You are looking at a man you know nothing

about—who knows nothing about you. You both stand there a long, gasping second in silence, and then you both start talking at once ! Have a little stock to fall back upon in such emergencies.

The most obvious topic of conversation is that which is close at hand. Therefore, you might discuss what you have in common, your mutual hostess, her home, some floral arrangement close at hand, a picture, or the party. It might go like this :

YOU : I always enjoy Mary's parties. I used to work with her at the library.

HE : Oh, did you ? I'm a better friend of her brother's than I am of Mary's.

YOU : Oh, how is Jim ? (Meaning the brother.)

HE : Just fine. I understand he likes the East.

YOU : He's just like Mary—very adaptable and makes friends easily—don't you think ?

HE : Yes, doesn't he ? Your mentioning that Mary worked at the library with you, makes me understand why she's so interested in books. You know, the other night I just happened to drop in and she was reading Maugham's *Of Human Bondage* for the third time. I thought it was so interesting that . . . .

It looks as though you're off on a reasonably nice conversational bout. Discussing your hostess's personality can be dangerous or often boring, and you might run into luck like this :

YOU : I always enjoy Mary's parties. You know, I used to work with her at the library.

HE : Is that so ?

YOU : Yes, we had a grand time. We were in the research department.

HE : You'd never connect Mary with a research department now.

YOU : (Ignoring his sarcasm.) That's one nice feature about research . . . it's so easily concealed. What do you do ?

HE : Engineering.

YOU : Oh, that must be fascinating work, isn't it ?

HE : Oh, so, so.

YOU : Does your work get you out of doors ?

HE : Yes, quite a bit. I cover half the country.

YOU : That's quite a lot of ground. You must know all the gay spots then. I've been thinking of a holiday. Where would you suggest ?

HE : Well, if you really want a different holiday, I know just the spot . . . .

It was rough going, wasn't it ? But you followed a pretty well-established routine. You

started with your mutual interest, your hostess He bungled. You gave him a chance to ask you about your work, which he missed.

You gave him a further opportunity to tall about his business, which he refused. You tried to ferret a hobby out of him, and failing all of these, you fell back on that feminine ace of asking his advice about something upon which he was qualified to speak authoritatively. Maybe he'll be fun after all !

I'm Nancy Jones. Often you find yourself in a spot where you have to make yourself known. The moment you step inside your hostess's door you should speak to, or be gracious with, all the other guests, whether or not you have been introduced. It's quite a feat for a busy hostess to see that everyone meet everyone else.

You should not walk into the cloakroom, take off your wraps, and remain silent just because you haven't been introduced to other guests there. You will say, " How do you do ? I am Nancy Jones—Mrs. Jones."

You needn't carry on any further conversation, because it is not good form to linger in the cloakroom. Or you may say only, " Good evening."

Later during the evening you may be standing or sitting beside a man whom you do not know. It is your place to present yourself to him. If you fail to do so, and the situation is uncomfortable, he may take up the reins.

YOU : I'm Nancy Jones—Miss Jones. (If you're married, you might say, " I'm Mrs. Bacon—Mrs. Walter Bacon.")

HE : How do you do, Miss Jones ? I'm Norman Blake. I've been admiring this coastline.

YOU : It looks familiar somehow.

HE : Yes, doesn't it ? That's just what I was thinking.

That should get the two of you talking about holidays—and then back to where you work.

You remember me. What throws you faster than the complete stranger who walks up and says, " For heaven's sake, if it isn't Marguerite Mullins ! It's so good to see you again—how have you been all these years ? " *Never assume that a person will remember you.* There are too many people in the world ! Tell him your name, how you happen to know him and when.

For instance, you might say, " Marguerite, I am Louise Daly and I was in Dr. McCallum's class at the University with you." Even if the other person knows you, and recognises you instantly, it's better to give too much information than too little. Even when a person says, "Marguerite, I am Louise Daly. How have you been keeping ? " her name alone may not place her in your mind.

Oh, thank you. Very often the beginning of a conversation is thrown askew because of a compliment. For many generations it was considered poor form to inject a compliment into the initial stages of a conversation.

A little personal research to-day, however, shows that a man almost invariably compliments a woman very early in the conversation. This holds just as true between two women. Custom makes it acceptable.

The person receiving the compliment can either manipulate it so that it acts as a smooth transition to further conversation, or she can miss her cue completely and hit a conversational blind alley. Contrast these techniques :

HE : I was admiring your hat from across the room.

YOU : Oh, this old thing ? Don't tell me that. I stuck a couple of feathers on last year's felt. I didn't know whether I should wear it or not.

HE : Well, it looks awfully good to me. But then I'm no judge of hats.

YOU : I bet you tell all the girls that, but *I'm* wise to your kind !

HE : Well, no. I'm just a man trying to get along. Be seeing you . . . .

Here's another try :

HE : I've been admiring your hat from across the room.

YOU : Oh, thank you. Now I'm glad I bought it. Hats are one thing you men don't have to worry much about.

HE : I suppose that's right. But we have other problems.

YOU : What, for instance ?

HE : Well, I have to make a living.

YOU : Now, that's a nuisance ! What are you doing ?

HE : I'm a wholesaler, and I have to be down at the produce market at four o'clock every morning, six mornings a week . . .

I know of no other single conversational skill which is more generally bungled by both men and women than that of giving and receiving compliments. Regardless of the compliment, you are called upon to say, " Thank you," at least.

Don't apologise, as the first young lady did here. Don't disagree. Don't get flustered. If you are really up on your conversational toes, you will try to find a transition from the compliment to a general topic of conversation. In the second instance, the young lady did this very nicely with just a few words.

The compliment that is so often embarrassing to a girl or woman of taste is the one that's too personal. *But if your outstanding feature is your hair, your teeth, your figure, you might as well be prepared to hear about it from the men.* And more important, have some rejoinders on the tip of your tongue. I think one of the smartest replies I have heard to a personal compliment came from Virginia Mayo, lovely Samuel Goldwyn star, when she first came to Hollywood from Broadway. She was in my class at the Goldwyn Motion Picture Studio, and Mr. Goldwyn had stressed the importance of conversational ability. One day I said to Virginia, " What are you going to say when some man says, ' Not bad legs there, Virginia ! ' ? She spoke up immediately, ' Oh, I've had a stock answer for that since I was fourteen. I say, ' Thank you, Tom. They get me around.' I laugh and then say seriously, ' Speaking of legs, did you know that Barnum's sister, even at sixty-seven, was supposed to have two of the most photogenic legs in the world ? ' The tie-up never fails, Miss King, because almost everybody has some comment to make about Barnum, his circus, his sister, or legs in general."

I decided right there that Virginia was one very clever girl who would go far. Her reply incorporates every principle of accepting a compliment graciously.

First, she thanked the giver. She followed with a statement which showed she was very levelheaded about her beauty. She was not apologetic, embarrassed or derogatory. In almost the same breath, she linked the compliment with a subject of general interest. And she did all this on one of the most personal subjects.

You look heavenly. Men are particularly embarrassed with a compliment which is too gushing, especially in the presence of others. Your compliments can be as extravagant as you like when you are alone with your man, but when others are around, he is inclined to be a little sensitive.

Often the manner in which a compliment is given makes a gracious acceptance difficult. My column in the newspaper is the focal point for many pet complaints from men.

Here's one of their common complaints, in their own words : " A woman invites you to her home for dinner. She may even ask you to pick up a friend of hers. Then when you arrive at the door, you are surprised and a little embarrassed by the enthusiasm with which she says, ' I'm so glad to see you, John,' as though I'm a complete surprise ! What else can a man do, but lamely say, ' Well, I'm glad to be here.' Can't she greet me less enthusiastically, so that I don't get embarrassed ? "

What is your first reaction when a man says to you, " You know, Molly, you're the best-looking redhead in this part of the world " ? Of course, you don't believe him. You resent his belittling your intelligence to the extent that he thinks you believe him, so that you are tempted to hurt him by saying, " How do you know ? " No matter how exuberant or insincere you consider the compliment, *you must remember that two wrongs do not make a right.*

A sarcastic, withering reply only puts you in a bad light. Should you act upon your instincts and say, " Just who do you think is going to fall for that kind of talk ? " he must become defensive immediately and say, " But that's right. You name another redhead as pretty as you." Then you are in a spot, because the situation has lost every semblance of dignity. Instead, you will say something like this, " Oh, thank you, Tom. That's the best news I've heard all week. I suppose that's one reason I like you. You always give me such a build-up. But tell me, speaking of redheads, did you see Rita Hayworth the other night ? " Give him credit for trying to say something nice. It was his gesture.

From a woman's standpoint, I suppose the compliment that really throws her most goes something like, " Dora, that is the best-looking suit you ever had on ! " You weakly go through your social paces with a disheartening attempt at " Thank you, Mary, I don't know when I've ever enjoyed wearing anything more. Incidentally, did you see the white suit that Esther Williams wore when she arrived at the 'plane ? "

Underneath you get the idea that Mary thinks that all the other suits you have worn look like sacks ! In this case, you're more at fault than she. She didn't mean to be unkind. You are overlooking her generous compliment, and thinking unkind thoughts about her.

Don't think that people want to hurt you ! Realise that it's more apt to be their lack of ability to express themselves well. I think the best lesson on overcoming sensitivity is this law of psychology : people are not interested enough in you to want to hurt you. And if they do go out of their way to make you uncomfortable, you gain nothing by giving them satisfaction.

Learn to appreciate the good will involved in the gesture of a compliment even if it's stated tactlessly. If you are short-tempered, embarrassed, or flippant in your reply, you will soon find that you have no compliments to worry about.

One of a woman's best indications of her feminine allurements can be estimated quickly by totalling her compliments for the past month. They needn't be extravagant, extreme, or too exalting, but good will should be coming your way as your womanly due.

In general, try to state your compliments with sincerity. Use such approaches as :
1. " Mary, it seems to me you get prettier every year."
2. " I like grey on you, John. What do you call the material in your suit ? "
3. " I heard so many nice things about your work on the committee this last year, Marguerite."

Do not try to give other people compliments by belittling yourself.

For example, haven't you heard a conversation like this ?

YOU : Say, you're brilliant at mathematics, aren't you ?

HE : Oh, thanks—it's just a matter of practice.

YOU : Maybe so, but I don't think I could ever learn. I never was any good at arithmetic and I took geometry three times before I passed.

HE : It can't be that bad.

YOU : Oh, but it is. I can't even add up my cheque book. I always have to get someone else to do it for me. I just can't seem to . . .

HE : That's too bad. Well, if you'll excuse me . . .

And about time ! Give the other fellow his due, but you can do so without taking yourself down a peg. Why couldn't this conversation be handled this way ?

YOU : It must be a satisfaction to juggle figures that way.

HE : Well, as a matter of fact, yes. At school I never could understand why so many of the fellows had trouble with it because . . .

You see ? You've helped him establish his

feeling of importance without injuring your own standing.

The Short Conversation

The long and the short of it. There is a very definite difference in technique between a short and a long conversation. Since all day long, most of your conversations are short, let's take short ones first by observing some of the following principles :

1. Let a thread run through your short, casual conversations.

2. Recall something you have heard about your friends since you last talked to them.

3. Don't mention a topic which will take longer than half a minute to tell. You are encroaching upon his time.

4. Don't discuss operations, ill-fortune or gossip.

5. The short conversations especially must be stimulating and create goodwill.

6. Don't be on the defensive.

Contrast these chance encounters in the street :

MARY : Well, hello, John.

JOHN : Hello, Mary. How are you ?

MARY : I'm just fine. How are you ?

JOHN : Can't complain. What's the latest ?

MARY : Oh, the same old grind, day after day. Nothing new or exciting. You know how it goes, just work, sleep, eat. What's new with you ?

JOHN : Not much new with me either. How's your mother ?

MARY : The same. There's not much hope for her, John. She gets pretty despondent. And it doesn't make it easy for the rest of us. So hard to live with her.

The other day she had another heart attack and the next-door neighbour had a *time* getting all of us. By the time we all got home from work she was better, but it's quite a worry, never knowing from day to day what's going to happen. Do you realise she's been ill for almost three years now ? Seems to me I've forgotten what good times are.

JOHN : That must be tough. Say " hello " to her for me. Well, I must be shoving off . . . . Goodbye, Mary . . . .

MARY : Goodbye, John . . .

Do you think Mary or John felt better after this chat ? Obviously they are not very good friends, or they would have seen each other more recently. But even had they seen each other quite frequently, it would still have been poor form for Mary to discuss on the street her mother's last heart attack. At best she aroused his sympathy, maybe pity, but she takes a chance, too, that he will think of her as down-in-the-mouth, complaining and unable to take it. Now let's see what she might have said.

JOHN : Hello, Mary.

MARY : Why, hello, John. I haven't seen you since last Summer when you were going on holiday. Did you get away ?

JOHN : Yes, I made it. And it was a good holiday.

MARY : I'd love to hear about it. Did you take any snaps ?

JOHN : Yes, as a matter of fact, I did. I got some beauties, too. I'm planning to enter one of them in an amateurs' photo contest. But let's talk about you—how's your mother ?

MARY : About the same, John. She was asking about you the other day. And laughing about the time you tried to carry her up the stairs and your own legs gave out !

JOHN: That was a night to remember. Is there a chance of dropping in one night soon ?

MARY : I think so if you promise to be on your good behaviour.

JOHN : How about Friday ?

MARY : Friday's perfect.

JOHN : I'll 'phone you on Thursday night, then.

If you analyse this conversation, you will see that Mary very cleverly employed *each* of the conversational rules mentioned here for short conversations.

Suppose a friend you meet on the street asks :

HE : Have you seen " The Other Girl " ?

YOU : No, I haven't—I'm working late these nights and by the time I get home, change my clothes, and have dinner, it's too late to do anything. Don't even know when I last saw a film.

HE : That's too bad.

The conversation is now up against a wall. No wonder you're getting nowhere fast. Now let's see how you might have used his interest to advantage.

HE : Have you seen " The Other Girl " ?

YOU : No, I haven't—but I hear it's wonderful. Did you like it ?

HE : Yes, it's one of the best musicals I've seen on the films.

YOU : Is that so ? I understand that dance of

Gene Kelly's was really worth seeing.

HE : Yes, it was. I laughed when he scolded himself as he danced.

YOU : (Laughing). Oh, how clever. I've had to talk to myself hundreds of times like that, haven't you ?

HE : Yes, I have. You should see that picture. Are you free any night this week ?

You see how it works ? The underlying rule is this : when people mention a book, exhibition, play or film—they don't actually care whether you saw it or read it. They want to *talk* about it. It's something they will mention during a chance short meeting. So encourage them to tell you why they liked it. In that way you make them see you're interested, alive, fun. You sound like more !

THE LONG CONVERSATION

The long way home. It's helpful to understand that when you know you are going to be with a person several hours, your conversational technique can be much different from that employed in your short conversations. The time element makes your contributions unhurried and deliberate.

A long conversation can be likened to a slow, meandering stream, as it makes its way around bends and curves across the fields. There may be places where the impetus is speeded up, and other minutes of extreme leisureliness. Let's go over a few rules for your long conversation :

1. Don't try to say everything you want to say in the first fifteen minutes.

2. Be a good listener if the other person seems to have something to tell you. Be able to hold up your end of the conversation if he seems inclined to be quiet.

While he is talking, listen to what he has to say. Don't rehearse what you are going to say next so thoroughly that you stand the risk of being discovered. There may be a woman clever enough to listen well and think about something else at the same time, but I have never heard of her.

3. Don't be in a hurry to change the conversation. If everyone else in the group seems to be enjoying the discussion, it's rude to switch it abruptly. Your time to make your contribution will come, and if it doesn't, you're none the loser.

4. However, when you sense the first slackening of interest in the topic under discussion, jump

in enthusiastically with a switch. Even then you must watch how you change the subject.

Writers speak of blending one sentence into the next. Make-up artists speak of blending base and rouge. The more skilful the blending, the better the job. So it is in conversation. You must be aware of linking one topic with another—of blending your comments with those of others. This is a conversational transition. The old stand-by is, " Speaking of . . . . "

Some conversational authorities are scornful of the triteness of this transition and recommend very elaborate ones. That's perfect if you can juggle with them, but since the most pleasant conversation is effortless, you want to be perfectly natural when introducing a new subject.

You might vary the " speaking of " gambit by saying something like, " Dorothy, as you were talking about your mother's collection of pictures, I thought of an eccentric uncle of one of my friends. He lives in America and goes in for swimming pools. I understand he had three on his estate. I visited his home on my trip and I don't think I ever saw a place more beautiful than it. "

Be sure to give credit to the other person's anecdote, story, contribution, before you introduce your own. You are thus paving the way for at least an unprejudiced reception. You know the bore who says, " I heard a better story than that," or " Here's a tale that will top yours."

Change a subject swiftly, when it becomes obnoxious, distasteful, or may hurt anyone present. People who use their pet grievances at the expense of other people deserve to have a conversational door slammed in their face. Simply say, " Pardon me for changing the subject. . . . I hope you won't mind my switching the subject but I am so anxious to tell you about Louise's good fortune."

In the long conversation, don't be afraid of silences. There is something congenial and united about silences. Especially if you have been contributing more than your share of the conversation, a silence often will force someone else to rise to the occasion.

Many people are lazy conversationally, and will sit back and let you take the lead indefinitely. You will always be respected more if you let others know that you refuse to be taken advantage of conversationally or otherwise.

Of course, often to help your hostess or save an embarrassing moment for everyone involved, you feel obliged to cut a silence immediately—especially, when you know the hostess better than some of the other guests, or when you know you're better acquainted with the group as a whole than some of the others.

One of the most challenging long conversations is during that important first date. A poll of three hundred single girls from fifteen to twenty-one admitted that they were most successful when they didn't like the young man too much. As one girl phrased it, " If only I could be with those I like—as I am with those I don't, I'd be a howling success ! "

The same poll showed that when you don't like a young man too well, you're gay, impersonal, and go out of your way to make the " poor man " feel important. The minute you get a date with someone you especially like, what happens? You overdo or underdo. Thus to him you appear either too eager or too self-satisfied. The most popular woman I've had in my class in personality training at the University admitted " I'm an actress with the boys I really like on the first few dates. I try to imitate the light, good-humoured mood I naturally assume with boys that I know are just dates."

Believing that the male's side of the date question would be helpful here, I'm listing verbatim reactions from seven hundred males between the ages of eighteen and fifty-two.

The following remarks are worded just as they came to me in answer to the question, " What don't you like in the girl you date ? "

I DON'T LIKE A GIRL WHO : " Interprets everything in a peculiar light ; is too emotional ; can't accept a gift gracefully—if a man goes out of his way to give a girl a present (and especially if he taxes his resources to do it), he reacts violently when it's received with, ' It's beautiful, but you SHOULDN'T have done it ' ; [Now, this is a slight, isn't it ? How many of us have said JUST this !] ; is always hungry ; has to hear a joke or some witty remark before she smiles.

" The girl who is obviously making an effort to please ; kisses you good-bye without seeing that all of the lipstick is off you ; is unable to hold up her end of the conversation on national and international affairs ; swears ; has no religion or philosophy of life that she practises ;

continually expounds her equality with men ; talks about herself too much ; explains or amplifies everything I say ; follows a set line of thought ; is too, too gushing ; grins like a Cheshire cat ; waddles ; wears too much jewellery and make-up ; has an extreme hair style ; wears dark lipstick and fingernail polish ; wears perfume that knocks you out ; falls all over every new man ; uses coarse language ; has crooked stocking seams ; has two pairs of lips—her own and those she plasters on ; uses red toe-nail polish ; makes me sick with heavy mascara on eyebrows and eyelashes.

" Is untruthful in small matters ; is too generous ; has too little respect for women in general ; is too lazy ; is too familiar with other men ; flirts ; does not know the value of money ; insists on arguing over every issue ; never helps at parties after she has volunteered ; acts like a juvenile ; is constantly wondering what other people think about her .

" The girl who beats me at badminton, tennis, golf ; shows jealousy and acts possessively ; tries to run her husband's business; has a grating, high-pitched, piercing voice ; flirts with men after they're married ; is too sophisticated ; laughs at my stories, encourages me to tell them, and then says ' I don't like Jack's brand of stories ' ; tries to improve me, my speech, appearance and ideas ; fixes my tie, adjusts my pocket handkerchief ; pats my hair into a curl, and takes charge of our programme ; is over-eager ; thinks her husband is trying to improve on her cooking when he wants some freedom around the kitchen ; always wants me to take her somewhere but finds it inconvenient to go when I need company ; shows her superiority in knowledge or skill ; has bad breath ; is immodest—we usually like things better when they are not too easy to get ; seems to think whatever I do or say is perfect—I made an error once in 1916 ; uses a continuous ' come-on ' attitude, ending in a slap in the face and unjust accusation ; forgets to let her escort handle the difficult situations that often arise in public."

I LIKE A GIRL WHO : " Gets along with her mother ; makes me feel needed ; can control her emotions in the event of sudden scary events ; has personal ambitions as well as being a wife and housewife ; has intelligent suggestions for an evening's entertainment ; builds up my ego by complimenting me on my clothes, etc.

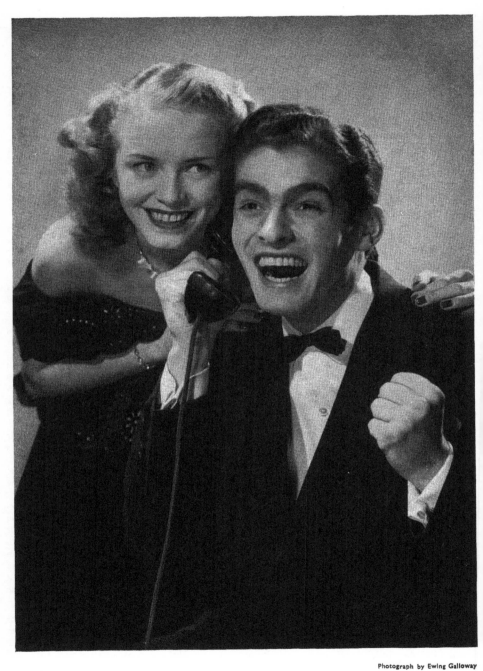

Photograph 15.—Go out of your way to make him feel important.

" A girl who knows how to cook ; is a good sport and will enter into most activities willingly, even though she might enjoy something else more ; is sincere and doesn't give the impression that she is an entirely different person under her mask ; carries herself erect without stiffness ; doesn't attract attention too much in public ; is informed upon topics that are of interest to men ; a girl who has 'pep' and enthusiasm ; smiles a great deal ; can accept last-minute changes in plans occasionally with a cheerful smile instead of a growl about how she is expected to do this on such short notice ; considers my friends and relatives just as important as her own ; can act as well at a formal dance as at a beach party ; is sweet and sincere without being artificially pleasant ; doesn't drop those subtle hints that make a man feel like a cad for not remembering some insignificant (to him) event or occasion ! "

Well, they're " eye-openers," aren't they ? You may wish to write down how your conversation and actions stand up against these.

CONVERSATIONAL DO'S AND DON'TS

Once you understand the psychology underlying pleasant conversation, it's up to you to apply it. Since conversation is a habit, it's wise to review conversational do's and don'ts every few months. Here are some of the most important which apply to either a short or long conversation :

1. DO be pleasant. Whatever else you may or may not be conversationally, be an ambassador for harmony.

2. DON'T be too abrupt with your opinion. If you must disagree, ease into your belief with, " Yes, I have heard that side of it several times and know there's a lot in it, but I also feel . . . " And go easy on the " but " ! Then when you have stated it, you might ask for your partner's reaction. No matter how vehemently you disagree with him, don't say, " No, I think you're all wrong there," or " There is no evidence to back an opinion like that," or " You'd better read the facts in the case." Men might get by with this, but not women !

3. DON'T ask people if they have children. If they have, you'll hear about them soon enough.

4. If you can carry on a conversation all evening without a personal reference, you are good. And if you can't, practise it and notice the new interest you attract. The best conversation-

alists can talk about impersonal subjects for hours at a stretch and still be stimulating.

5. DO read the newspapers daily—at least one columnist thoroughly—the advertisements, a magazine on current events, and remember your facts. Listen to a variety of radio and television programmes. You have to know what's going on about you.

6. DO read books in several fields so that you have at least an asking acquaintance with a number of subjects, such as the theatre, art, paintings, artists, sculpture, architecture, history, fiction, biographies.

7. DO be sure to hide your fatigue or boredom. If you have accepted an invitation, then you owe your hostess the courtesy of seeming interested and awake. If you are tired, excuse yourself and go home ; fatigue may be misinterpreted as superiority.

8. DO be kind in everything you say. You can't overdo this principle.

9. DON'T admit you are self-conscious, have an inferiority complex, or are sensitive. It's like talking about your operation.

10. DO keep an approachable, pleasant look on your face, especially if you're the quiet type.

11. DON'T make exaggerated statements, such as, " It's the finest book I ever read," or " It's the lousiest film I ever saw." You weaken your opinion and you destroy the listener's faith in your opinion !

12. DO imply that you assume your listener is as well read as you. Therefore don't say, " Have you ever read ' David Copperfield ' ? "

13. DO mention beauty in all the little things about you. Don't wait for something stupendous to bring forth your admiration.

14. DON'T say belittling things about yourself. By doing so, you simply demand that the other person come to your rescue.

15. DON'T start an argument. If you get in one regardless, insist that the subject be changed. You may have to say, " I refuse to argue with you, Don—let's talk about your new boat." If he refuses, excuse yourself, and leave.

16. DON'T direct your conversation to only one person in a group, especially if there are less than six in the group.

17. DO bring a neglected person into the conversation by looking at him or asking him a question.

18. DON'T be a faddist or a crusader. Conversationally, you are skating on thin ice.

(For advice on developing conversational ability, write to Miss Ethel Cotton, Psychology House, Marple, and mention "Glorify Yourself".)

19. DON'T dwell on gloomy subjects.

20. DON'T introduce politics, religion or race. If these subjects are brought up, refuse to be intolerant or make or encourage slurring remarks.

21. DO make others feel at ease.

22. DO inject humour into your conversation. Read the comic strips. You needn't be the life of the party, but you can cultivate a light, happy manner of speaking.

23. DON'T explain the point of your story.

24. DO speed up the tempo of a story by omitting irrelevant details.

25. DO learn to tell jokes, but don't laugh while you're telling them.

26. DO tell jokes on yourself.

27. DO remember that the self-assertive person is often timid and unsure of himself.

28. DO remember that the boastful person or the one who tries to sell himself is likewise unsure of himself. Go out of your way to make him feel important and he will stop bragging. (See Photograph 15).

29. DON'T be loud in public.

30. DON'T ask that a story be repeated if you're late getting in on it. One way to be a bore is the habit of saying, " Start it over again."

31. DON'T overdo pet expressions, such as " I'm telling you," " My word," " A case in point," " Well, I mean," " In other words."

32. DON'T ask too many questions. True, they are helpful once in a while. Be sure your questions are not of a personal nature.

33. DON'T ask a second question until you have given the other person a chance to ask one.

34. DON'T start each sentence with " Er " or " Well."

35. DON'T complain, especially in male company. You sound and look your worst when you complain. This means that you shouldn't complain about your health, your husband, your finances or your job. It's easy to speak of the things that go wrong. Form the habit of speaking of pleasant aspects of your life.

36. DO learn to distinguish between sympathy and destructive curiosity. Be wary of the person who says, " You poor little girl, I don't see how you do it all." She may be encouraging dangerous confidences.

37. DON'T "talk shop" unless you know the other person is genuinely interested. The other person

may be trying to forget shop responsibilities.

38. DON'T be stingy with your praise. Acknowledge a job well done. Your mother would say, " Give credit where credit is due."

39. DO pause frequently when speaking. Men particularly dislike nonstop feminine voices. Vary the tempo of your speech to avoid monotony —and frustration for your listeners !

40. DON'T interrupt. Don't supply words. Everyone does this to some extent. Be sure you're not overdoing it, because it is highly irritating.

41. DON'T be a troublemaker. Troublemakers are unkind ; they hurt others. Don't carry stories or repeat unkind comments or unpleasant remarks.

42. DON'T be envious. Learn to get pleasure out of others' pleasures—to be able to actually rejoice in their successes.

43. DON'T be a martyr. Don't get a resigned and wronged tone in your voice.

44. Most important of all, DO BE KIND.

AND SO GOODBYE

In expressing your appreciation to your hostess, tell her that you enjoyed the evening, the dinner, the guests, the music, the speaker ; but never say, " I enjoyed MYSELF," or " We enjoyed OURSELVES ! " What's nicer than " Thank you, Jane, for including me " ?

When circumstances prevent your thanking your host or hostess for including you, call the very next morning to explain the reasons surrounding your hurried departure.

Occasionally, illness or an emergency may necessitate your leaving early, and you do not wish to cause an obvious break in the gathering. And be sure you always express your appreciation to both the host and the hostess.

Once you've decided to leave, stick to your decision. You needn't rush, but don't linger. Don't keep your hostess in a cold hall or doorway with prolonged good-byes. Husbands and wives should get together on their departure signals, so that one isn't waiting while the other delays.

I hope you've enjoyed this conversational jaunt with me, and I know that if you apply even 50 per cent of the suggestions here, you'll be pestered for life with, " But we NEVER see enough of you ! "

Self-Test Questions Based On Lesson Eight

We all have a certain natural reserve when meeting new people. It often causes others to get a wrong impression of us from the start. We ourselves lose opportunities socially and professionally. This Lesson will at least have started you on the road to achieving charm in your contacts with other people. Further studies will help you still more.

After you have studied this Lesson, you should be able to answer the following questions. If you have any difficulty in doing so, refer to the Lesson for further study and revision. Your answers should not be sent to the publishers of this Course.

1. What is the secret of success in your contacts with other people ?

2. Describe in 15 — 30 words what your attitude should be to any person to whom you may be introduced.

3. With whom does the decision lie as to whether to shake hands or not when meeting a member of the opposite sex ?

4. What rule should you follow in introducing people to each other ?

5. How should you accept a compliment ?

6. What should you always be, whether a compliment is acceptable or not ?

7. Sum up in six points the do's and don'ts of a short conversation.

8. What is the underlying rule you should remember in carrying on a short conversation successfully ?

9. To what could you liken the gist or course of a long conversation ?

10. Are silences permissible in long conversations ?

If you wish to determine the progress you are making, give yourself 10 points for each question you answer correctly. If the total comes to 90 or more, it is excellent; 80 or more, good; 70 or more, fair.

Notes:

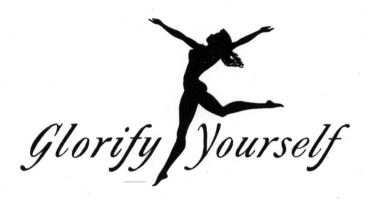

Glorify Yourself

★

A Complete and Up-to-Date Course on
Beauty and Charm by One of the
Most Famous Beauty Specialists
and Consultants in the World

★

LESSON NINE
by

Sally Young

★

STUDIO TALK •

Issued only for Student
of the Eleanore Kin
Course on Beauty. Char
and Personality.

Number Nine.

Dear Student,

This Lesson has been prepared by my colleague
Sally Young, who is known to millions of women as the
Beauty Editor of a widely-read women's weekly magazine.

Miss Young herself admits that she was not born
a beauty. All through her school years she was considered
not just pleasantly plump, but chubby. You might say she
had as little or as much to start with as the average
woman, but she had determination - she made up her mind
to be better looking each year. Because she has succeeded
so well, she is exactly the person to co-operate with me
in helping other women on the way to beauty.

Lesson Nine is a complete guide to woman's crowning
glory.

"Fair tresses man's imperial race ensnare,
And beauty draws us with a single hair".

Those words are as true to-day as they were when
Alexander Pope wrote them nearly 250 years ago. He was
writing about the great ladies of Queen Anne's court, and
was doubtless smiling to himself about the elaborate hair
styles of that era. In those days it was not uncommon to
see a jewelled galleon in full sail on the waves of
milady's tresses.

We live in easier times. You do not have to be a
great lady to achieve a fashionable hair style. Beautiful
hair is within the reach of any woman who will give just a
reasonable amount of time and care to this all-important
feature of feminine allure.

The first essential is to promote the general
health of the hair; and so the opening pages of the Lesson
give you a number of simple routines and techniques which
will ensure that your hair is always soft and silky with a
brilliant sheen. These routines are for regular applicati
Do not on any account neglect them.

(over)

216

Once you are satisfied with the general condition of your hair you can have fun choosing the particular style which will suit your own individual features. The second part of the Lesson is lavishly illustrated. From the pictures you can select a style and copy it exactly; or better still, use its general principles as an outline for creating your own hair-do. Your hairdresser will be glad to help you to produce an exclusive styling to highlight your individual personality.

Yours sincerely,

Eleanore King

EK.9.

P.S. A large variety of interesting hints and tips are awaiting your attention in Lesson Ten.

Hair

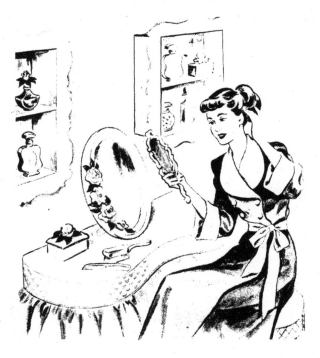

FOR beautiful hair you need more than a wave.

Do you know that the hair is something like the skin ? The same life-giving elements that help make beautiful skin also help make beautiful hair. So see to it that you remain vibrantly healthy. Watch your diet, get plenty of fresh air and sleep, and don't give in to depressing blue moods.

Your hair needs to be healthy if you wish it to look its best—beautiful, gleaming and glamorous, sparkling with life and lustre.

If you know your health is tip-top, there's no reason why your hair shouldn't be lovely—if you give it proper care.

All the new hair styles in the world will not do much for your glamour unless you begin with gleamingly clean hair and a healthy scalp. Basic to clean hair and the healthy scalp is your regular shampoo, which, to be done correctly, should consist of five definite steps.

STEPS TO A PERFECT SHAMPOO

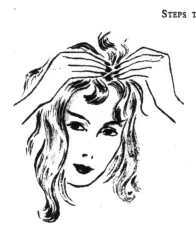

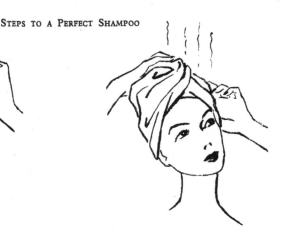

1. The first step consists of firm massaging of the scalp with the fingertips. This should be done daily, as well as before the shampoo, for it brings the blood up where it can readily do the hair some good.

3. To make dirt removal easier, wind a hot towel around your head. Prepare the towel by holding it under hot water and wringing it out almost dry.

If you have very dry hair, apply warm oil to the scalp with a cotton pad. Then apply the hot towel.

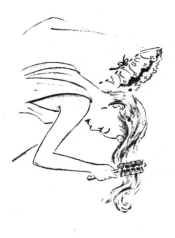

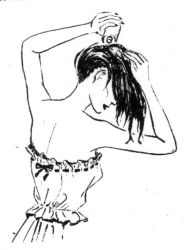

2. The second step is vigorous brushing to further stimulate the scalp and to distribute natural oils along the hair shaft.

4. Step four is the actual shampoo. Wet the hair thoroughly with warm water and apply the shampoo. Massage it into the scalp and hair,

working up a rich lather. Rinse and repeat the lathering. Then rinse, rinse, rinse with cooler and cooler water, until your hair is free of lather. Towel dry, rub briskly.

To help keep blonde hair blonde, an egg-yolk rinse can be used with good results. Beat the yolk of a strictly fresh egg and add it to a cup of cool water. After the hair has been washed and rinsed thoroughly of all soap, pour the egg mixture over the entire head and hair. Rub it well into the scalp and on the hair. Rinse it off with clear water. Some girls who use this egg treatment further highlight their hair by giving it a final rinse with witch hazel, and some just substitute half a cup of witch hazel for the cup of water when adding it to the beaten egg yolk.

5. The last step is to comb out your hair, one strand at a time, starting at the ends of the hair and working up toward the scalp inch by inch, disentangling the hair as you go. Set it in pin curls, according to your favourite hair-do.

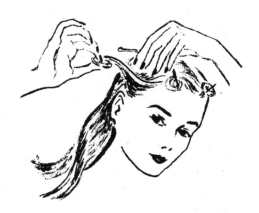

DAILY ROUTINE HAIR CARE

GENERAL

1. Brush hair daily to remove accumulated dust.

2. Cleanse daily, or on alternate days, with a special hair lotion for cleansing and removing dandruff.

3. Apply pomade sparingly with fingertips.

OILY HAIR

1. Cleanse scalp and hair with an oily-hair lotion, using daily until improvement is noted and thereafter on alternate days.

2. For added cleanliness, apply a special hair lotion at least twice weekly.

3. Brush daily, using a soft, flexible-bristled brush.

DRY HAIR

1. Cleanse and lubricate with a dry-hair lotion.

2. Apply scalp pomade daily, working into scalp and through hair.

3. Use a cream-type hair dressing for finished grooming. Brush daily.

METHOD OF APPLYING LOTIONS

Part the hair at intervals. Apply lotion directly to scalp, massaging it over scalp surface and through the hair. Brush. Clean brush on soft, lintless towel. Repeat brushing.

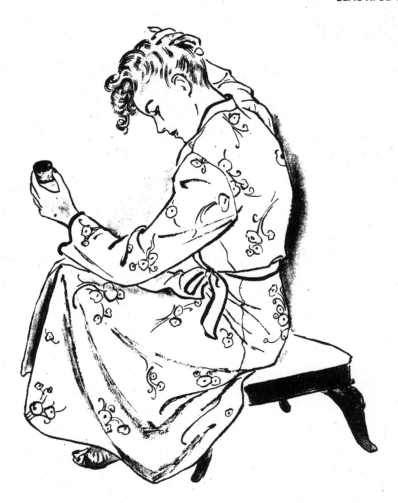

CODDLE THOSE LOCKS

So often I hear the complaint, " My hair grows slowly, and is dry and brittle." In a great many instances, the complaining party herself is at fault.

CAUSES OF DRYNESS

One of the most prevalent causes of brittle hair is too-tight permanents.

Having a new permanent too soon also make the hair dry and brittle. The ends break off, an the usually healthful brisk brushing of scalp an hair causes further breakage. As the ends brea off, the growing process seems to be slower.

Often a woman will insist upon having permanent, even though her Hairdresser advise against it. If scalp and hair are too dry or to oily, and the operator recommends a check-up by a doctor, she is protecting the patron.

Another factor to consider is home shampooing. Insufficient and careless rinsing without thorough removal of soap or shampoo eventually causes unhealthy hair and scalp.

It is important to remember that all forms of ill-health are directly reflected in your hair. General poor health, nervousness, organic diseases leave your hair undernourished.

While surface care, such as reconditioning treatments and shampoos, helps in combating unhealthy scalp and hair, the logical aim should be to get at the cause, and cure through medical diagnosis and treatment.

HOT OIL TREATMENT

The care of the scalp must be considered as part of your complexion programme, for the scalp, like the skin on your face and body, can only be fed by the bloodstream. It is elementary knowledge that massage stimulates hair growth that thorough brushing twice daily is important even for a healthy scalp. If you can bring a warm rush of blood to the scalp, increased circulation will normalize an excessively dry, flaky or oily condition.

A hot oil treatment, the best method of stimulating scalp circulation, can be taken at home. Simply warm to body temperature a small amount of hair oil, olive oil or baby oil and, parting the hair off at one-half inch intervals, apply the oil to the scalp with a cotton pledget. Then take the fine end of your comb and comb the length of your hair from scalp to ends to ensure even distribution. Dip a bath towel in hot, steaming water, wring it out and wrap it around your head, allowing it to remain until tepid. Apply the hot towel four times. Then shampoo in the usual way.

After the oil treatment your head should be soaped and lathered thoroughly at least three times to remove all oil. Massage briskly, and use warm water. Rinse in clear tepid water four times.

COLOUR CHANGES

Hair colouring is an integral part of your personality and hair-do. And just because nature blessed (or unblessed) you with the colour you now have is no reason to think that colour best for you. Often hair fades because of physical or acid conditions. And then, not to do something about it is to fail to make the most of your potentialities.

Maybe your hair needs only a good shampoo to bring out lovely highlights. Or a rinse.

Naturally, if you want to change the colour of your hair, a rinse is not enough and at this point you should have only the best expert advice available from a hairdresser in your locality. Remember this : Blonde or red hair does not go with all complexions, and in such cases shades of brown may be preferable.

There is a new attitude to-day about grey hair. Women are less and less inclined to touch it up because they know that natural hair is more becoming. However, there are many good tints and rinses on the market which wash off with each shampoo. This is a personal problem to be decided by you and a good hairdresser or specialist.

Vigorous brushing is, of course, important to keep hair healthy and lustrous. Brush it conscientiously every day, from the scalp to the very ends—and let the bristles of the brush touch the scalp to rouse circulation.

KEEP WHITE HAIR WHITE

There is no longer any need to have drab looking or yellowish grey hair. Hair cosmetics have made great strides recently, especially in the field of colour rinses.

A rinse is not a dye. It washes out at each shampooing. When used properly it brings out highlights and adds lustre as well as a little colour.

A blueing rinse is recommended for white or greying hair.

The blueing you buy at your chemists usually comes in powdered form and is diluted with water before use.

The colour that goes into your hair is controlled by the amount of water you use—more water for a milder blueing, less water for a stronger solution. A lighter tone is usually recommended on white hair ; a darker tone on grey hair.

Several shades of rinses come under the heading of blueing. For white hair, a platinum, light blue or violet shade will neutralise yellow streaks and make your hair look still whiter.

A steel-blue rinse will blend the colouring of grey hair more evenly.

It is, however, much better and wiser to leave the application of tints and dyes to a skilled hairdresser. But if you do decide to treat your hair at home, to get the best results from your rinse you must, of course, first shampoo your hair thoroughly.

Apply the shampoo and work up a lather. Rinse and apply more shampoo. Manipulate the shampoo through the hair at least five minutes and then rinse thoroughly with water. This last water rinse is very important, for it must remove all soap so that no film is left on the hair.

Then apply the colour rinse, preferably with a small brush. Part your hair down the centre of the head, then dip the brush in the rinse solution and brush it up from the roots halfway to the ends of your hair. (Hair ends are usually porous and take on the colour faster than the rest of the hair, so in order to keep the rinse application even leave the ends till last). Part the hair again about one-quarter of an inch from the first part and repeat this process until you have covered your whole head. Then run your comb through your hair down to the ends.

Dilute the unused portion of the rinse with water and pour it on your hair. Leave it on for a few minutes, then rinse with clear water.

Apply a cream hair dressing for that final shiny, well-groomed look.

TIP ON TINTING

Nowadays, many women consider a hair tint as much a cosmetic as powder. They see no reason for having drab hair any more than they want drab faces.

If you're thinking of changing the colour of your hair, it is usually best to go to a salon—at least for the initial tint. The hairdresser should give you a patch test for allergies, and she should help you choose a shade most becoming to you.

If it is grey hair you want to cover, make sure to pick the right colour. Many women think they should match their original hair colour. That's not always wise.

If you're 10-20 per cent. grey you should choose a colour three shades lighter than your own hair. This will blend in with the grey hair, but won't add too much colour to your original hair shade. Adding more colour to the part that isn't grey would make your hair too dark.

If your hair is 20-50 per cent. grey choose a colour two shades lighter—because you have more grey hair to colour, less that will turn darker.

For hair over 50 per cent. grey, choose a colour to match your own hair. Apply tint to greyest portion first.

If you want to do your own touch-ups where your hair has grown out, note these points.

1. Tints work faster in a warm room than in a cold one.

2. Your touch-up should not take longer than 12 minutes to apply. Use toothbrush or a cotton swabstick for application.

3. Count your application time in with the over-all time. If you're going to leave your tint on 30 minutes, remember 12 minutes have been used up.

4. If you change the type of tint you've been using, the old colouring should first be removed with a colour-removing substance.

5. Once a bottle of tint has been opened, it must be used up within four weeks or it will have lost its strength.

6. Hair does not need to be washed before a touch-up unless it is very dirty.

7. Retouch at least once a month.

8. Hair that has been newly permanently waved takes a tint faster. Therefore, dilute your mixture with an equal part of water.

Don't confuse bleaching and tinting. A bleach takes colour out of hair—makes hair lighter. A tint adds colour—makes hair darker.

For those who don't want to cover grey hair completely, there is a colour blender. The blender lightens your own hair a little and darkens the grey hair to a certain extent. The result is a blending of the two shades of hair, making the grey hair less noticeable.

PROFESSIONAL HAIR CARE

Do you ever wonder what the hairdresser who sets your hair and gives you permanents thinks of your hair?

You come in for a permanent. Of course you want the best permanent available. The latest contribution to *permanent* hair beauty is the *Superma* Tepid Machineless Wave. Yet if your hair has been neglected, is dry and brittle, sun-bleached and wind-whipped, do you listen when an honest outspoken hairdresser recommends several scalp treatments before the permanent wave? You know that no permanent can be better than the health of your hair.

Proper hair brushing is most important to hair elasticity, cleanliness and polish. Your excuse is that brushing makes your hair split. But do you take your hairdresser's advice about getting a softer-bristled brush, which will allow the brushed strands to spring back into place?

Many hairdressers, if you ask them, will tell you that your hair can be re-set and arranged just as neatly without the water shampoo and the electric dryer, if you will just give them a chance.

Come in for a weekly set, certainly. But instead of allowing the hairdresser to wash out the natural hair oils each time, let her give you a " waterless shampoo " with a cleansing lotion and have her brush your hair clean.

The lotion leaves just enough moisture for setting the hair. At most, you'd need five minutes under the dryer before combing it out.

A special hair tonic for extra-oily hair, rather than constant shampooing, gives best results, we are told. The oil glands should be relaxed and treated instead of stimulated.

Your hairdresser should know these various methods of treating hair. Go to her for advice. Consider her suggestions fairly. Give her co-operation in caring for your hair.

PREPARE FOR PERMANENT

We all know that the condition of your hair has a great deal to do with the success or failure of your new permanent wave. So about a month before your date with the hairdresser, work at putting your hair into tip-top condition and health.

Keep your hair especially clean during this period. Shampoo weekly—two sudsings—each time. For stimulation and more thorough cleansing use a small brush.

When your hair and scalp are clean, massage with a little oil, especially into the dry tips of the hair, to banish any brittleness. And the day before the permanent rub in the oil and leave it on the hair overnight for final conditioning.

Protect the sheets and pillow slips on your bed by putting a towel around your head. Next day have the "permanent" and feel assured that you'll get the best possible results and a head of hair that's healthy, alive and shiny.

A new thrill . . . a new pleasure awaits you at your Hairdressers if you ask for and gently insist on a *Superma Machineless Tepid Wave*, the new professional " permanent " destined to charm feminine hearts. Its cool comfort will delight you ; its soft natural beauty will evoke envious admiration and its easy-to-manage responsiveness will give you many months of lasting hair beauty.

ARTISTIC HAIR STYLING

Hair styling as an art has much in common with sculpturing, it seems to me, for the inspired coiffeur must outline and balance his creation as skilfully as the sculptor.

Are you broad-hipped, narrow-shouldered ? Then never, never, style your hair high so that you look like a triangle. Are you petite and dainty ? Keep your hair in character. Consider the hairline and the set of the ears. Make the most of interesting points and peaks. An irregularity, properly handled, may become an asset. Try the part in various places, none of which needs to be orthodox.

Most important of all, let your coiffure express your personality. Gay ? Curls perhaps. Serious ? A more formal hair-style. Sophisticated ? Make it severe. What is your occupation—housewife, office or factory worker, politician, film star ? Whom are you trying to please—the mirror, the neighbours, your husband ?

ROLL YOUR OWN CURLS

Rolling your hair up in curls is a nightly beauty routine in homes all over the country, for most women realise they look much better with a well-placed curl.

There are two general methods of placing that curl—the roll-it-up-in-a-curler method and the pin curl. Each gives good results if you know which to use for which hair style. Generally, curlers give a tighter curl, pin curls a more natural wave.

There are certain " do's " and " don'ts " to using curlers properly. For instance, don't roll up your hair when it is dripping wet. The curls will be too tight.

Part your hair off in sections and make sure you place the curler at the tip of the strand of hair. To do this, start with the curler mid-way on the strand of hair and push it down to the tip. The reason you roll from the very tip is to avoid " fishhooks."

Using a " rat-tailed " comb, tuck in all stray ends around the curler as you wind up the hair. Wisps of hair sticking out here and there do not make for a neat coiffure.

Roll loosely to avoid any frizzing.

Now, if you wish to make pin curls the hair may be somewhat damper than for curlers.

In making pin curls it is important to divide the hair into smaller sections than you do when using curlers. The strands of hair to be used for the curls must be uniform in size, and each strand must be cleanly separated from the rest of the hair.

You can make natural looking waves with pin curls if you start each curl near the scalp and wind in ribbon-like fashion. By that I mean wind the hair around the finger without twisting or turning the strand.

Roll each curl with the hair ends in the centre. Don't let stray ends stick out.

Pin each curl close to the head, not on top of the next strand you must pick up to form another curl.

Pin each curl carefully so as not to spoil its roundness.

And for best results all the curls in one row should face the same way—in the direction you want the hair to go when you comb it out.

Curls can be held in place with one bobby pin or two hairpins. Naturally, if you take thick strands of hair you may need more pins to hold the curls. If you plan to sleep on the pin curls, bobby pins probably will hold more securely.

Everyone's hair reacts differently and almost everyone has a different idea of the degree of curl she wants. Therefore, the way you put up your hair depend on the effect you're after, and the only way to learn which method is best for you is by experimentation. Try both methods before you decide.

Begin your combing-out technique by combing hair in the direction in which it's been set, section by section. Then brush to remove the stiff " set " look. This helps your curls fall naturally in position. Use both your brush and your fingers to swirl your hair into place. For a finishing glamour touch, spray your hair with a little of your favourite perfume.

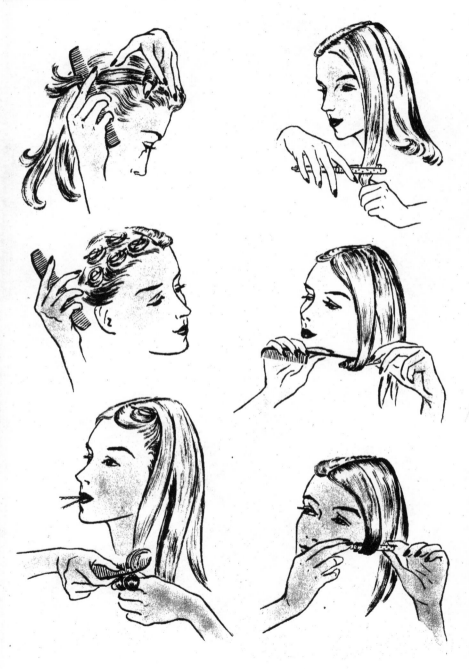

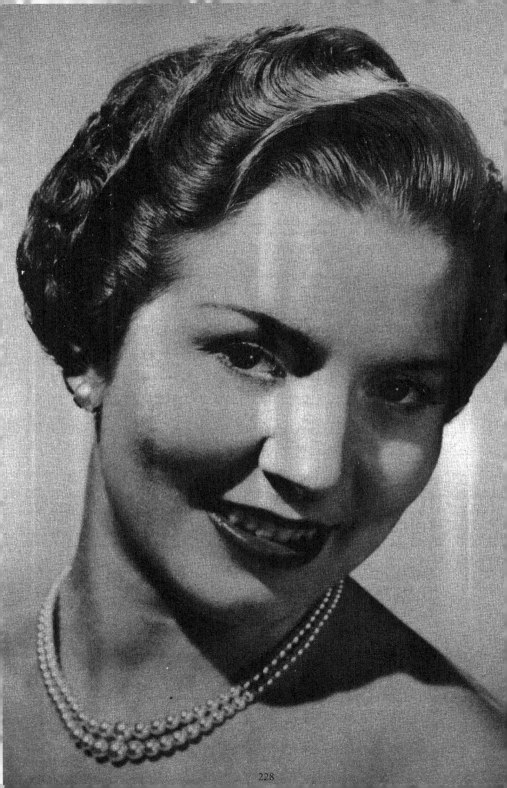

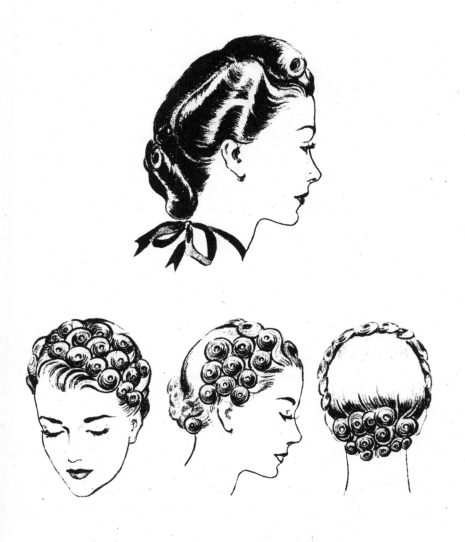

SAMPLE SETTINGS

To look especially smart for that big date or for just everyday wear, here are easy hair settings of pin curls that won't take much of your time. Simply use these sketches as guides, following the direction of the pin curls in setting them. Comb your hair carefully and you will be amazed at the expert hair-setting job you can do.

For longer hair, this setting will give pleasing results.

229

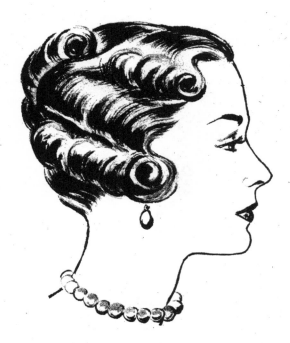

Try this different arrangement
for the short effect.

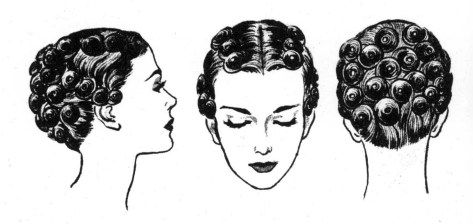

BETTER PROPORTIONS

Somewhere along the line we learn that everything is relative. Perhaps your house is considered large when compared with a tent, but it is small if compared with a skyscraper.

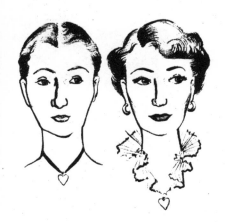

The same rule applies to good looks. A nose, for instance, is large only if the other features are small. But when you enlarge the other features by emphasising the eyes and embroidering on the mouth and fluffing the hair, the prominent nose recedes into better proportions. To emphasise the eyes use eye-shadow and mascara. To give the mouth a better outline use a lip pencil or brush.

Too-large ears can be treated in a similar way. You can, of course, cover the ears entirely with hair or you can enlarge the surrounding features, especially the hair, add big earrings and thereby push the ears into the background.

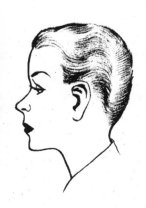
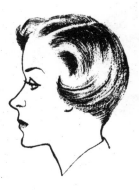
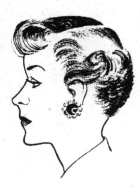

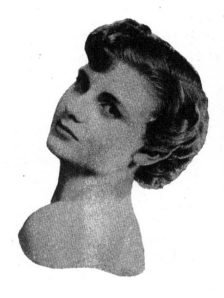

The perfect face is oval in shape, but who's perfect ? Those of us who aren't can disguise our feature faults with clever hair arrangements. Take the long, narrow face at right, the hair puffed out at sides gives width to the face.

A very practical modern coiffure which can be easily and readily converted to evening wear. The large downward wave over the ear terminates in springy curls at the back. The front portion is dressed low on the forehead to form a pleasing fringe.

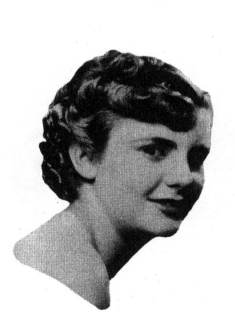

In many instances, curls give you the needed height. You can vary this style by letting the back hair down into a chignon or pageboy.

Note the forward loosely waved curl which dips over the forehead giving a pleasing frontal movement. An array of curls dressed high preserves shape and balance. A coiffure eminently suitable for one in the early twenties.

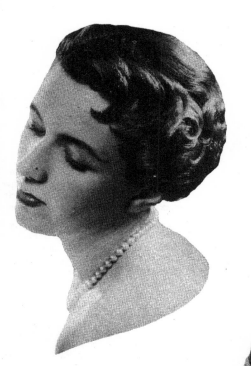

A modern version of the "flicked curl" front with a triangle parting on the right.

Back view of the dressing above. The sides are taken back and the back set in loose curls lightly brushed out.

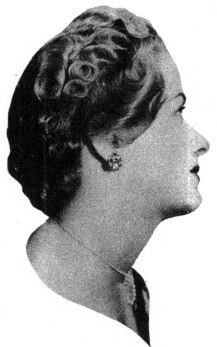

For wide cheekbones and narrow forehead and chin, wear a hair-do that will give you width in the places needed. At left is a suggestion that may solve the problem.

This style designed for evening wear or for special occasions. The coiffure shows a combination of waves and curls interspersed to give an unusual movement where the hair partly covers the right ear.

This photo shows a pompadour style of dressing, with the sides waved back, and dressed loosely out in curls to the nape of the neck, giving a shingle effect.

This is an example of the side effect.

Young women, especially those with natural curls, often prefer the efficiency of a short hair-do.

At right is the basic line.

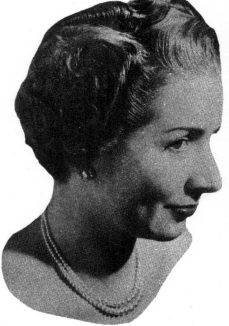

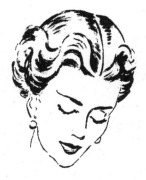

There are many ways to wear this basic style. For instance, parted in the middle and waved back as shown above.

For those who prefer even shorter hair—here are two versions : one swept upward, the other smoothed down.

Bangs are everywhere.
There are side bangs moving off the face and bangs turned the other way.

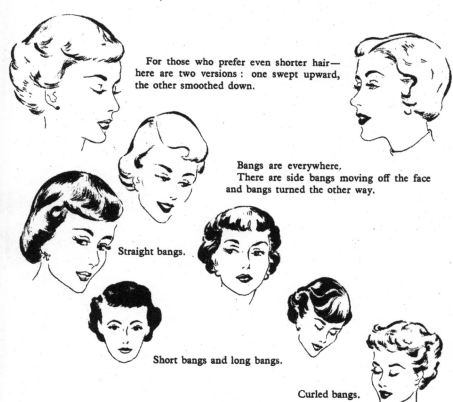

Straight bangs.

Short bangs and long bangs.

Curled bangs.

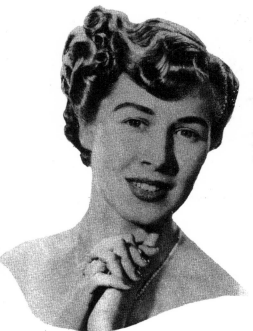

This dressing makes an ideal style for the woman with a high, wide forehead.

Note the unusual treatment of the curls dressed high on the left side and the smoothly waved front section dipping low on the forehead.

Shows the reverse side to the dressing illustrated above. A large wide wave sweeps down from the parting and is merged into a soft cluster of curls at the back.

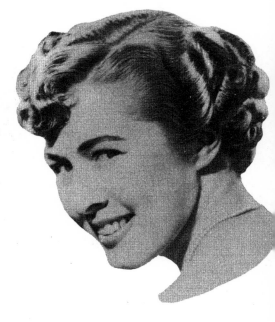

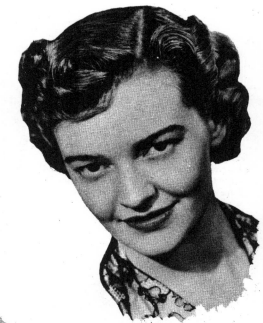

A more formal style suitable for both day or evening wear. The accent here is on the softly waved " bang " or fringe which can be brought forward on to the forehead, as shown, or brushed into a backward wave. The sides are swept back in waves to meet a softly curled back.

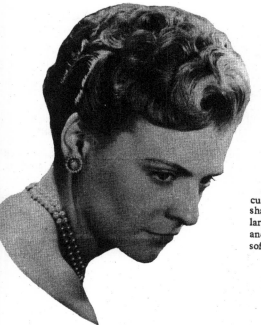

A practical interpretation of the " poodle " cut which depends largely on its cutting and shaping to achieve balanced beauty. The large curl over the forehead is loosely dressed and merged into the deep waves to give softness to the front hairline.

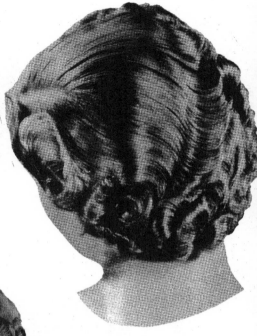

A medium short hair style, easily manageable, for the out-door or sport-loving girl. A simple yet practical dressing that will stand a good deal of brushing and yet retain its shape with very little bother or trouble.

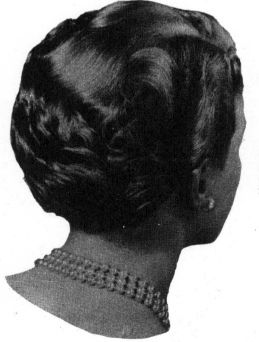

Back view of a modern dressing, distinctive in design yet easy to manage. Note the wide smooth wave swirling over the right ear, and also the back of the head dressed out in feathered curls. A style much in favour to-day.

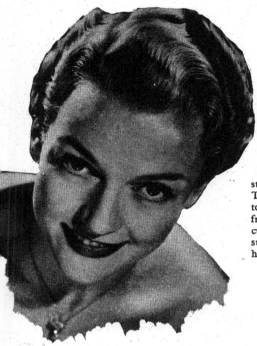

For the woman with a low forehead, this style is again both pleasing and practical. The dressing from the parting sweeps towards the back in large deep waves and from the crown to the nape is set in loose curls. Easy to keep neat and smart, yet ideally suited for the busy business woman or housewife.

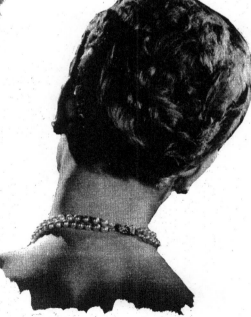

The dressing showing the back view of a head is set clock and anti-clock wise. The lines travel upward at back and sides, concentrating on the crown of the head. The hair is brushed out thoroughly to complete a practical yet pleasing dressing.

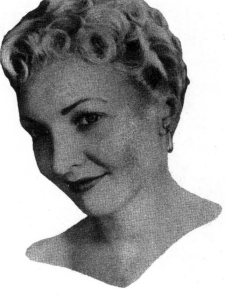

The four illustrations on this and the opposite page show four separate views of the same hair style on the same model, thus giving a complete dressing from all angles. They depict a modern, casual, elegant style.

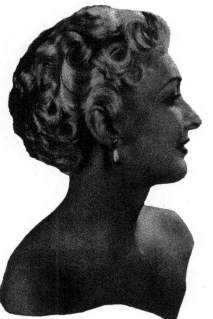

Here is seen the right side-view with curls all over, natural-looking but smart.

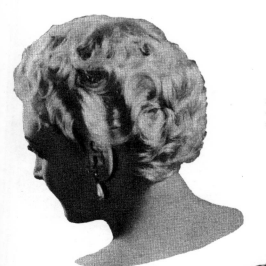

The top is kept fairly low. The front is set in loosely-waved curls which are carried on all over the head to the back by brushing, as shown here.

The left view is as attractive and smart as all other angles of this complete and modern dressing. This is a coiffure that is easily adaptable to various styles of hair to suit different types of people. The method of brushing is important.

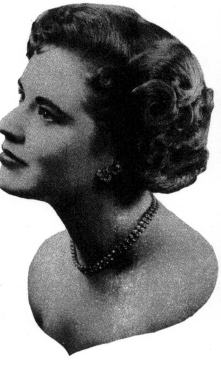

This is the very latest style and is considered by women who have seen it, to be a very lovely style. Hair all over is of even length, about 2 inches, with a flat crown and the sides dressed out with large movements and dressed back. The hair in the nape of the neck is also loosely brushed out.

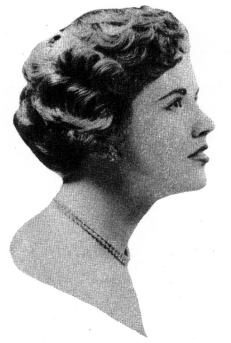

These two photos show different views of the same hair style on the same model. Note the complete difference in the two sides which is partly what adds to the attraction of this new style called the ALEXANDRA Style. They might be dressed out on two different models.

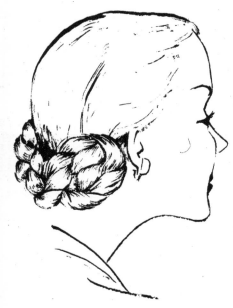

Simple but effective, the chignon braid can lend distinction to very plain and otherwise unattractive hair. As illustrated here, it makes an ideal career-girl special.

If you're not satisfied with your hair as it is, add a hair-piece. A good hair-piece is made of real human hair, most of which comes from the Balkans.

How successful is "artificial" hair to-day? That's up to you as a buyer. Be sure to have colour and texture matched exactly. A master blender can match it expertly, if he has a sample strand before him. Drab blonde is hardest to match.

White hair is rarest and most expensive, because such hair is usually too fine to be used in artificial hair-pieces.

Most switches have specially designed devices that pin them on to stay forever.

BACK TO BRAIDS

Artificial braids are versatile. They adapt to your way of life, your hat, the time of day, the nature, length and thickness of your hair—

possible combinations are numerous. As for style, look below :

Take good care of your braids. They need cleaning as often as your hair needs shampooing. And if hair is light, more often then when dark. At any rate, don't treat the braids like a hat which may not get cleaned for seasons on end.

" Artificial " hair should be dry-cleaned with a reputable dry-cleaning fluid, we are told by a well known manufacturer of hair-pieces. The braid should be opened, combed and then dipped into the solution. Dry-cleaning revives lustre. Tints should not be used.

Daily combing removes surface dust.

With proper care you should get good wear from " artificial " hair, though the actual life of a braid depends on the owner and how often it is worn.

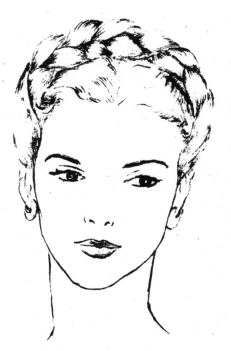

The classical halo braid is good almost any time. Longish faces, please note.

Self-Test Questions Based On Lesson Nine

Beautiful hair has always been of vital importance to women. Everyone to-day, with care and treatment, can acquire this asset to beauty and charm. By following the instructions in this Lesson you can be sure of more lustrous hair.

After you have studied this Lesson, you should be able to answer the following questions. If you have any difficulty in doing so, refer to the Lesson for further study and revision. Your answers should not be sent to the publishers of this Course.

1. What is the first essential if you wish to cultivate a beautiful head of hair?

2. Write here four important points to watch in your search for health and beautiful hair.

3. After attention to health what is the next most important matter to consider if you aim at beautiful hair?

4. What exactly must you do to carry out proper hair care?

5. What MUST you do every day to keep your hair healthy and lustrous?

6. Write a short account of the preparation you should give to your hair, if you decide to have a permanent wave.

7. Write down four causes of dry and brittle hair.

8. Have you found the hair style which suits your face and personality? Study the examples given in the Lesson.

9. Describe briefly how to make pin curls.

10. In what way should you comb your hair after setting?

If you wish to determine the progress you are making, give yourself 10 points for each question you answer correctly. If the total comes to 90 or more, it is excellent; 80 or more, good; 70 or more, fair.

The illustrations shown on pages 12, 16, 17, 18, 19, 20, 21, 22, 23, 24, 25 *and* 26 *are reproduced by courtesy of Superma Ltd., Originators of the Machineless Wave.*

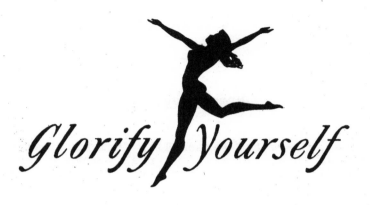

Glorify Yourself

★

A Complete and Up-to-Date Course on
Beauty and Charm by One of the
Most Famous Beauty Specialists
and Consultants in the World

★

LESSON TEN

by

Sally Young

★

STUDIO TALK •

Issued only for Student
of the Eleanore King
Course on Beauty. Charm
and Personality.

Number Ten.

Dear Student,

Beauty, Charm and Personality form an ideal at
which every woman should aim. I really mean every
woman - including those over forty - including mothers
and mothers-to-be!

That is why I have called Part A of this Lesson
"Life Begins at 40", and why it includes a number of
simple, health-giving postural exercises, grouped
together under the title "Be a Model Mother".

Of course, you are still advised to do these
even if you are in your teens or if you are a career girl.
They are guaranteed to improve the posture of all women;
and if they are practised regularly they will give you
a tingling, vital glow of good health.

Part B is entitled "Seasonal Advice". The
information it gives will help you to be cool in summer,
warm in winter and poised and attractive at all times.

There are even more hints and ideas in Part C,
including a specially useful section on etiquette. This
section should preferably be studied in conjunction with
Lesson Seven, to which it forms a particularly valuable
supplement.

Part D of Lesson Ten shows how you can safeguard
two important, but often overlooked beauty assets - the
hands and feet. It has been said that a woman's hands
are more revealing than her face. Certainly, they come
under constant scrutiny, and they can help to express
your personality. So here are ten simple exercises for
hand grace which will yield rich dividends if you
practise them regularly in your spare moments. You will
learn, too, how the proper care of your feet can safeguard
their health and beauty.

Yours sincerely,

Eleanore King

EK.10.

LESSON TEN
Part A
Life Begins At Forty

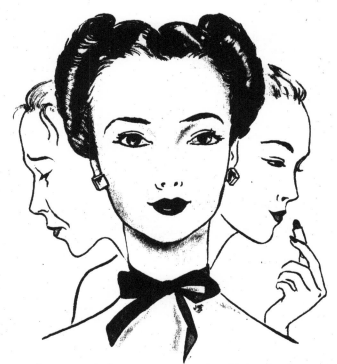

Poise seems to be even more important to charm in a woman of forty and over than for her younger sister.

Serenity is primarily a state of mind, but the body, too, needs to be relaxed. These exercises will help you :

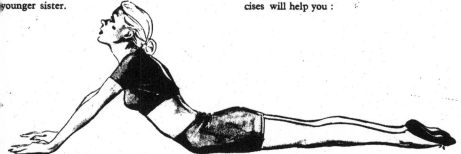

1. Stretch, keeping elbows straight, push the torso from the floor.

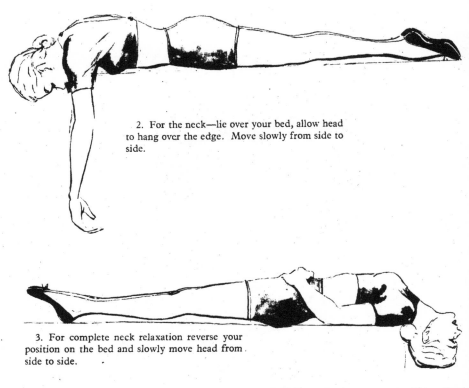

2. For the neck—lie over your bed, allow head to hang over the edge. Move slowly from side to side.

3. For complete neck relaxation reverse your position on the bed and slowly move head from side to side.

4. Relax and rejuvenate yourself by allowing the blood to flow to your head. Lie on the floor, on your bed or on a couch with your feet higher than your head. Relax at least fifteen minutes a day.

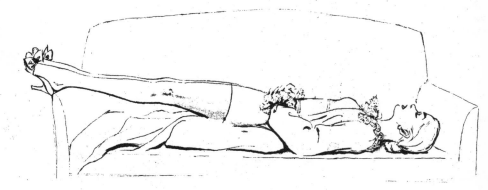

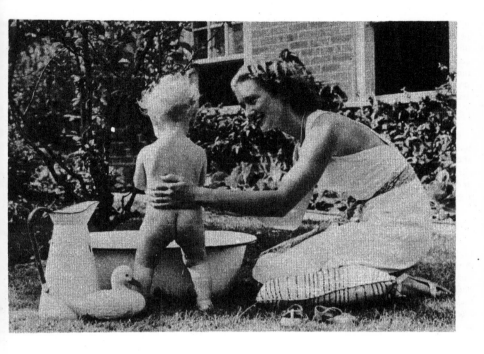

Photograph 16. Be a Model Mother

Do you know that motherhood can improve he average woman's figure ? Physicians have ound that if an expectant mother wears a properly fitted and scientifically designed oundation garment, follows dietary instructions nd gets a normal amount of exercise, the xperience should not leave her any the less ttractive in appearance.

Many obstetricians recommend maternity orsets for the control of abdominal muscles and or back support. You may need this aid for proper body balance. It takes balance, you know, o rest the weight of the child in the pelvic basin /ith a minimum of strain on you.

If a maternity girdle or corset is worn, it should be put on early in pregnancy, so that ab-dominal muscles will not over-strain.

Designers in the foundation-garment industry, with the co-operation and assistance of leading obstetricians, have created a variety of scientific maternity garments for to-day's expectant mother. They include the all-in-one as well as separate girdles and brassieres.

Their construction varies ; many are not unlike ordinary foundation garments in appear-ance, while others are constructed with lacings in the back or at the side, or both, depending upon the figure requirements.

No one type of garment will be equally suitable in all cases, since figure needs vary greatly. Extreme care should be taken in the selection of a maternity garment. It should be fitted by a specialist, guided by advice from the physician handling the case. Changes in the condition of the mother-to-be usually require monthly adjustments by the corsetiere to keep the child's weight balanced properly in the pelvic basin.

Well-designed maternity foundation garments build a wall around the pelvis and support the abdomen without compression at any point, give aid to the lower spine and muscles of the back and thighs. This relieves the strain on the neck, legs and feet.

Care of the figure after delivery of the child is highly important too and should not be neglected. A woman's welfare depends on adequate protection of weakened muscles for many weeks. Frequently a mother may wish to have her maternity garment adjusted to fit her figure after the birth of her child. This arrangement has proved satisfactory in certain cases.

However, gynaecologists often recommend a different type of support after childbirth to protect the walls of the abdomen, which tend to relax for a period of at least eight to ten weeks. Once the mother is on her feet, it is important that she have a properly-fitted support to aid the abdomen and steady and protect, but not compress, the pelvic joints.

Following this period, she should then return to her regular foundation-garment wardrobe.

When Baby Dear has left you for the pram, you can't wait to try on your pre-baby size dresses. Do they fit ? Or does the zipper strain at the waistline ? Before you go into an emotional tailspin over your ruined figure, remember it took months to stretch. Be patient in reshaping it. If you didn't start exercising before baby came, lose no more time (unless, of course, your doctor has advised against it for some special reason).

If your doctor hasn't outlined your post-natal exercises for you, here are are some that will do the trick.

1. TORSO LIFT : Sit up, arms out in front, toes pointed. Lie down. Repeat these exercises 15 times for 15 minutes a day.

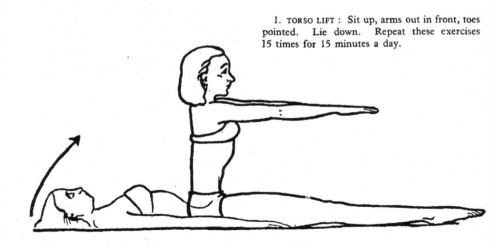

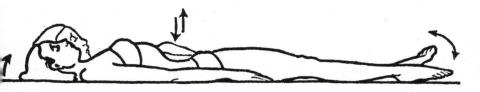

2. HEAD LIFT : This exercises the *rectus abdominis*, the long vertical muscle which spreads apart during the bulge growth. This muscle needs attention for six months or so to bring it back to perfection again.

TUMMY PUSH-UP : Breathe deeply with your diaphragm.

FOOT WIGGLE : This helps leg circulation.

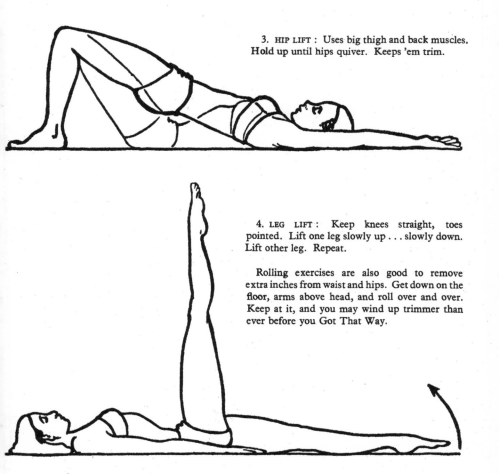

3. HIP LIFT : Uses big thigh and back muscles. Hold up until hips quiver. Keeps 'em trim.

4. LEG LIFT : Keep knees straight, toes pointed. Lift one leg slowly up . . . slowly down. Lift other leg. Repeat.

Rolling exercises are also good to remove extra inches from waist and hips. Get down on the floor, arms above head, and roll over and over. Keep at it, and you may wind up trimmer than ever before you Got That Way.

LESSON TEN

Part B

Seasonal Advice

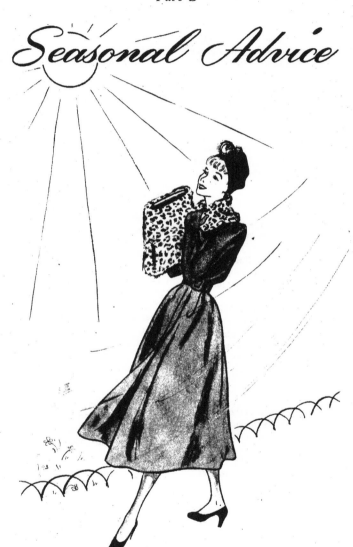

LOOK TOWARD SPRING

When spring stares you in the face, is your face ready to stand the scrutiny? Or have you had such a strenuous winter that your energy is at low ebb, with the result that your complexion looks drab and sallow?

255

Perhaps your face needs a spring cleaning. A soap-and-water washing isn't enough. You've got to scrub, and a friction wash or mealy beauty grains are a good thing to scrub with. Make the scrubbing work for you. Stimulate circulation, wash away dead cuticle, banish winter from your face.

Follow the washing with an application of cream to soothe, protect and beautify.

Now is the time to rouse and stimulate your circulation, that complex and wonderful process that goes on just beneath your skin surface. An effective way of doing this is to apply a beauty mask. You simply stroke on this cooling substance and lie down for twenty minutes' relaxation while it does its work.

MAKE-UP

Spring make-up, as you know, is subtler and more feminine. Faces should be made to look younger.

If the skin itself is clear and translucent, as it will be if you give it proper care, make-up is no problem. The soft dewy-fresh, Dresden look is what you want.

Soft shades of true red and pink, delicate shades in face powder, with rouge ever so carefully blended to simulate natural colouring, will help give you the pretty-lady look with which to greet the new season.

Refer to Lesson Two for advice on make-up.

SUMMER BEAUTY

In summer your hair style should be the utmost in simplicity. A sleek line looks cooler, is less trouble to keep neat. Short-cuts couldn't be more tailor-made for summer.

If your hair is long, there are still cooling devices at your command. Try a smooth roll, braid or neat ringlets atop of your head. If you prefer your hair worn severely drawn back and away from your face, anchor your mane at the nape of your neck with a colourful ribbon, barrette or flower and bobby pins. Refer back to Lesson Seven for further ideas on hair styles.

There is nothing so warm-appearing as a gleaming face with smeared make-up : so watch it. If your skin has a tendency to be oily, wash your face at every chance. Plenty of soap and water is needed, followed by an application of a skin astringent to tighten the pores. Instead of leaving face cream on overnight, wear it during your bath and wash it away with skin freshener or water afterward.

Lighten your application of make-up in summer, else a pasty look will result. Change make-up more often, too. Whisk off the old with soap and water or special tissue or pads that remove dirt and shine. Try gossamer-light liquid foundations, or airy cream foundations and a light coating of powder. Refer to Lesson Two.

If your skin is sun-tanned, accent eyes and mouth : otherwise your features would blend together without distinction.

Mascara should be " double-brushed " (first, when applied, then with a dry brush to remove clotted mascara). Lipstick application must be checked and double-checked. On with your first coat, then a dusting of face powder. Another application of lipstick, a blotting with face tissue and you have the perfect, longer-lasting lip outline.

Cool blue or green eyeshadow is especially right for summer and extra care should be taken in application to prevent " melting eyelids " after two hours in the sun or heat.

One trick to keep make-up looking fresh longer is to apply foundation and powder ; then splash cold water on your face to " set " the make-up. Or, if you like, spray on a mist of your favourite Cologne with an atomizer.

Make-up colours in lipstick and rouge should be on the true red, coral or pink side to give anyone that " sea breeze " feeling on beholding you. Purples and oranges are definitely not wanted in midsummer.

Deep tan, rose-tan or any of the tawny shades are preferred in foundations and powders for girls with a tan.

HOW TO KEEP COOL.

Cool, calm and collected—with the emphasis on cool—that's the way we should all look on a hot summer's day.

And you won't get that way by taking a cold bath. Far from it. However, there are definite measures to take to look and feel cool.

Start with the inner woman. Watch your diet and concentrate on " cool " food. Mixed salad greens with thin dressing, raw vegetables, fruit and vegetable juices, meat and fish and jellied consommés are all steps in the direction of keeping cool in summer-time.

Take cool or tepid baths. Pat, don't rub, yourself dry, with a thick towel. Then apply your favourite underarm deodorant and splash a flower-scented Cologne or toilet water over your body. And last, powder-puff yourself completely dry with a silky afterbath powder.

Talcum, incidentally, is a wonderful preamble to donning your girdle in summer. Makes it slide on without tugging or puffing.

In the interest of daintiness and comfort, change under-garments often. Though light stockings, leg make-up or have tanned legs. Looking neat is part of the art of keeping cool.

A touch of Cologne is a quick refresher when you're away from home and can't indulge in a cooling bath. Dab it on the wrists, inner elbows, the back of the neck and under the chin. Fragrant sachets can be used to advantage tucked inside the neckline of your dress, clipped to your lingerie, pinned to the lining of your bag or simply smoothed on your wrists, arms and palms of your hands. Several two-minute refresher

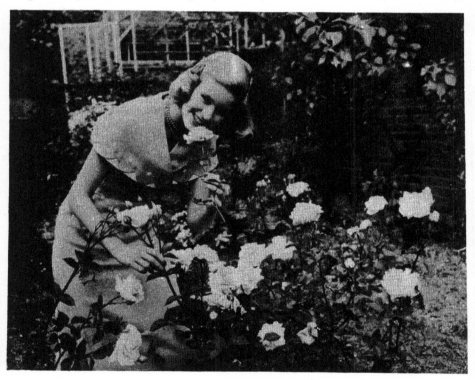

Photograph 17. Looking neat is part of the art of keeping cool

weight, your summer foundations need frequent and thorough washing.

Summer heat becomes almost unbearable if feet hurt and swell, so remember to shake foot powder into your shoes. Treat feet to a soapy foot bath at the end of the day to take down any swelling. Then soothe feet by massaging them with foot lotion.

Keep legs fuzz-free whether you wear periods a day are a good idea for summer.

Cologne as a refresher is especially effective around the hairline and the nape of the neck. Use a handy cotton square saturated with the essence. Squeeze it until there is just enough moisture to cleanse and refresh the skin. Your hair will remain sweet and fragrant and you will look and feel as cool as a lettuce leaf.

Try the two-minute refresher on your arms

and, when you are not wearing stockings, in the curve at the back of the knee. Always pat gently and leisurely.

The colour and fabric of your clothes are important in attaining the cool look. It goes without saying that clothes should be freshly laundered, loose fitting, crisp looking. Shy away from reds and oranges ; instead try green, lavender, grey, beige, turquoise, lemon yellow, blue, and, of course, white.

Your hair requires more attention in summer. so surely turns a permanent wave into a frizzy failure as continued neglect of " holiday hair." Try to restore its resilience by scheduling shampoos at longer intervals than ordinarily. Between shampoos, use a special preparation to cleanse scalp pores of dust, oily deposits and flaked-off scalp tissue—so that the oil glands won't be blocked.

On alternate days, depending on your particular problem, apply a preparation for dry or a preparation for oily hair, parting the hair strands

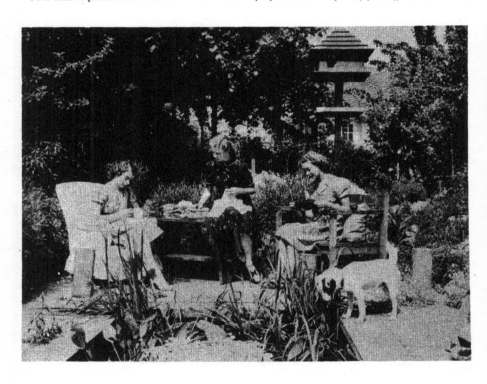

Photograph 18. Cool, calm and collected. Try to be occupied but unhurried on a hot day

Protect it from the sun to prevent drying and discoloration ; hair oil or a light hair cream will shield your locks from the sun's rays. Your scalp perspires, too, so shampoo locks more frequently in hot weather. Regular brushing helps keep it clean and manageable and gives emphasis to highlights.

If yours is sunburned, over-exposed hair, start some intensive remedial treatments. Nothing so that the entire scalp may be reached with a bit of cotton, moistened in the corrective lotion.

Rub the hair dry, lightly, with a soft, lintless towel ; then finish by brushing.

Just before your permanent (home or salon) give your hair the benefit of a rich, protective cream hair pack or a special-purpose permanent wave shampoo that lends hair a safety margin against drying effects.

If your hair remains dry or seems drier still after the permanent, be sure to take every precaution against emphasizing the scalp's lack of natural oils. Set waves and curls with a solid brilliantine-type cream, which should also be used daily as a hair dressing or make-up for dry, brittle, split hair ends.

SUMMER FOOT COMFORT

Summer months are foot-discomfort months. Feet tend to swell, perspire, ache and burn. What can be done to make them comfortable at this time of the year ?

First of all, wear shoes and stockings which fit your feet. Shoes should allow for foot expansion. Shoes which create pressure points and cause corns and bunions are too short, too narrow or otherwise ill-fitted. Remember, a shoe has to carry you !

Wear Oxfords, high-cut pumps or closed back sandals with Cuban heels most of the time. The heel counter of the shoe should enclose the heel snugly and comfortably. Half the hot pavement battle is won when you wear the proper shoes. Check your stockings, too. Toes must have sufficient wiggle room at all times.

MASSAGE : Oil, bathe, brush and massage the feet daily. First soak them in an antiseptic foot bath. Using a stiff-bristled brush, scrub thoroughly, especially hard-skinned areas. Dry feet briskly and thoroughly.

Apply a foot massage cream between the toes, along the foot and sole, and around the ankle with firm strokes.

1. Bend one knee and grasp each toe between thumb and forefinger, rotate to right and then to left.

2. Curl the toes down with one hand, and massage deeply with the thumb of the other hand in continuous circular motion all along the base of your toes.

3. Place thumb and forefinger at top of toenail and massage between the toes, toward the base.

4. Place the fingers on the anklebone and massage around your ankle joint.

ON THE BEACH : When you are on the beach give your feet freedom and sunshine. Take off your shoes, walk on the sand barefooted.

Correct walking on the sand exercises and massages the muscles of feet and legs.

Walk erect with your feet parallel, shoulders well back, chin up and abdomen in ; first step

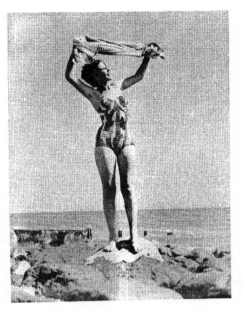

Freedom of movement on the beach is healthful
Photograph 19.

on your heel, roll to the outer side of your foot and thence across the ball to your big toe and roll back to your heel.

BEAUTY ON THE BEACH

In summer let's not stick our necks out nor our faces, arms, backs and legs, without proper protection. You can't get a deep tan in one day. So don't try. Tanning—the healthful kind—is a gradual process.

Basically, the whole process of acquiring a sun-tan is one of increasing the colouring element in each of the several layers of the skin. However, the skin, in addition to this pigmentation or darkening to protect its deeper layers, reacts further to protect itself by building a thicker, heavier layer of the outer skin.

To prevent this dry look, you should get yourself a sun-tan lotion or cream that filters out the short burning rays but admits the desirable tan-producing rays.

Your sun-filtering lotion or cream should be applied to all parts of your body not covered by clothing. It should be re-applied at short intervals or whenever the skin feels the slightest bit drawn, and again each time after you go

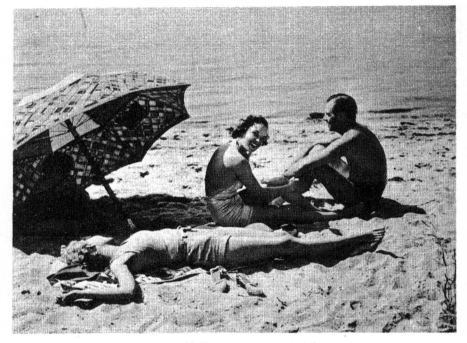

Photograph 20. Take care not to get too sunburnt.

swimming. After your day's sunbathing take a warm shower or bath. Dry thoroughly and re-apply the preparation, massaging it well into the skin.

Many people are under the false impression that dark-complexioned individuals are immune to sunburn. This is not true. No one is immune to sunburn. Dark-complexioned people often do show a characteristic tan colour very quickly or after very short periods of exposure. But this can be illusory, and a severe sunburn may still result.

While the extra pigmentation of dark-complexioned people protects the deeper layers of the skin, it does not protect the sensitive outer layers. This explains why the apparently well-tanned fellow often complains of painful sunburn. Without a dependable " filter " preparation to protect the sensitive outer layer anyone can, and will, burn.

BEACH MANNERS.

I'll admit it. I've been eavesdropping. The boys were discussing bathing " beauties," rather some of their glaring faults, and in the interests of womanhood I kept my ears unfurled. Like most eavesdroppers, I came away with a blushing brow and some very straightforward information.

What did the lads say? One of them said all women were silly on the beach. They come loaded down with sun hats, sun oils, sunglasses, blankets, lotions, combs, hairpins and anything else they can get some poor escort to carry for them. They spend their whole day in the good sunshine shying away from the sun. As for going for a swim—not these hothouse flowers !

Hefty legs came in for the most booing. Let them diet or exercise them away before displaying them, was the general opinion.

Next pet criticism was the extreme bathing suits on girls who had no business wearing them. In other words, let the "cuddly chicks" wear the next-to-nothing versions. The rest of us with merely passable figures, will look much better clad in a standard one-piece model that's not too short and not too flashy.

Ungainly beyond words, said one of our male gossips, are women wearing high heels with a bathing suit. That also goes for high heels with slacks But this objection is easily remedied.

Strangely enough, none of the boys minded the appearance of stringy wet hair after bathing. They thought it looked cute in a refreshing sort of way. Nevertheless, if your hair doesn't curl naturally after such a ducking, it's probably better up in braids. The boys all thought bathing caps were pretty sensible things to wear.

They were outspoken, too, about make-up on the beach—outspoken against it, I should say. A little lipstick of a light, bright shade was permissible, they felt, but none of this caked, heavy make-up. They want to see a girl looking fresh and dewy when she comes out of the briny deep—not with a plaster of Paris face.

A sun-tan rates "tops"—but not the peeling, lobster version. Even if the tan isn't dark, as long as the girl looks pink-cheeked and shiny-nosed and healthy, the boys are happy.

Another annoying thing about women on the beach—and you'd never guess this one, because it doesn't show on the surface—is the shouting and calling that travels back and forth over the sands. As one hoarse-voiced chap in the group put it, " I can take almost anything—fuzzy legs, tight bathing suits, sunburned noses—but deliver me from a screecher."

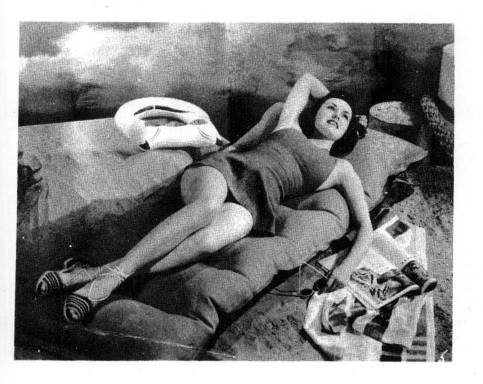

Photograph 21.   Beauty on the Beach.

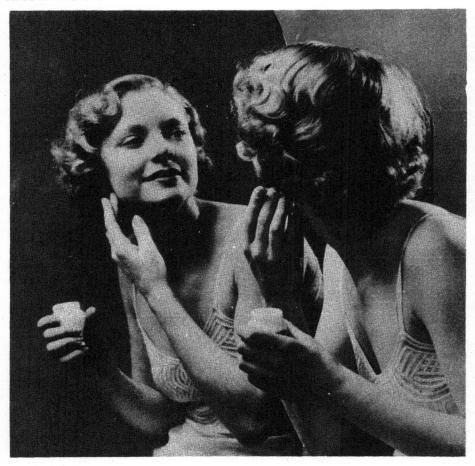

Photograph 22. Back to Peaches and Cream.

At the beginning of the summer season we always make good resolutions that this year we're not going to let our skin be turned to leather by sun and wind. But that was at the beginning of the season and here we are with lines around the eyes, furrows in the forehead, untanned rims on a tanned face.

Now what?

Let's start with a cleansing cream, which refreshes and lubricates the skin. Wipe away the cream and grime and repeat until your face is absolutely clean, then apply a skin lotion.

Or coax a blush into your cheeks with a heavy cream and small electric patter which works up circulation while you relax.

For daytime your complexion needs protection. Probably at this time you'll want something beneficial to dry skin, perhaps a creamy fluid make-up foundation, a light, sheer foundation which leaves a silky second skin on which to base your make-up. You need it to blend in untanned lines and further to protect your skin.

Naturally, dirty make-up will do more harm than good, so it is advisable to remove it midway during your day and re-do it.

Make-up removal during the day can be quite simple. Take out the cleansing cream again and the tissues. Follow up with a piece of cotton saturated with skin refresher. Go over your face thoroughly with upward strokes. Then you're ready for the new foundation and make-up.

If you follow this routine faithfully for a few weeks, you'll be ready to face the autumn and winter season with a shining pink-and-white complexion.

FACING WINTER WEATHER

There are several special skin-care rules for cold, blustery days.

Our great-grandmothers thought that taking a bath every day in winter was a risky procedure. Now we know that daily baths are essential. Regardless of temperature, baths may safely be taken just before going out provided they are taken correctly. That is in the following way :

Don't use water that is too hot. Extreme changes of temperature tend to make the skin chap and crack. Take a cleansing bath in comfortably warm water using plenty of soap. Rinse yourself well ; then take a cool-off shower or sponge yourself with tepid water.

If you prefer, an all-over massage with rubbing alcohol will serve the same purpose. Any one of these three methods will close the opened pores of your skin so that you will not be chilled when you go out.

Rub every single square inch of your body briskly with a turkish towel. Rub until the skin tingles and glows. If your face is extra sensitive—and many of us do have tender skin—then cover your cheeks with a very thin veil of wind-and-weather cream just before you leave the house. Most women find that a make-up base and make-up over it give protection against the weather.

If you feel chilly when you get home, take a nice warm bath to stimulate your circulation. Relax in rich soapsuds and find how wonderfully revived you feel.

Be sure to change and launder all your underwear frequently. A vast amount of perspiration is collected by clothing worn next to the skin even in cold weather. We dress for the cold outdoors and then sit in heated rooms, so naturally we perspire.

Especially in winter, proper washing and drying are important for hand health and beauty. After washing well with warm soapsuds, rinse your hands in clear, warm water and dry them carefully with a clean, soft towel. If your hands tend to chap, pat them dry against the towel instead of rubbing them dry. A protective layer of hand lotion or cream should be worn at all times. And never forget gloves—rubber gloves for housework, warm gloves for outdoors.

"WINTERIZE" YOUR FEET

As with clothing, men and women tend to confuse the weight of shoes with warmth, and believe that bulky coverings will somehow keep out cold.

During the winter it is very important to give your feet room to breathe, since impeded circulation will bring on chilblains. So be sure your shoes are of a size that fits the larger of your two feet (everyone has one foot bigger than the other, you know) and that your stockings are at least half an inch longer than your big toe.

As a general aid to winter comfort, leather shoes are best since they permit ventilation, doing away with cold, clammy feet that result if foot perspiration cannot evaporate.

The use of two pairs of socks instead of one extremely heavy pair is generally beneficial. A light-weight pair of cotton under woollen socks, or even cotton feet under nylon or silk, helps to keep the feet at an even temperature. When heavier shoes are worn out-of-doors they should be removed when coming into a warm room and a pair of dry shoes put on instead. Rubbers should never be worn indoors or in a warm bus, car or

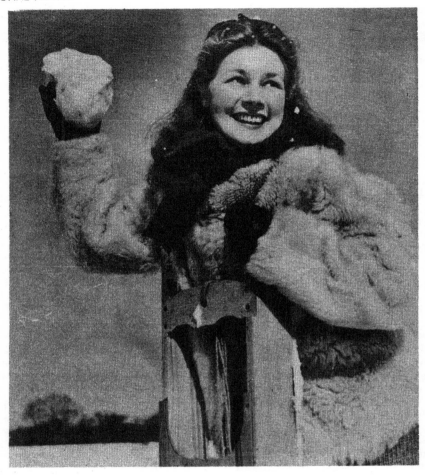

Photograph ... Facing Winter Weather.

train.

Make a habit of giving your feet plenty of exercise in winter. Even with your shoes on you can do some toe-wiggling and keep circulation moving.

Another winter complaint of many women is excessive dryness of the skin of the legs caused by icy winds. This "chapped" look shows up through sheer nylons and detracts from the well-dressed look.

Treatment of rough, raw and scaly legs is simple. It consists of rubbing lanolin or baby oil (which contains lanolin) on to the legs each night before bedtime. In stubborn cases the use of a hand-shower spray on the legs has been found to be of immense benefit. Spray the length of both legs from the thighs to the toes with comfortably hot water for about three minutes, then change to one minute of cold water.

If you're bothered by chapped skin around the heels of your feet, try applying a soft cream every night as a preventive. Don't forget your foot exercises such as toe-wiggling, foot-flexing and rubbing the soles of your feet briskly with a dry towel.

LESSON TEN

Part C

Hints and Ideas

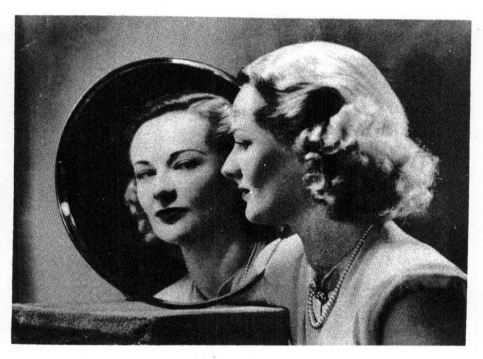

Photograph 24.   Analyse Yourself.

One of the most difficult things for a woman to do is to see herself as others see her. No sooner has she decided on a new hair style than her husband says, " Why do you wear your hair like that ? I don't like it."

The poor, heckled wife looks into her mirror and what she sees doesn't displease her. Yet her husband gets a full view of her, whereas she can only see one side or section of herself. So she wonders, is he right or just awkward ? How is she to know the answer if the mirror won't tell her ?

A bright leading photographer has come up with a solution to the problem. She makes a business of arranging various hair styles and make-up on women, and photographing them from all angles—front, three-quarter, profile view and back view. In this way the camera can become the impartial arbitrator in any husband-and-wife dispute. What this smart photographer does in her studio in a professional way, you can simulate at home, with time and your own camera.

Naturally, you need a collaborator in this

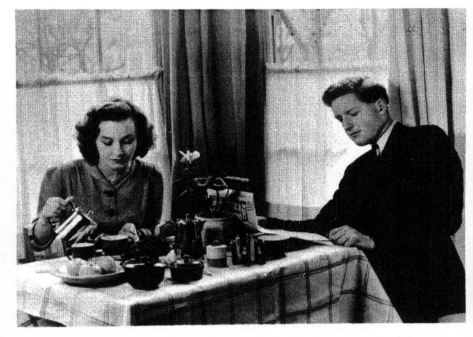

Photograph 25. Be Pretty at Breakfast.

beauty venture. If hubby won't help you out, why not get together with a friend or neighbour and do the analysing for each other? It's a profitable way to spend some quiet afternoon.

At the studio you are first photographed in your usual hair-do and make-up.

After all views are taken you are given a professional make-up. You are shown the best line for your lipstick, the proper application of rouge and eye shadow and the shape and intensity of eyebrows.

If you are doing this at home, you would naturally experiment with your own make-up. Draw your lipstick on in a new way, experiment with eye make-up.

At the studio you have your hair rearranged in several styles—perhaps one formal and one casual. In these you are again photographed from all angles.

At home you can go on indefinitely experimenting with hair lines and styles. Try putting the hair up, or back. Try parting it in the middle or in the back. Try buns, try curls, try it straight.

You can also experiment with necklines. Do you know whether a V-neckline looks better on you than a rounded one? The possibilities of photographic analysis are numerous.

The beauty of a photograph is that it is a lasting image to which you can refer when you want your hair arranged, not a mere fleeting memory of something you saw in the mirror.

We have no statistics on how many husbands rush off to a day's work without breakfast. But we'll bet we know who's to blame. His little helpmate—that glamour girl who became a scarecrow after he married her.

You can't blame the poor man for losing his appetite if he has to face a drab, sleepy-eyed, hair-in-curlers woman over the breakfast table. No secretary ever looks like that to him.

Of course you don't have to go to extremes in the other direction, like the bride who never removed her make-up until the lights were out and got up an hour before her husband awoke to have time for a complete make-up.

You can have your beauty treatments, without frightening your spouse out of the house. The trick's to do it when he's not around.

At night, certainly you must remove all make-up, but you don't have to go to bed with a repulsive face.

Then there are pin curls and curlers. They're necessary, quite true, but if you must wear all that metal work to bed wrap a piece of veiling turban-fashion around your head. Not only will you look pert and neat that way, but you'll save your bed linen from being torn.

There are other ways of putting up your hair that are not as short on glamour as is the usual hardware in your hair. You might try ribbon curlers, for example. With each ribbon a different colour they make for an attractive setting.

In the morning, get up a little ahead of time ; give yourself time to don a clean, unwrinkled morning coat or house-dress. Brush your teeth. Give your face a wake-up treatment. Brush out your curls, or retie the veiling, or straighten out the butterfly bows. And the least you do in the interests of a well-nourished husband is apply lipstick.

Fix a hearty breakfast. You'll find his appetite has suddenly improved.

SLEEP, MY LADY

Without a proper amount of sleep, no one can be healthy, and without health there's no beauty.

Experimenting with sleep, a certain physiologist found that lack of sleep affected his thirty-five subjects like strong drinks. After two nights without sleep, subjects' eyes were dry and irritated. They often saw double. There were deep circles under the eyes. Skin became parched-looking and gave way to wrinkles more easily. A general listless attitude, which even affected the hair, was noticeable.

In general, all subjects showed hyper-irritability and irascibility. Mild-mannered persons became ill-tempered. Hallucinations occurred. Co-ordination was seriously affected.

So you see, unless the required amount of sleep is obtained regularly, one's level of accomplishment is lowered, his lack of co-ordination makes him prone to accidents, his mental outlook and disposition are impaired, and his general state of health is affected.

In order to get the most benefit out of the hours devoted to sleep, the experts advise setting the stage with the most restful conditions possible.

First, have a comfortable bed. Muscle tension cannot be relaxed on a bed which sags or is lumpy. Proper rest depends to a great extent on level, resilient mattresses and springs which will properly support the head and neck muscles, as well as the entire body.

Second, don't worry. Train your mind to dwell on the pleasant things that have happened to you. Lock up uneasiness, anxiety and unpleasantness in an obscure corner of your brain once the lights are out. Save your problems until morning when you are refreshed and clear-headed—you'll find that the solutions will be more quickly and easily reached then.

Third, use sheets and blankets that are long enough, and learn to make a bed correctly, with hospital-style corners.

Fourth, don't wear tight, binding nightclothes.

Fifth, watch room temperature and ventilation. Cool air tends to deepen sleep, provided the feet and rest of the body are comfortably warm. Open windows at both top and bottom so that all the air in the room may be replaced at least eight times an hour, but guard against a draught if you've a cold. Place your bed so that you will not be in direct line of sudden cold blasts that may zoom into the room from time to time.

Sixth, open the windows on the darkest side of the house. Place your bed so that possible light from the outside will not stream in directly on your face or use a screen to deflect the light.

Seventh, minimise the noise element. Even slight sounds raise your blood pressure and affect the quality of your sleep.

Eighth, manage to work in some physical exercise during the day.

Ninth, indulge in a half-hour or so of mild recreation before bedtime.

Tenth, take a tepid—not hot—bath. Sitting in a bath of lukewarm water is delightfully relaxing.

What is real beauty without the final touch—etiquette ? Lovely as your voice, your carriage and make-up, your hair-do and figure and specially-selected wardrobe may be, they lack meaning without manners.

GUEST IN THE HOUSE

For instance, how are you as a hostess ? Do you greet your guests with genuine cordiality ?

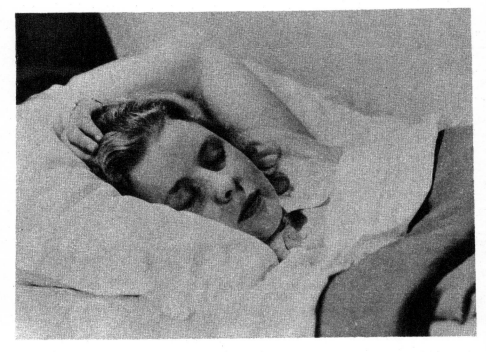

Photograph 26. Without a proper amount of sleep there is neither health nor beauty.

Do you make them feel at home ?

Manners are merely forethought. Are there plenty of towels in the bathroom, a face cloth, a new cake of soap for your guest ? An added nicety for the feminine guest would be a supply of bath salts, talcum powder, hand lotion, Cologne and similar toilet accessories.

The guest's bed should be comfortable, with clean sheets and pillow-cases, warm blankets. There should be a lamp of sufficient wattage for reading in the guest-room, with a plentiful supply of books and magazines. Plenty of hangers in the wardrobe are generally appreciated.

The perfect hostess respects the privacy of her guest, but informs him of entertainment possibilities if he cares to participate.

Now turn the tables. Suppose you're the guest. Good manners and good sense should tell you you'll be more popular if you cause as little work and trouble for your hostess as possible. It's always courteous to bring her a box of chocolates or flowers, or a basket of fruit or a book. If she has children, bring a toy or some small article for them.

Condense the amount of luggage you bring, both in quantity and size. A week-end case should be sufficient for a period of two or three days. Pack one or two hangers to keep your dresses neat and your hostess's room tidy.

The guest nobody ever invites again is the offender who " dog-ears " books, burns furniture with cigarettes, stands wet glasses on tables, leaves her room in cyclonic condition, is late for meals, leaves lipstick stains on napkins and towels, and so forth. A little consideration—another name for good manners—wouldn't let you do such things. The ideal guest is ready for anything—or nothing. She fits her life to the plans of her hostess.

If your hostess has no servants, don't burden her with extra duties. Keep your room in order and help out around the house. If she's fortunate enough to have a maid or domestic help, tip the maid for your week-end stay. Do the tipping privately before leaving the house.

If you're the guest at an evening party, always greet your hostess first. Here's how to enter a room : Pause imperceptibly on the threshold to get your bearings. Your hostess should come to meet you, but if she doesn't you go to her. Don't make the entrance a big stage production, but on the other hand don't rush headlong into the room, pausing in confusion later.

The well-mannered guest never becomes boisterous at a party. Though good-natured participation in the party activities is due to your hostess, you need never lose your poise.

Your good-bye should be as well planned as your entrance. You thank your hostess for the pleasant time you have had. Don't keep her standing in the open doorway while you think of last-minute chit-chat. Be off with you.

OFFICE ETIQUETTE

There's more to office etiquette than saying a bright " Good morning " to the boss. Harmony between you and your co-workers depends on a lot of little traits of behaviour.

Certainly you're not going to be a very popular member of the office staff if you comb your hair over the washbowl. Not only is it injurious to the plumbing, but it leaves the bowl in an unsanitary condition for the next user.

Are you the offender who wipes her lipstick off on the roller-towel ? Would your family stand for that sort of thing at home ? Then why inflict it on your office "family" ?

How's your aim ? Does the waste paper you pitch at the office wastebasket really reach its mark ? Or if you missed do you let it lie where it fell ?

Again, an inkstain on your dress is a major calamity. But a stain on the office furniture—well, do you take the attitude that it isn't your furniture, is it ?

At home, you close the windows before you leave the house for fear it may rain in sometime during the day. What about the office windows when you leave for the night ? Are they left wide open ?

And where you pay your own electric bills you turn out the lights when they're not needed. Perhaps your boss could raise your salary sooner if you did the same for him.

You may leave your home in a cyclonic condition if your rush to get to work on time ; that's a private affair. But leaving your work—or your implements, such as pencils, scissors, papers, paste—scattered all over your desk when you leave at night labels you as more nuisance than help.

Office etiquette, like all other social behaviour, is merely thoughtfulness. Put yourself in the boss's place. How would you feel if you had an employee who utterly disregarded the comfort of others ?

Answer that one honestly and then practise the Golden Rule.

LESSON TEN

Part D

Hands and Feet

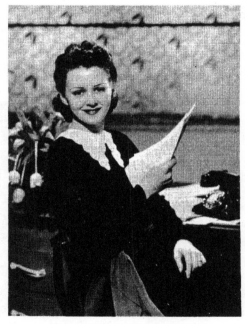

Photograph 27. Hands—a Beauty Asset

The one American actress whose greatness is commemorated in the Hall of Fame, Charlotte Cushman, once said that a woman's hands are more revealing than her face. This is no quaint observation of a hundred years ago.

Your hands—the look of them, their grooming and movements—come under constant scrutiny; and people use them as an index to your whole personality.

Learn to safeguard your hands, therefore, in the many little commonplace duties of daily living. Use the cushions of your fingers instead of your nails when typewriting. Use tools, no fingertips or nails, to pry off lids and open cartons. Protect your hands with cotton gloves for heavy housecleaning. Don't subject your hands to very hot water for long periods of time. Be sure to rinse them in clear, cool water after each soaping— —and dry them thoroughly.

Any shape hand may develop a grace and character of its own with regular care. Such care implies, first of all, keeping the skin on hands—and wrists—smooth and supple. One inflexible rule is to use a good hand cream, preferably a greaseless one, after washing, before going out, and at night. Apply it to your upheld hand in long downward strokes, or in " wringing " motions. This type of massage will tend to make any prominent veins and tendons less conspicuous.

Ragged cuticle is best conquered with cream or oil. Cuticle should not be clipped ; it should be trained into place. Cream should be massaged into the cuticle to make it soft enough to push back from the nail. Push cuticle back, too, each time you dry your hands.

The cream or oil you massage into your cuticle is also good for your nails—to keep them from splitting or peeling. Occasional hot oil treatments are also good. Heat a small amount of olive oil, castor oil or nail oil and dip your fingertips into the warm oil. Massage the oil into the nails, and if you're not doing anything for a while, leave it on.

Another prettifying "must" for lovely hands is the weekly manicure. Here sleight-of-hand will pay nice dividends. For instance, if nails are too broad, leave a tiny margin at the sides free of varnish. For very long nails, apply varnish so that the moon is well defined. Short nails, on the other hand, look best with moon and tips covered.

Between manicures check up on such foibles as chipped or peeling varnish. We consider this a worse offence than no varnish at all ! And inspect your hands for tiny calluses at the sides of the nails, and nicotine stains. Pumice stone will help to get rid of both.

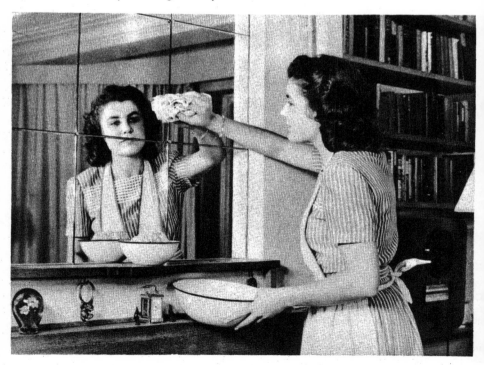

Photograph 28. Learn to safeguard your hands

272

EXERCISE FOR GRACE.

Neither jewellery nor highly tinted nails will make ugiy hands beautiful. What you want is hand grace. Gracefulness, if you're not born with it, can be acquired for your hands as well as for the rest of your body. Hands can be slenderized and strengthened, made more flexible and expressive.

1. FOR SLENDERIZING : Draw your fingers up until your hand resembles a claw. Tense fingers until they vibrate. Then relax. They will tingle and glow with circulation.

2. FOR FLEXIBILITY : Sit on floor cross-legged. Place palms flat on floor. Rock hands forward to tips of the fingers, down to the middle of the hand and back on the heel of the hand again.

3. TO RELAX AND ENCOURAGE CIRCULATION : Shake the hands vigorously from the wrists, as if you were trying to shake them off.

4. FOR DEFTNESS : Take each finger separately with the fingers of the other hand and bend it backward until it aches.

5. FOR GRACEFULNESS : Hold the hands out in front of body, palms down ; clench them tightly, then relax the fingers, letting the hands hang from the wrists.

6. FOR STRENGTH : Stretch the fingers back as far as possible with the fingers of the other hand.

7. TO LIMBER THE WRISTS : Kneel on the floor, palms flat and fingers pointing forward. Without moving your hands from the floor hump the spine, then pull backwards until you feel the stretch all through your arms and shoulders.

8. ALSO FOR FLEXIBILITY : Double your hands up into fist, keeping the thumb outside and bent back as far as possible. Clench the fingers hard. Now unfold first joint, then second, then the entire fingers until they are bent backwards as far as the thumb. After you have learned this movement, practise it quickly for extra dexterity.

9. TO STRENGTHEN MUSCLES : Stretch arms out sideways straight from shoulders. Push them as far back as possible. Keeping your hands tensed, fingers far apart, palms away from body, push your hands up. Relax. Repeat until tired.

10. FOR FINGER DEXTERITY : Do piano-playing motions on a table. Keeping all fingers slightly curved, rest the tips lightly on the table. Then lift one finger at a time up as high as possible. Hold it as long as possible : put it down and go on to the next.

One more hint to make your hands count for you. Be on your guard for any nervous mannerisms. Drumming on the table, fiddling with the corner of napkins, picking at crumbs (you may add your own peccadilloes to the list !) only detract from your hands and your poise. Gestures which are easy and relaxed—neither flamboyant nor affected—will call the most flattering atten.-tion to your hands—and to you !

THE HAND " FACIAL "

Neither you nor any other woman can be truly beautiful unless your hands are as lovely as your face. As you well know, a woman's hands invariably reveal her age, though her face, because of the loving care it gets, looks years younger. A clever woman, of course, knows what to do about such tell-tale hands.

She cares for her hands as meticulously as she does her face. As a matter of fact, she regularly gives her hands a treatment that corresponds to a good facial.

This once-a-week " facial " for your hands is accomplished with a mask cream, which stimulates the local circulation, thus helping to refine dry, coarse and crinkled skin. Apply this cream to your hands liberally and leave on fifteen minutes. Remove with tissue. After the mask has been removed, saturate a piece of cotton with astringent lotion and go over the skin. If your hands are in a really deplorable condition, apply a thin film of hand cream or warm olive oil, put on thin cotton gloves and keep on overnight.

For a regular night treatment, use a hand smoother and softener to help replenish natural softening oils, thus retarding coarseness and wrinkles due to skin dryness. Put on a pair of lightweight cotton night gloves to help keep those softening oils close to your skin.

For daytime protection of your hands, use a hand cream. Smooth it well on to your hands every time after they have been in water. This will help to guard them against chapping and ageing skin dryness.

If, in spite of this home care, your hands do not respond as you might wish, or if you have a case of long neglect, go to a hand salon and get professional care, such as a paraffin treatment.

The special oils in the paraffin do wonderful things for hands grown red and neglected-looking. The nails are also greatly benefited by these softening oils. This type of paraffin treatment is so beneficial to the skin that the

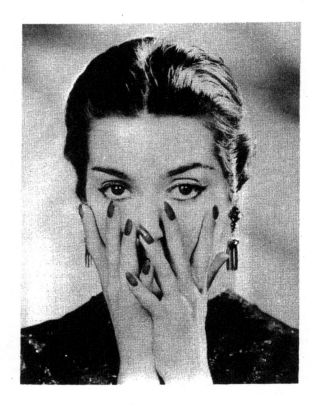

armed forces used it in caring for frost-bitten hands and feet.

FLAWLESS HANDS

Colour on the nails is important to lovely, feminine hands. Colour makes ordinary nails lovely, and disguises inferior ones.

Coloured nail enamel distracts the eye from defects of the hands, from freckles, large knuckles, redness and prominent veins. So use colourful nail varnish—it's your hands' best friend.

Take time with your manicure. A manicurist allows an hour for it in her shop, and plenty of time to dry. No rush job, please, as you follow these steps :

1. File nails. Do not file deeply into corners. For strength give nails oval shape with each side.

2. To remove varnish, press cotton wool saturated with remover on nail for thirty seconds to dissolve old varnish. Wipe off nail.

3. Buff nails for stimulation. It peps up circulation and helps to make a healthier nail.

4. Soak right hand in soapy water about three minutes. Scrub and wipe dry.

5. Massage nail cream around base of nails with firm rotary motion.

6. Press cuticle back gently to loosen, using orangewood stick tip wrapped in cotton wool, dipped in cuticle remover. Repeat steps 4, 5 and 6 for left hand.

7. Go over nails with polish remover again to remove all traces of oil, thus ensuring longer-lasting varnish.

8. Apply base coat to right hand, then to left.

9. Apply one coat of nail varnish. Re-dip brush after each nail. Don't shake the varnish bottle before you use it. This makes air bubbles which come out in blisters on your nails. Don't thin your varnish with remover, because it is likely to change the chemical staying power of the varnish.

10. Wipe hairline edge from tip of nail to prevent chipping.

11. Apply protective seal.

12. Dry your varnish at ordinary room temperature. Intense heat keeps the varnish soft, while a fan draught is likely to cause the varnish to blister.

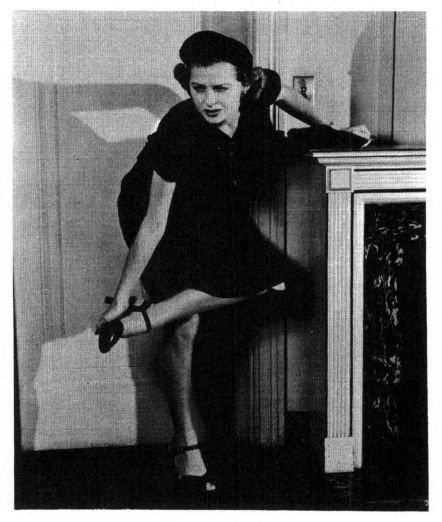

Photograph 30. Foot Problems

Although women must walk with the crowd—to and from trains, up and down stairs—and pound the normal office or homemaking beat, they're also supposed to wear frilly feminine footwear, and devil take the metatarsals ! Women who work often forgo the down-to-earth comfort that men derive from wearing good solid Oxford shoes.

But it is not hopeless. Here are pointers :

1. When you get through the day's work, switch into house shoes. This does not mean slippers of the sloppy variety, but well-made

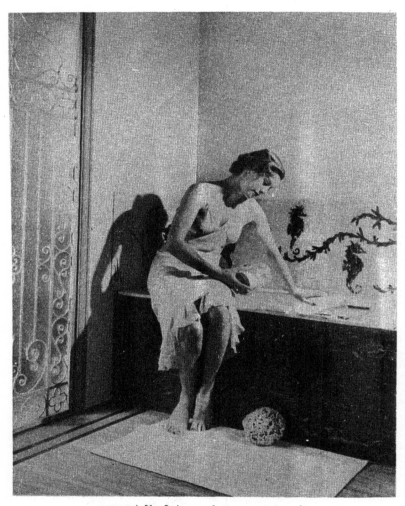

rnotograph 31. Bathe your feet once or twice a day

lace Oxfords, with roomy toes, lightweight kid or calf uppers that are soft over the tips, with flexible leather soles, and with heel heights one and a half inches or under. Change shoes daily. This may seem expensive, but it is really a money-saver. Tests show that shoes last three times as long if changed frequently.

2. For business wear, podiatrists recommend the lowest heel height allowed by the particular job environment. We know there is no use recommending low-heeled shoes to a girl whose job requires high-heeled glamour. A mid-heel is better than no heel at all, and also better than a miniature stilt.

3. Avoid short shoes as you would the plague and insist on a snug heel fit. Fewer corns and foot deformities will result if you make sure of a proper fit.

4. Leg exercises, such as bending the knees sharply, encourage the muscles to work smoothly in assisting the circulation. Any form of constriction, such as tight elastic in the legs of knickers, should be avoided. General fitness and adequate rest play their part in promoting the health of the feet.

5. Wash frequently. Bathe your feet once or twice a day, dry them and dust on foot powder. With a little hand shower, spray your feet three minutes with hot water, one minute with cold. Keep alternating for ten minutes. Stimulates circulation.

6. Walk right. Cultivate good posture. Don't have " stenographer's stance," the habit of hooking feet in back of chair legs. It's bad ! Shortens calf muscles and distorts arch structure, Do keep feet squarely in front of you.

7. For salesgirls and others who stand, here's one : Don't stand in one spot too long. Do keep feet in motion. Reason : Blood has to travel a long way from heart to feet. Standing makes heart work harder, veins overstretch, ankles well. Foot action helps pump the blood.

8. Exercise. Here are four you can use to limber up your feet at intervals.

TOE CURL : 'Bend toes under several times, stretching legs as you do so. Good for strengthening muscles that support the metatarsal structure.

TOE WIGGLE : Grasp the big toe and rotate it—round this way and that way. Good for high-heel cramps.

FOOT FLEX : Sit on edge of bed or chair, xtend legs and flex feet up and down, knees straight. Helps to stretch calf muscles which ave been shortened by high-heeled shoes.

SOLE ROLL : Stand barefoot, feet six inches par. Roll the feet outward twenty to thirty me so that body weight is supported on outer dge of feet. Good for arch, ankle and calf,

THE PEDICURE

Here are directions for home foot-massage and pedicure done in a professional way :

1. Remove old varnish from nails of left foot.

2. File nails straight across, never into corners, as this may encourage ingrown toenails. Smooth corners of nails.

3. Buff in one direction only. Back-and-forth buffing may overheat and injure the nails.

4. Soak foot in, warm soapy water for five minutes, while repeating steps 1, 2 and 3 on right foot.

5. Dry left foot and massage nail cream around cuticle. Soak right foot.

6. Dampen end of orange-stick, wrapped with cuticle remover. Push cuticle back very gently. Repeat steps 5 and 6 on right foot.

7. Scrub toes of both feet thoroughly to remove all traces of nail cream and cuticle remover. Dry carefully.

8. Weave cleansing tissue in and out between the toes to separate them for easy application of varnish.

9. Apply base coat and two coats of coloured varnish to all ten nails.

10. Apply hand Cologne for a final luxury touch. Don't get it on the freshly applied varnish just on the foot itself.

Notes:

Self-Test Questions Based On Lesson Ten

This Lesson gives beauty advice for the Seasons, with a special note for women over forty. While hands are important because they are noticed so often, feet are rarely given the attention they deserve; they well repay you many times both in smartness and comfort for any extra care you may give them.

After you have studied this Lesson, you should be able to answer the following questions. If you have any difficulty in doing so, refer to the Lesson for further study and revision. Your answers should not be sent to the publishers of this Course.

1. What should you learn to do in order to attain poise and serenity of mind?

2. Give four rules or suggestions for keeping cool in summer.

3. Quote, in short, ten conditions essential to refreshing sleep.

4. What is the secret of a good hostess or a good guest?

5. How would you sum up office etiquette?

6. Describe shortly what you should do if your hands have been neglected and are in a very bad condition.

7. What point should you keep in mind when choosing shoes, especially for summer wear?

8. How can you protect your feet and your shoes, especially if your work necessitates your wearing smart serviceable shoes all day?

9. Quote four things you may do daily in order to ensure foot comfort in hot weather.

10. Should you suffer at any time with rough, raw or scaly legs, what treatment should you give them?

If you wish to determine the progress you are making, give yourself 10 points for each question you answer correctly. If the total comes to 90 or more, it is excellent; 80 or more, good; 70 or more, fair.

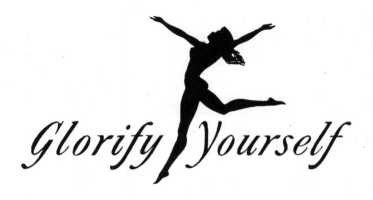

Glorify Yourself

★

A Complete and Up-to-Date Course on
Beauty and Charm by One of the
Most Famous Beauty Specialists
and Consultants in the World

★

LESSON ELEVEN
by
Terry Hunt

★

STUDIO TALK •

Issued only for Students
of the Eleanore King
Course on Beauty. Charm
and Personality.

Number Eleven.

Dear Student,

Lesson Eleven contains a comprehensive and lavishly illustrated selection of exercises designed to benefit every part of the figure.

We start with the neck line, and proceed to routines for developing - or reducing - the bust. Next, the waist line receives attention, then the abdomen. Further exercises help you to streamline your hips and to slenderise your thighs.

These exercises must be performed regularly if you are to derive full benefit from them. But they are not only work - they are fun, too! And just think of the benefits you will obtain. You will shape your figure, you will give your skin a new lustre and vibrancy. You will overcome overweight, underweight, bad posture and chronic fatigue.

Fifty beautiful pictures specially posed by Miss Kathleen Hughes, the famous film star, show you _how_. Clear concise directions tell you _where, when_ and _how much_. You can't go wrong.

All you require is a little determination and patience. Don't overdo the exercises - ten minutes a day is sufficient for a start. Don't expect miraculous results after a few days. But make the exercises a regular, conscientious habit. After a week or so there will be no temptation for you to neglect it.. Your daily exercise period will pay a rich dividend. Physical and mental fitness give you new zest in tackling the problems we face every day.

This Lesson has been compiled by Terry Hunt, the famous Hollywood conditioner of such film stars as Rita Hayworth, Olivia de Havilland, Shirley Temple and Ingrid Bergman. The recommended exercises represent, in handy

(over)

282

page 2.

form, the results of years of research and experience
at Mr. Hunt's Health Club in Beverley Hills. The simple
routines selected are designed to meet the needs of
to-day and are regularly practised by the stars of
to-morrow.

But the principle is an old one. Over two
hundred years ago James Thomson said:

"Health is the vital principle of bliss,
And exercise of health."

How right he was!

Yours sincerely,

Eleanore King

t.11.

PS. Lesson Twelve ties up all the loose ends and will
help you put the finishing touches to your new personality.

LESSON · ELEVEN

KEEP FIT—STAY BEAUTIFUL

I HAVE been employing the selected exercises demonstrated in this Course with hundreds of women over a period of many years in my Health Club in Beverly Hills. These exercises are yours to use now with complete confidence.

Film stars including Olivia De Havilland, Jean Arthur, Jeanne Crain, Shirley Temple, Lucille Ball, and dozens of others have performed them religiously, to guard and preserve their glamour, and for the fitness of body which goes hand in hand with mental well-being.

Doctors have sent me hundreds of their patients suffering from overweight, underweight, bad posture, and chronic fatigue. My greatest compliment is that these doctors not only recommend my system, but use it themselves.

There is no easy way to the beautiful body. No one hands you a pill or waves a wand and, voila, Betty Grable ! You must adhere faithfully to the proper regimen of both exercise and diet.

You must face frankly the simple fact that exercise is a form of hard work. But there are rich rewards. Exercise-and-diet give your body eye appeal, shape your figure, and give your skin a lustre and vibrancy. And physical conditioning is the first requisite in mental and emotional capacity to cope with the professional, social, and personal problems which we all face every day.

MAKE A HABIT OF IT

Exercise must be a completely conscientious habit. It must be as regular—for it is intrinsically as important—as sleeping and eating.

These exercises are no mere theory, nor are they effective only with certain cases. Anyone who puts them to consistent practice over a sustained period will show marked improvement.

Let me give you this brief, basic outline : First of all, you must have a definite technique, performing your work-out with interest, rather than listlessly.

On the other hand, moderation is important. It's wise to begin slowly and easily with a few warm-up and deep-breathing exercises before starting.

WHAT TO DO

The following exercises are presented in the order of increasing difficulty. Begin your programme with the first two exercises of each set. Gradually add to your routine until you can do them all.

Note: *Read the advice given on Page 27 before commencing an exercise programme.*

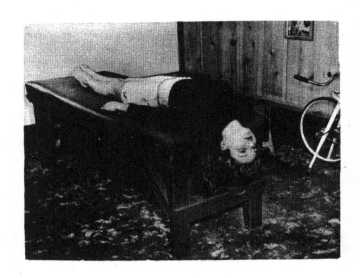

These exercises leading to figure perfection are demonstrated by Miss Kathleen Hughes, 20th Century Fox star.   Starting with the neckline—

POSITION: As illustrated in photograph No. 1.

EXERCISE: Bring head forward slowly until chin touches chest as in No. 2. Slowly return to original position. Hold for a few seconds. Repeat.

BREATHING: At will.

REPETITION: Start programme with 10 exercises. Gradually increase to 20.

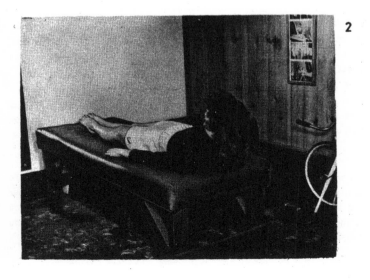

2

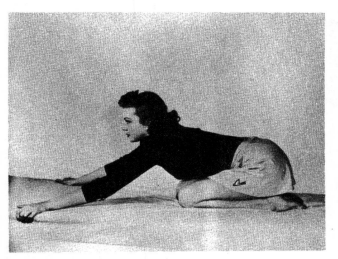

A-I

The following exercises are beneficial to
the bust—also to the shoulders and arms.

A POSITION: As illustrated in photograph No. A-1.

EXERCISE: Slowly lower body to table (or floor) as illustrated in photograph No. A-2. Then slowly return to your original position.

BREATHING: Inhale through nose as you raise body, exhale through mouth as you lower body.

REPETITION: Start programme doing 5, increase to maximum of 10.

A-2

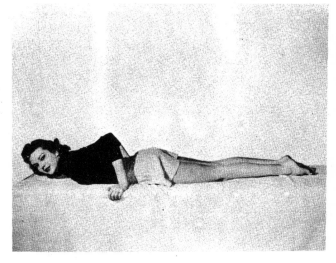

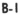
B-1

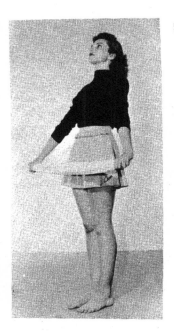

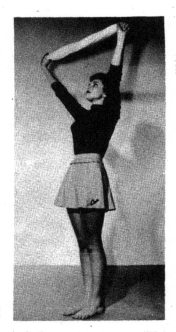
B-2

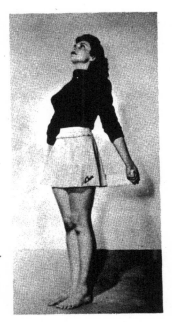
B-3

B POSITION: Stand erect grasping towel in both hands as illustrated in photograph No. B-1.

EXERCISE: Raise towel over head and behind back as in B-2 and B-3. Return to original position.

BREATHING: Inhale through the nose as you raise arms up and over head, exhale through mouth as you return them.

REPETITION: Start with 6, increase gradually to maximum of 10.

NOTE: Do this exercise slowly, keeping elbows rigid. The closer the grip, the harder the exercise.

CD-1

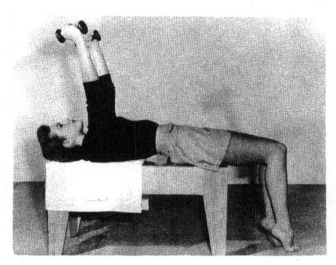

C On this and facing page are two exercises for improving the bust.

POSITION: As in CD-1. Hold dumbbells or books of equal weight.

EXERCISE: Lower arms forward as in photograph CD-2, keeping elbows rigid. Make complete circle and return to your original position.

BREATHING: Inhale through your nose as you start the circle forward, exhale through your nose as you complete it coming up from the back.

REPETITION: Start by doing 5, increase to a maximum of 10 circles.

NOTE: To reverse, start as in photograph CD-1, lower arms backward as in CD-3 and return. Inhale as you start, exhale on completion.

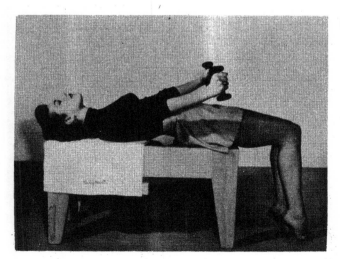

CD-2

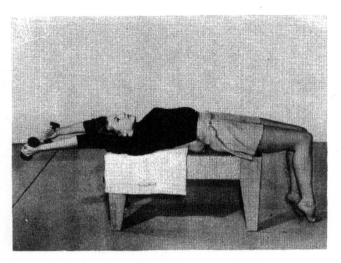

Here is another beneficial exercise for toning up the bust: D
POSITION: As illustrated in photograph No. CD-1.
EXERCISE: Slowly lower the arms to the sides as illustrated in photograph
No. CD-4, then return to original position shown in CD-1.
BREATHING: Inhale through your nose as you lower arms, exhale through
your mouth as you raise arms.
REPETITION: Start programme doing 5 exercises, gradually increase to 10.
NOTE: These exercises should always be done very slowly. If a bench is
not available you may do them just as well from a standing position.

CD-4

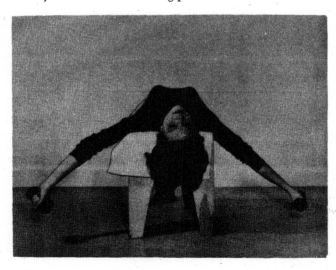

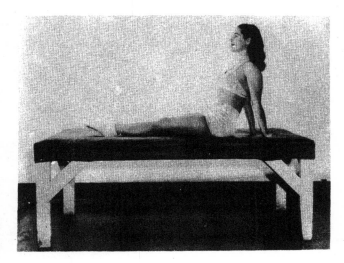

E-I

E POSITION: As illustrated in photograph No. E-1.

EXERCISE: Slowly raise the body until the elbows are rigid, as illustrated in photograph No. E-2. Then lower the body to original position.

BREATHING: Inhale through nose as you raise body, exhale through mouth as you lower it.

REPETITION: Start programme doing 5 times, increase to a maximum of 10.

E-2

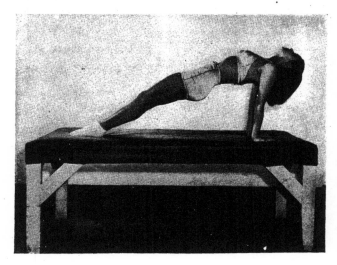

THE BEAUTIFUL BUST

POSITION: Stand with your back to the
wall as illustrated in photograph No. A-1.

A

EXERCISE: Stretch left arm up as high as
possible as illustrated in photograph No.
A-2. Repeat, raising right arm, relaxing
left.

A-1

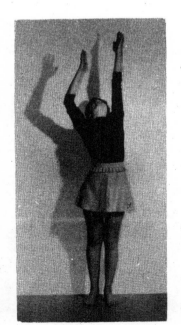

BREATHING: At will.

A
(cont.)

REPETITION: Start programme with 6
stretches, increase to a maximum of 10
stretches.

NOTE: The important thing in this exercise is to really s-t-r-e-t-c-h.

A-2

B

POSITION: As in photograph No. B-1.

EXERCISE: Bend forward, twisting body, and touch left foot with right hand as in photograph No. B-2. Return to original position. Alternate by touching right foot with left hand.

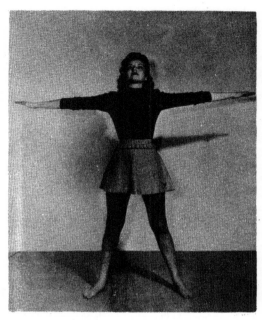

B-1

B (cont.)

BREATHING: At will.

REPETITION: Start programme with 5, increase gradually to a maximum of 15.

NOTE: It is important in doing this exercise to keep the knees absolutely rigid.

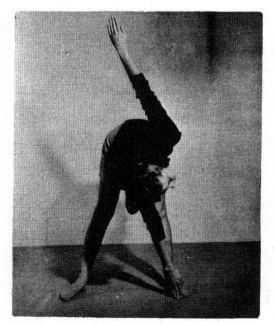

B-2

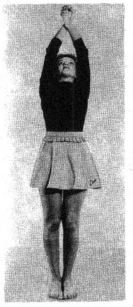

C-1

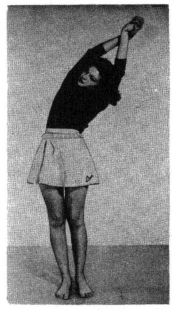

C-2

C   POSITION: As illustrated in photograph No. C-1.
EXERCISE: Bend body sideways to left as illustrated in photograph No.
C-2. Bend to right without pausing at original position. Return to original
position.
BREATHING: At will.
REPETITION: Start programme by doing 5 bends, increase to maximum of 10.

D   POSITION: Lie on back, knees bent, feet slightly raised.
EXERCISE: Swing legs from left to right touching table (or floor) with
thigh on each swing, but keeping back and shoulders flat on table.
BREATHING: At will.
REPETITION: Start programme with 8 swings. gradually increase to 15.

D

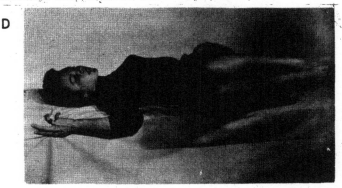

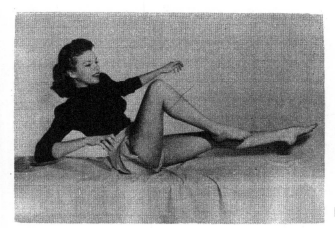

E

E POSITION: As illustrated.

EXERCISE: Twist upper body from left to right, first raising right knee and touching it with left hand, then raising left knee and touching it with right hand. Keep legs, shoulders and elbows off table (or floor).

BREATHING: At will.

REPETITION: Start programme with 6, increase gradually to maximum of 15.

T
H
E

S
M
A
L
L

W
A
I
S
T
L
I
N
E

F POSITION: Hang on bar as illustrated.

EXERCISE: Swing from left to right, pushing heels down as you swing.

BREATHING: At will.

REPETITION: Start programme doing 6 swings, increase gradually to a maximum of 20 swings.

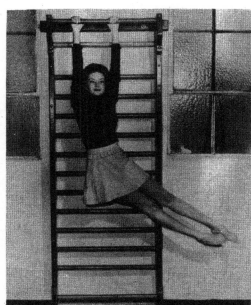

F

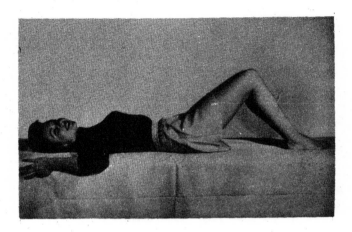

A-1

A POSITION: As illustrated in photograph No. A-1.

EXERCISE: Bring knees up to chest as illustrated in photograph No. A-2, then return to original position.

BREATHING: Inhale through nose as you lower knees, exhale through mouth as you bring them up.

REPETITION: Start programme by doing 6, increase gradually to maximum of 10.

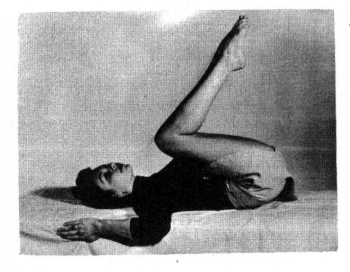

A-2

THE FLAT ABDOMEN

B

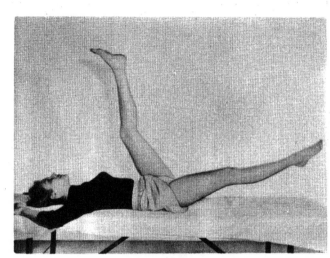

B POSITION and EXERCISE: Lie on back. raise legs about 8 eight inches off table (or floor). Bring left leg up as illustrated. keeping knees rigid. Lower left leg. bringing right leg up. Alternate rapidly in scissors motion.
BREATHING: At will.
REPETITION: Start programme with 8, increase to maximum of 15.

C POSITION and EXERCISE: Take position as illustrated. Slowly lower the legs to table (or floor), keeping knees rigid. Return to original position.
BREATHING: Inhale through nose as you lower legs. exhale through mouth as you raise them.
REPETITION: Start programme with 6. increase gradually to maximum of 12.

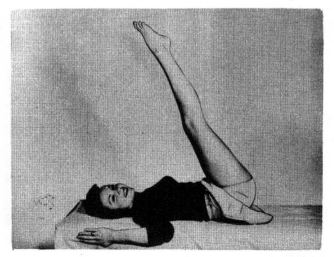

C

D

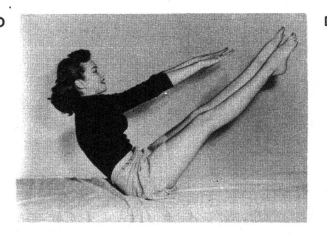

D POSITION and EXERCISE: Lie flat on back. Lift shoulders and legs off table (or floor) as illustrated. Hold for a few seconds. Return to original position.

BREATHING: Inhale through nose as you lower shoulders and legs, exhale through mouth as you lift them.

REPETITION: Start programme with 5, increase to maximum of 10.

E-1

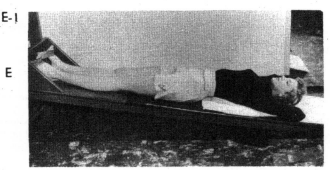

POSITION: As in photograph No. E-1.

E

EXERCISE: Raise upper body and bring it forward as illustrated in photograph No. E-2. Return to original position.

BREATHING: Inhale through nose as you go back, exhale through mouth as you come forward.

REPETITION: Start programme with 6, increase to 15.

NOTE: This exercise is easier if done with arms stretched overhead instead of locked behind neck.

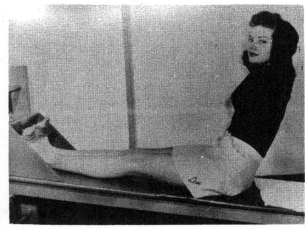

E-2

F

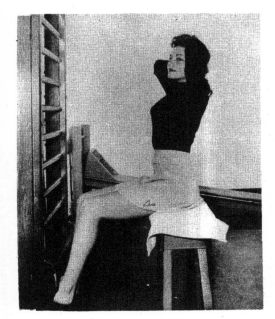

POSITION: As in photograph No. F-1.

EXERCISE: Bend upper body back as illustrated in photograph No. F-2. Return to original position.
BREATHING: Inhale through nose as you go back, exhale through mouth as you return to position.
REPETITION: Start with 5, increase to maximum of 15 bends.

F-1

F-2

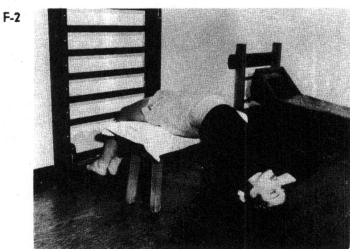

A

POSITION: As illustrated in photograph No. A-1.

EXERCISE: Lift right leg and right arm as illustrated in photograph No. A-2. Return to position.

BREATHING: Inhale through nose as you lower arm and leg, exhale through mouth as you raise them.

REPETITION: Start programme with 6 with right leg and 6 with left, and increase to maximum of 12 with each leg.

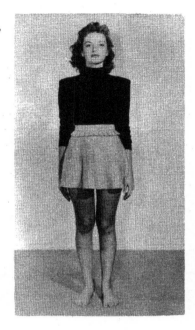

A-1

A-2

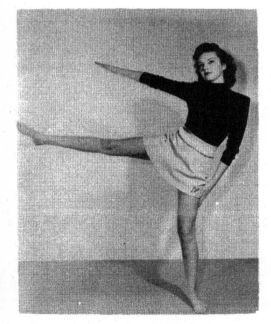

B

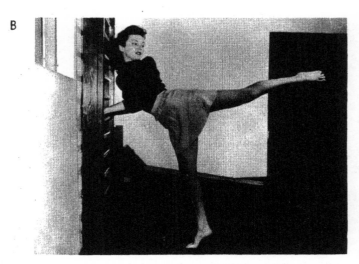

B POSITION and EXERCISE: Take position illustrated. Lower left leg to floor, keeping knee rigid. Return to original position. Repeat.
BREATHING: Inhale through nose as you lower leg, exhale as you raise it.
REPETITION: Start with 6 with left leg, 6 with right, increase to 12 each.

C POSITION and EXERCISE: Lie flat on back. Swing left leg up and over right leg as illustrated. Return to position. Repeat with right leg.
BREATHING: Inhale through nose as you swing leg back, exhale through mouth as you swing it over.
REPETITION: Start with 6 swings with each leg, increase to 15 each.

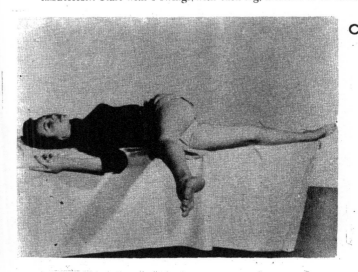

C

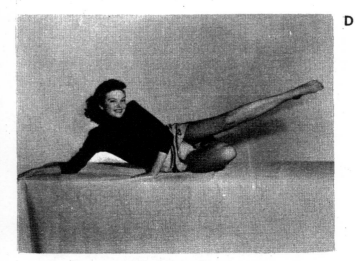

D

D POSITION and EXERCISE: Take position on one side as illustrated. Perform a regular bicycle movement with your legs.

BREATHING: At will.

REPETITION: Start with 10 revolutions, gradually increase to 20.

E POSITION and EXERCISE: Take position as illustrated. Perform a regular scissors movement with legs, keeping knees rigid. Make long strides.

BREATHING: At will.

REPETITION: Start with 10, increase gradually to a maximum of 20.

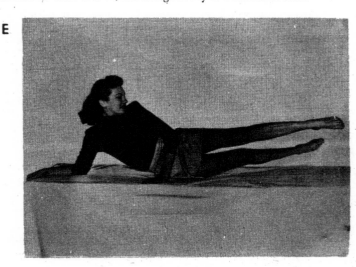

E

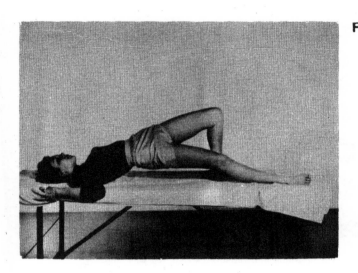

F

POSITION and EXERCISE: Take position as illustrated. Bounce up and down on fleshy part of right hip. Repeat on left hip.

BREATHING: At will.

REPETITION: Start programme with 6 bounces on each hip. increase to 20.

CAUTION: Bounce on fleshy part of hip only. Be careful not to strike any part of lower spine.

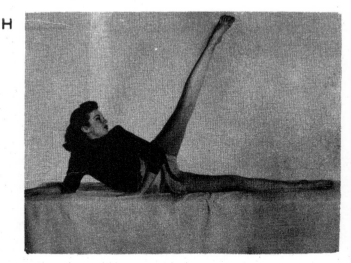

H

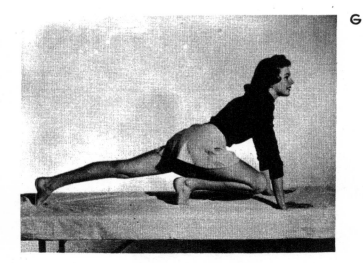

G

POSITION and EXERCISE: Take position illustrated. Kick right leg back and bring left leg up, then kick left leg back and bring right leg up. Alternate in this fashion to create a "stationary" running movement.

BREATHING: At will.

REPETITION: Start with 10 times, increase gradually to maximum of 15.

H   POSITION and EXERCISE: Take position in photograph at left. Make series of continuous circles with left leg, keeping the knee rigid. Change position to other side and make series of continuous circles with right leg.

BREATHING: At will.

REPETITION: Start by doing 6 circles with each leg, increase to 15 each.

A

POSITION: Take stance as illustrated in photograph No. A-1.

EXERCISE: Lower body to squatting position as in photograph No. A-2, keeping back rigid and heels flat on floor. Return to position.

BREATHING: Inhale through nose as you rise, exhale through mouth as you take squatting position.

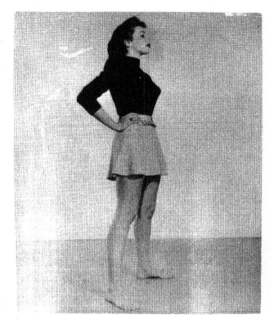

A-1

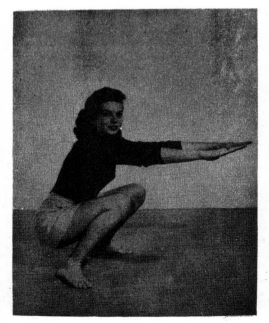

A
(cont.)

REPETITION: Start with 6, increase gradually to maximum of 15.

NOTE: Do same exercise on your toes, to streamline calves of legs.

A-2

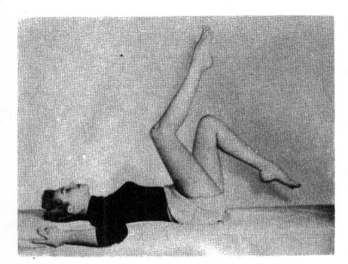

B

POSITION and EXERCISE: Take position illustrated and perform a regular B
bicycle movement with your legs, while lying on back with knees raised.
BREATHING: At will.
REPETITION: Start with 10, increase gradually to a maximum of 20 times.

C POSITION and EXERCISE: Lie on right side and raise left leg as illustrated,
keeping knee rigid. Return to original position. Repeat.
BREATHING: Inhale through nose as you lower leg, exhale through mouth
as you raise it.
REPETITION: Start with 6 with left leg, then 6 with right, increase gradually to maximum of 15 with each leg.

C

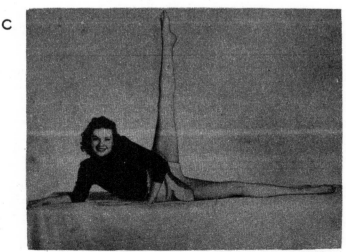

D

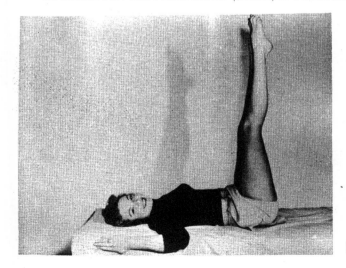

D   POSITION and EXERCISE: Lie on stomach, hands clasped over buttocks.
Raise shoulders and legs off table (or floor). Hold. Return to position.
BREATHING: Inhale through nose as you raise shoulders and legs. Exhale
through mouth as you lower them.
REPETITION: Start programme with 6 times, increase to maximum of 15.

E   POSITION and EXERCISE: Take position illustrated. Separate legs as widely
as possible, keeping knees rigid. Return to original position.
BREATHING: Inhale through nose as you separate legs, exhale through
mouth as you return them to position.
REPETITION: Start with 6 times, increase gradually to a maximum of 15.

E

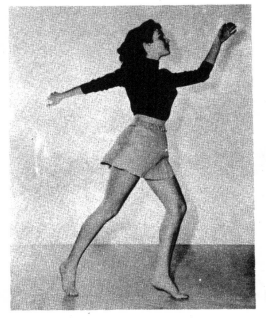

F

POSITION and EXERCISE: Stand on tiptoes, left foot forward. Kick left leg back and bring right leg forward. Then kick right leg back and bring left leg forward. Alternate rapidly to create a "stationary" running movement.
BREATHING: At will.
REPETITION: Start programme by doing 10, increase to maximum of 25.

F

G POSITION and EXERCISE: Take squatting position with hands at waist and walk around floor in a ducklike manner.

BREATHING: At will.

REPETITION: Start doing exercise for 5 seconds, increase to 10 seconds.

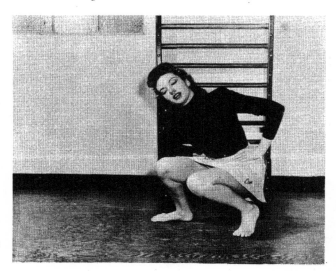

G

H

POSITION and EXERCISE: Take position as illustrated. Pedal at a good speed until legs begin to tire.

BREATHING: At will.

REPETITION: Start pedalling for one minute, increase to 5.

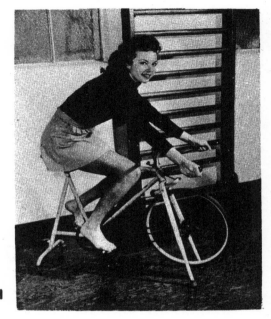

H

If you can't get a "Beauty Board" like the one shown here. use a plain board 6 feet long and 18 inches wide and prop one end up on a piece of furniture about 18 inches high. Take position illustrated. This relieves fatigue, strengthens abdominal muscles, improves appearance of bust, face, and neck. Lie on the board for 15 minutes daily.

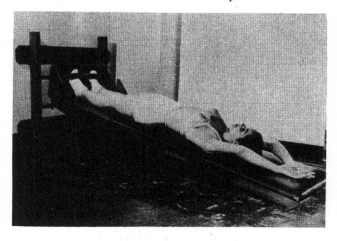

How to Do It

1. **HOW OFTEN?** Daily, for reducing. Alternate days for rebuilding.

2. **HOW MUCH?** Begin with a routine of ten minutes, gradually expanding it to a maximum of thirty minutes.

3. **WHEN?** At any time during the day, but always at least two hours after eating.

4. **WHERE?** In a clean, properly ventilated room (draughts are dangerous). Use a large table, or the floor.

5. **TEMPO?** For reducing, exercise rapidly. For rebuilding, very slowly.

6. **CLOTHING?** Play or gym suit that permits free movement and circulation. For reducing, the warmer the apparel, the better.

What Not to Do

1. Don't begin an exercising or dieting programme before first consulting your family doctor.

2. All exercise should be limited according to the age and physical condition of the person exercising.

3. Don't take a shower or steam bath directly after exercising—wait until your heart has slowed to normal.

Notes:

Self-Test Questions Based On Lesson Eleven

This Lesson is very practical. Most of us, under modern living and working conditions, get insufficient exercise to keep us in tip-top health. Practically every student will find in this Lesson exercises for her particular needs.

After you have studied this Lesson, you should be able to answer the following questions. If you have any difficulty in doing so, refer to the Lesson for further study and revision. Your answers should not be sent to the publishers of this Course.

1. How often should exercise be taken ?

2. Having studied this Lesson for two weeks—how much exercise do you take now per day ?

3. When should you take exercise ?

4. Have you studied your figure in relation to the groups of exercises given here and decided which group or groups you are most in need of ?

5. After two weeks of exercise, do you feel better, more alive, perhaps calmer ?

6. Do you look better, slimmer or more shapely—firmer ?

7. What will regular exercise do for you apart from improvement to the figure ?

8. Describe the best conditions under which you should exercise.

9. What benefits can you derive from the use of a "Beauty Board" ?

10. What difference will your age make to the nature of your daily exercise ?

If you wish to determine the progress you are making, give yourself 10 points for each question you answer correctly. If the total comes to 90 or more, it is excellent; 80 or more, good; 70 or more, fair.

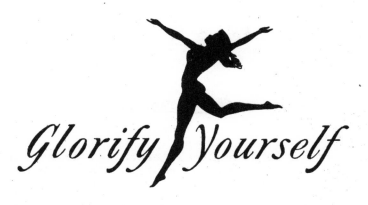

Glorify Yourself

★

A Complete and Up-to-Date Course on
Beauty and Charm by One of the
Most Famous Beauty Specialists
and Consultants in the World

★

LESSON TWELVE

by

Terry Hunt

★

STUDIO TALK •

Issued only for Students of the Eleanore King Course on Beauty. Charm and Personality.

<u>Lesson Twelve.</u>

Dear Student,

While this is your final Lesson, it is not, I hope, the end of your keen interest in charm and beauty. On the contrary, I trust that you will continue your progress towards even more splendid achievements.

The pursuit of beauty is supremely worth while. What could be more thrilling than the constant discovery of new ways to high-light your personality? What better tonic is there than the knowledge that you can make yourself ever more attractive? And amid the problems and perplexities of our difficult days, what better morale builders are there than immaculate grooming and confident poise?

If you have done all the things recommended in the Course so far, you will have already profited by it considerably. But don't let complacency overtake you in this last Lesson. Study the first section entitled "How Old Are You?" and make a frank appraisal of your physical and mental assets. If you find that you are doing the things that make you old before your time - such as over-indulgent eating, burning the candle at both ends and neglecting the exercises - then make it a point of honour to apply a little more self-discipline in your pursuit of beauty. Take to heart the teachings of Part B, and resolve to be yourself - not an inferior copy of any other personality.

Learn all about perfume from Part C and then study the fifty streamlined beauty hints which comprise the final part of this Lesson, and make it a point of honour to <u>act</u> on each and every one of these hints.

I cannot over-emphasise the value of revision. I would suggest that you revise all the Lessons regularly and conscientiously. In doing this you will discover many points which you may have underrated at first reading. Beauty can be marred by tiny faults and shortcomings which may seem trivial to you. But they are not trivial if they lessen your attractiveness and prevent the full expression

(over)

of your personality. Aim at perfection. You may not
achieve it, but you will gain immeasurably from the
noble effort of holding fast to an ideal.

I would like you to know that I and my colleagues
of the Academy of Charm and Beauty take a personal
interest in you. We would like to know how the Course
has helped you, and would sincerely appreciate your writing
to us. Everything you say will, naturally, be in strict
confidence, since the names of Students are never divulged
except by specific permission.

I know that you are now even more beauty-conscious
than you were when you opened your first Lesson. I hope
you have gained something more as well. I hope that the
Course has led you to a more vital awareness of beauty
not only in your own personality, but in the finer things
of life in general - art, nature, music. Most of all, I
hope that you now realise that you owe it not only to
yourself but everyone around you to GLORIFY YOURSELF.

If we have conveyed this to you, my colleagues and
I are more than happy. On behalf of them and myself I send
you my continued good wishes for a richer, happier, more
rewarding life.

Yours sincerely,

Eleanor King

EK.12.

Part A

How Old Are You?

THEY say a woman is as old as she looks and a man is old when he stops looking. To this, you might add, "And so is a woman old when she stops looking—for romance."

Many women are imbued with the strange idea that love and romance are for young girls only, that if a woman does not make a glorious match in her twenties, when she is budding, flower-like, and lovely, she might just as well tear this page out of the book of her life. What an insane thought ! Why, at thirty and beyond, a woman has just reached the point where she can truly appreciate the real thrills of romance.

Isn't it significant that the greatest story of our age, one which thrilled millions, the world over, involved the Duke of Windsor, who forsook his throne for a middle-aged woman, *past forty* ! When he stood by the radio and told an amazed world that he could go on no longer without the love of Mrs. Wally Simpson, mature women the universe over must surely have thrilled with hope born anew for themselves.

LET'S FALL IN LOVE !

The young girl is interested in love, of course. She is filled with energy, vitality, and curiosity. As often as not, she falls in and out of love a dozen times before the real thing comes along. Moreover, there are other interests in her life— college, social groups, films and plays, and a score of attractive things to do. In most cases, she isn't ready to settle down and make a home, to become a loving housewife, devoting her very existence to the comfort and happiness of one man. She is too interested in personal accomplishment, in living, in exciting experiences. As a matter of fact, because such young girls who have not had their fill of living do marry early, many of these marriages do not last. The girl is often too restless and animated to vegetate in

a suburb—she wants to " live."

Unless they have really found the man of their heart and want to settle down with him, early marriages are not especially good for young girls. Otherwise, they should get a job, go out a great deal, travel as much as they can, and tire out their sense of adventure and their curiosity about living before taking the final step. This isn't for all young women, of course. We have our youthful, maternal types who are interested in children and homemaking at eighteen, and for them marriage is the ideal thing.

IT'S NEVER TOO LATE

But the mature woman, the woman past thirty, has lived in the outside world. Probably she has worked for her living in an office or factory or store. She has spent these intervening years at home with her parents, or in a girls' club, or at some boarding-house. She has seen other girls marry and find happiness. She has been lonesome for someone to love and very tired of her business routine. In other words, her goal is a happy marriage.

There are other cases where the woman did marry young, and something happened to that marriage. Perhaps the husband died or deserted her. Perhaps the relationship struck some snag and broke up. The girl may have been hurt, bruised, offended by that unhappy marital alliance. At the time, she may have said, " Never again ! " But, as the years rolled by, and she saw how empty her own life was, how happy her married friends were, she began to regret her own lonely spinster state. In other words, she was prepared for a second try at an institution which, when it is right and happy, has no equal for a man and a woman.

Well, you will say, what is to prevent such a woman from going out, finding a nice chap, and marrying him ? Ah, there's the rub ! Nothing will prevent her from doing this, if she is still attractive and charming. In that case, she'll not only find a nice chap, but, since he will undoubtedly be older than the callous suitors of her youth, he'll also be better situated financially. It's a perfect match, depending on whether or not she is still lovely enough physically to attract such a man.

There's a curious, though perfectly normal characteristic of men, which is described elsewhere in this Course. They are drawn to glamorous looking, physically attractive women. They need to be proud of the appearance made by the girl who, for them, is " the only one." The fact that a man has turned forty doesn't alter his mood—he still feels in tip-top shape himself and can see no reason why he shouldn't have a beautiful mate. Frankly, who can blame him ? Probably he has much more to offer such a woman than he had at twenty-two.

MAY AND DECEMBER !

This man will not want a " spring chicken," to use a colloquialism. He has the sense to know he would look somewhat ridiculous paired off with a girl young enough to be his daughter. He doesn't want people talking behind his back. Moreover, experience has taught him that he would have little in common with such a girl. Their interests would be poles apart, their friends of different and irreconcilable ages, their moods and fancies not the same. Actually, he is looking for a lovely, gracious, and charming woman who will enhance his home, share his problems, and love him as he wants to love her.

Unfortunately, one of the first things a woman does who is disappointed in love, or who feels that love is not for her, is to let herself go physically. It no longer seems important to be attractive, or at least to take extensive pains in order to retain a trimness of figure, a lovely complexion, a joy in living. So if love does accidentally find her, as is often the case, she is completely unprepared and without the necessary weapons to win her man.

LIVE ALONE—AND HATE IT !

Some women reading this Course will say,

" Humph, do men think that love is all we are concerned about ? " No, they don't think anything of the sort. But at least they're not hypocrites, and they know, as any practical psychologist knows, that love is a vital and important part of every human being's life. Without it, something in that person dries up and blows away—a potentially rich and wonderful part of his or her life. You cannot underestimate its importance in the general scheme of living.

For the girl who has passed her thirty-year mark and has not neglected her looks throughout those years, appearance is no problem. Undoubtedly, her well-cared-for skin will be smooth and lovely, her hair lustrous and beautiful, her teeth white and shining, her nails groomed to perfection, her body sylph-like and intriguing to the eye. The chances are that such a woman will not be single, unless she happened to enter the world of commerce early and was so fascinated by it that she had no time for romance. If she wants now to leave that world and compete in the romantic arena, she will be more than a match for her younger sister, for there is an undeniable fascination in mature poise and charm.

The other woman, the one who has let herself go for years, really faces a serious problem. Don't think that it can't be conquered—it can. But there is no denying the fact that she has a genuine battle on her hands, one not of a few days' duration, but of weeks of patient care and body rebuilding. If she is sufficiently interested in her own rehabilitation, she will triumph and emerge slender and beautiful as a result of her efforts. If not, she can attain only an indifferent appearance, which means an indifferent success.

THE FIRST HUNDRED HOURS ARE
THE HARDEST

It is difficult and takes much conscientious work to get into shape, but, once you have achieved this enviable state, it is simple and easy to remain lovely and attractive. The woman who faces such a prospect can solace herself with the knowledge that when her training period is over, when she has slimmed down her body, dieted, exercised and groomed herself to a stunning appearance, a few simple rules turned into habits will keep her always so. The hard work need be done but once. After that the job of maintaining her figure becomes second nature and passes almost unnoticed as a part of her daily schedule.

CAREER GIRL

There are some women who are not interested in romance. Say that you have made business your life-work, that you have thrown all your vital energies and strength into a commercial enterprise, that you are the executive type with nothing else on your mind except business. Now, if ever, you need to pay attention to the suggestions in this Course, and take the same course of treatments which is advocated for the woman who seeks a romantic mate.

How often one hears the saying, " This is a young people's world." In business, particularly, older persons are constantly being eliminated to make way for fresh blood. The employer becomes weary of seeing the same greying head at his reception desk, at his switchboard, by his side when he dictates. He's only human ; he'd be refreshed by having his work done by some smartly groomed, attractive girl. If he has an intensive loyalty he remembers your years of service and retains you in the job. But honestly, how many employers have such a loyalty ?

So, to advance yourself in a business career, to further your own interests, to keep pace with the trim, lovely, challenging younger generation, you would keep abreast of them in physical attractiveness. If you are lovely to look at, I'm sure your employer would rather keep you on than get someone else—you know his work so thoroughly.

You will ask how you can begin this physical rehabilitation, what you must do to achieve the necessary degree of perfection in physical appearance. The purpose of this Course is to help you find it, specifically to aid you in becoming a charming, gracious, and attractive personality. It was written not merely to be read but to be studied from cover to cover, painstakingly, carefully, so that you may wring every iota of good from the advice given. This you must do to get the best out of it.

DIET—BUT EAT !

Start at the beginning. Adopt a proper, intelligent diet—reducing or gaining—according to your type and weight. Combine this with the right kind of exercise, also shown here, to help pep up your circulation, relieve you of sluggishness, and generally tone up your system. Get your figure down to its proper weight. If you are troubled with particular heaviness in any one portion of your body, you'll find specific exercises here to help you with such problems.

YOUR SKIN

Now take every detail of your person and commence to improve it. Make a study of your skin and learn what creams and astringents will best serve to beautify it ; what powders, lipstick, and rouge will most enhance it. Become proficient in their application—pay real attention to this very important business of making yourself lovely. Let a competent beauty specialist help you shape your eyebrows, and keep them clean of extra hairs and well groomed. Learn how to apply mascara properly. All the directions are given in this Course.

YOUR NAILS

Learn to care for your nails. Become adept at doing them yourself, so that they need never look unsightly just because you have been unable to secure an appointment at your beauty salon. Study what has been written about the care of the teeth and the eyes, so that both these features will be assets, not liabilities, to your looks. Read the lesson on " Hair," and learn how to endow it with a soft and beautiful sheen, and once this has been accomplished, to dress it yourself.

YOUR CLOTHES

Don't go into stores and buy any kind of clothes that attract your eye—not unless that eye is trained to know what suits you, as well as what is becoming.

Make a study of your personal colouring and determine what shades and cuts of garments fit you in the most flattering fashion.

Buy clothes, not in hit-and-miss fashion, but with the thought of creating ensembles.

Be selective in your purchases, realising that a dress of the wrong shade or the wrong lines can make you look fat, dumpy, sallow-skinned, ugly, while the proper dress can create a positive illusion of glamour about your person.

YOUR PERFUME

Study the various perfumes to find the scents which suit your type and enhance your personal attractiveness. Use them continuously, to create a faint aura of allure, a magnetic quality.

That's the outer you. When you've accomplished all this—and it will take you a little time—then carefully peruse the Lesson, " Do Something About Yourself." This will inform you how to build a personality which the world will find attractive and charming, which will attract others to you. It is not an overnight procedure, but the dividends are so big that you should be glad to make the effort to achieve the glamour or personality which will be yours once you have completed your training course.

START LIVING

Get the thought out of your head that thirty, or forty for that matter, is in any sense old. It is really the peak of life for you—the peak in your mental, spiritual, and emotional development. Untold years of happiness stretch ahead of you, years of achievement, years of romance. Like a connoisseur who has learned her speciality, you now know enough about living to commence really enjoying it, to eke from it some of its richest benefits.

A CANDLE BURNS FASTER FROM BOTH ENDS

One thing to remember is this : you cannot carry on like the twenty-year-old girl, staying out until the wee sma' hours of the morning, then sleeping it off, and emerge clear-skinned and fresh as a daisy the next day. If you don't want bags under your eyes, wrinkles, and that awfully tired feeling in your bones, you must keep sensible hours, and never fail to get at least eight hours of sound sleep in a large well-ventilated room. Don't ever underestimate the tremendous recuperative powers of sleep ; it is the only thing which will help you bridge the gulf existing between you and the girl in her teens.

The dissipation I speak of doesn't necessarily mean carousing in night clubs and cafes, or excessive drinking. Hunching over a bridge table until two o'clock in the morning, fretting when you lose, worrying over scores, are also certain ways of getting lines in your face and vinegar in your disposition. An hour of that time spent walking through the park will do you a thousandfold more good. In fact, you should make a nightly walk habitual—it will clear the cobwebs from your brain and help you to sleep.

When you are past middle age, you should go in less heavily for meats and tend more to fresh and stewed fruits and green cooked vegetables. Plenty of milk and eggs to provide body-building materials are also suggested. Eat at a regular time—that will help also to maintain your body equilibrium. Don't take excessive amounts of sugars and starches—your body is inclined to heaviness as you grow older, and there is no need to help the cause along.

PUSH YOURSELF AWAY FROM THE TABLE

Remember that your digestion doesn't improve with the years. Don't load yourself down with food to the point where you can hardly get up from the table. This mistreatment of your stomach can result only in constipation, skin outbreaks, indigestion, and other troubles of this nature. You'll find, as you grow more mature, that you can do with just a little less food. Don't feel that you're starving yourself—you will feel the better for it. So will your stomach.

As a woman grows older, she becomes prey to a number of female complaints, irregularities of health which, if checked at their inception, will not assume serious proportions. Every woman should have a reliable doctor whom she can consult regularly. This is a splendid preventative, helping to avoid trouble in the future. If you are concerned about some ailment, the condition can possibly be improved, or other assistance rendered which will keep you active, healthy, and in the swim for many years to come.

Women, more than men, are the victims of all kinds of curatives. They are prone to buy anything that promises to make them alluring, beautiful, glamorous, or to help rectify some trouble which they are undergoing. Don't fall prey to this weakness. If you don't feel well, you should see a doctor and find out what's wrong with you. He'll prescribe something to help your specific condition—which is more than the prepared fancily scented hocus-pocus.

TRY A HEALTH COCKTAIL

Learn to relax. Take time off every day when you just " let go " in every nerve of your body, when you ease the pressure of nervous strain, of worry, of brooding, of business activity, and clear your mind of fretting thoughts. This is a health cocktail which you must train yourself to take, for it is the constant concern over business and personal problems that makes a woman old before her time.

By the time you are past thirty or have reached forty, your habits of living should certainly be fixed. If they are not, then go over these carefully, determine the things to do which are good for you, and make habits of them. I refer now to such practices as eating sensibly, exercising, bathing, walking, and the like. Regularity in each of these will reflect well upon your future health and fitness.

So just try to remember—a man prepares against old age by putting money aside and creating an estate ; a woman by dieting, beauty treatments and conditioning.

LESSON TWELVE

Part B

Do Something About Yourself

THE Americans have developed a pungent and colourful language of their own. Thus, when they characterise individuals as " phoney," they mean to say that they are not genuine, but an imitation of the real thing. And so many people are phonies, not in the sense that they are crooked or dishonest, but they just aren't themselves.

CARBON COPIES

If you put a piece of carbon paper between two sheets of writing paper, it's quite a simple matter to distinguish the carbon copy from the original. The original is fresh, true, and real.

There are thousands of " carbon copies," young girls and old, going about in imitation of this big star and that. Every town and village has its carbon-copy Hedy, Lana, or Rita, each a take-off on some screen siren, a purer-than-driven-snow film heroine, or the current " oomph " girl. It requires a lot of work to effect this take-off ; it's not as simple as slipping a piece of carbon between two sheets of paper. And where do their strenuous efforts get them ? Exactly nowhere ! They're immediately labelled as " phoney."

These women have an ardent desire to be beautiful and glamorous. They are honest enough with themselves to know that they are neither one of these things. They feel that if they ape an attractive actress whose type is similar to their own, they will become equally colourful and intriguing. So they copy her style of dress, her coiffures, her mannerisms, her little idiosyncrasies of character, and then think they have succeeded in making themselves as unique and different as that star.

Quite often the personality, manner, and mode of dress of the star they are emulating do not sit well with these women. Instead of being their own lovely, radiant selves, these women develop into third- and fifth-rate copies of the beautiful stars whose shadows they see flashing upon the silver screen.

Remember, people never look more absurd or ridiculous than when they imitate someone they can't possibly resemble. The sad part of it is that there is really no need to imitate. Believe me, your own personality, properly developed, will suit you infinitely better than the copied reflection of another. The whole fascination of a personality is in its originality. At least you will be gloriously yourself, not a second-hand copy of someone glorious. Isn't that a more enviable goal for which to strive ?

At this point, it might be worth while stressing a thought brought up elsewhere in this Course. No outstanding star on the screen today, however glamorous, sprang full-blown to this position. All you have to do is to look at pictures of them in their earlier years to realise how little personality, glamour, and magnetism they once possessed. No, what they have today, the glamorous personality you see upon the screen, was developed in these intervening years. They transformed themselves, through determination, self-study, and superlative grooming, into fascinating public figures they are.

So you can see that personality is a matter of development. It means taking your best qualities, your gaiety, ebullience, kindliness, understanding of others, tolerance, thinking mind, and fusing them to create a lovely and charming individual. But, let me repeat, it must be you, not a take-off on someone else, if there is to be greatness in that personality. There is no immortality in imitations. Elizabeth Barrett Browning, Mary, Queen of Scots, Madame Curie, Joan of Arc, Queen Elizabeth I, Florence Nightingale—these were women whose basic claim to fame is that they were original.

BE YOURSELF

" Be yourself " is a great lesson to learn in starting the uphill climb to developing a glamorous personality. If being yourself means that you will be dull, phlegmatic, unattractive, then change that self. Analyse your lacks and rectify them, but remember that you'll never be an outstanding personality unless you are genuine. If this means that you must do a thorough housecleaning on yourself, trans-forming yourself completely inside and out, that's fine. But always realise that if you should emerge a truly fascinating person, it will be because you have made yourself so—not because you are pulling a pretty good imitation of some other personality.

Now we're getting somewhere. We realise we have to be authentic. So let us take ourselves apart and see what it is we have on the credit and debit sides of the ledger. For example, are we greedy, envious, vengeful, selfish, deceitful, petty ? Such characteristics show in our faces— to achieve radiance and charm we must eliminate them. It isn't easy to rid oneself of ingrained habits, and any woman who can learn not to be these things is achieving a distinct triumph, one which will pay her dividends.

THE FORGOTTEN WOMAN AND . . .

All right—take another type. Are you an introvert, self-conscious, shy, withdrawn ? Do you often say to yourself, " I find it hard to talk to people. I'm just the kind of a person who was made to be by herself " ? This is false reasoning. If you continue to think in this fashion, you will be alone all your life.

THE UNFORGETTABLE WOMAN !

Force yourself to go out among people and converse with them ; make a definite effort to master the art of small talk. Learn to laugh out loud, rid yourself of your habit of reserve ; attend parties ; introduce yourself to those present whom you don't know, dare to be gay !

If you are shy and reserved and get a sort of stage fright when among strangers, set out

deliberately to conquer this feeling. Take a course somewhere in drama, in public speaking, in self-expression. The publishers of this Course market a good Course on Conversation and Public Speaking. Practise on everyone, making it your business to be entertaining, to charm people with your enthusiasm and buoyancy of spirit.

When a woman has nothing but charm and personality, she has everything. When a woman has everything but charm and personality, she has nothing !

Perhaps you're one of those nervous types, whose bubbling personality finds expression in a giddy, scatterbrained attitude. If you are, then make a serious effort at self-control, for this type of personality can be awfully irritating. Your personal vivacity and enthusiasm, when properly harnessed, can be utilised to make a charming personality of you, but you must be able to use just the desired quantity—you must be able to turn it off, too.

VIVE LA DIFFERENCE !

Someone once claimed that he'd analysed women and catalogued them, and found sixty-five distinct species. If this was so, he must have had acquaintance with *exactly* sixty-five women ! For every woman is different from her sister— every personality is unique. And if you make yourself charming, intriguing, lovable, and at the same time *just yourself*, there will be no one quite like you. Dare to believe that you, properly developed, are as interesting as any woman alive, and make yourself such a woman. It will prove your salvation. How you were yesterday, a year ago, is not important. But what you do from now on, is !

LOVELY TO LOOK AT

Of course if you want people to be attracted to you, you must supply some of that attraction— and in a woman, that attraction is physical.

It is up to you to attain that physical attraction. How to attain it, is all here before you in the lessons of this Course. Conditioning, proper diet, exercise, make-up, costuming—it's all here within these covers. Take advantage of it.

Make yourself a lovely thing physically, sylph-like in body, flawless of skin, luminous of eye, with a sheen to your hair, your whole being radiating superlative care and proper grooming, and you'll get everything you desire out of life.

There have been women in the past who, though crippled or physically deformed, have battled through to success, solely through the magnificent vitality and fascination of their personalities. But exceptions such as these merely prove the rule. If you are sluggish, weary, apathetic, dull, you can never attract anyone. The secret of fascination is vitality. People who glow with life, with vibrancy, with physical energy, have won half the battle already. They attract others to them as cream attracts a kitten, as honey the bee.

You could safely say that this is the outstanding characteristic of every great personality. We, here in Hollywood, who come in daily contact with the great and the near-great of the motion-picture industry, are charmed by their personality off screen as well as on. They're so alive, so filled with the ecstasy of living, so eager to preserve their supremacy in their chosen field, so much on their toes ! That is why they are stars while others remain obscure—because they communicate this " sock " to everyone who works with them, who sees them. And to audiences in the four corners of the earth, they are intriguing, fascinating, exhilarating, lifting them to a plane of breathless, romantic excitement !

There was a character actress in pictures called Zasu Pitts. She made a good living from exhibiting a personality that, seemingly, gives the lie to everything that's been said. This character was listless, apathetic, dull. Her fluttering hands revealed indecision and a complete inability to cope with the problems which confronted her. But let me tell you a secret : it was just a pose with Miss Pitts. Had she actually been such a character, she would never have got anywhere in pictures. Actually, she's a wide-awake, intelligent, sensitive artist, and the personality she portrayed was just a simulated character whom she successfully sold to the public and to the film moguls as well.

Your outward attitude must, of necessity, be somewhat of a calling card for you, introducing you to those who have not previously met you. Make this outward attitude, then, one of decision and confidence. Walk as though you believed in yourself, and let that confidence be' seen in your carriage. Walk with purposeful strides ; send out vibrations which indicate that you are a live, unique, and interesting personality. Believe in your high destiny, your guiding star.

SMILE, DARN YOU, SMILE !

Learn the power of your smile and use it to advantage. What have you got to smile about ? You're alive, aren't you ? Then show it ! Let your emotions show on your face—transform it from a lifeless mask into a sensitive instrument accurately recording your moods.

After you have transformed yourself into an interesting human being through study and self-application, then have faith in the fact that you will be attractive to others. Nothing inspires confidence more quickly than self-confidence, provided it is not cocky and offensive, but sure and real.

Keep your head up, your chin out ; face the world with assurance. Don't droop ; don't sigh mentally, physically, or spiritually. Don't constantly bathe yourself in a tepid, strangling bath of self-pity. Don't ever show despair at your chances of making good, or for any other reason. Always exude an air of strength and sureness of your own powers, of your own magnetic personality, of your courage. People flock to the strong, and ignore the weak. Remember that. As you evince strength of character, power of personality, so the world will be intrigued by you and cheer you.

Acquire poise. Get over being tense, apprehensive, unsure of yourself. Learn to, take life easily, gracefully, in your stride. Force yourself to be more casual in your contacts with people, friendly and pleasant, without stiffness, or coldness of attitude. Frankly, you'll find it easiest to obtain perfect poise when you have accomplished the requirements outlined in other parts of this Course. Yes, when you are physically trim and attractive, healthy, perfectly groomed, you will have the confidence in yourself to be easy and graceful in the presence of others.

You have probably sat in church and listened with a certain patronage while the minister spoke of "brotherly love." But you'd be amazed at how strongly your inner feelings toward your fellow men affect your personality. Emotions of warmth, generosity, friendliness—these attract people to you ; discontent, jealousy and malice avert people's interest and repel them.

So many people are actually ashamed to express an honest emotion. How silly is such prudishness ! If you are happy, exhilarated, gay, let the world in on your good mood—it loves to laugh, too ! And laughing with you, it is sure to like you.

Read books on how to attract and influence people. The publishers of this Course will supply you with suitable titles if you will write to them.

Make the business of " charming " every person you meet a fine art. I don't mean stupidly, obviously, by looking at them out of big, goo-goo eyes, and breathing, " Wonderful " to every statement they make. I mean to charm them by your intelligence, your vivacity, your interest in them. To charm them by your kindliness of attitude, your wholesome spirit, your sweetness of disposition. To make them feel the warmth of you and the sincerity of your interest.

You cannot be withdrawn in character or personality and still " register " with people, They do not feel the life in you, the vibrancy, the spirit which, in the more lively girl, is so pleasant and welcome. Being too shy or backward gives an impression of stupidity, or lack of interest. If people are not repelled by such an attitude, at least they derive no satisfaction from it and so turn away. You may have a heart of gold beneath that quiet-looking exterior—but how are they to know it ?

This brings up a vital point. Aren't you really interested in the welfare, the activities, the heartaches, and problems of other people ? Well, you really should be. There's much to be learned from such observation. Every human being has something of value to give his neighbour. If you do not possess this interest, how about imagining it is there ? Listen to your neighbour's conversation with real attention ; try to visualise yourself in his place ; make an honest effort to be helpful. If you actually do some good, it will leave you with a warm contented feeling inside ; if not, you'll at least be glad you tried.

No Business Like Show Business !

It's common knowledge that many a great talent has gone unnoticed in the theatrical world because of one thing—lack of personality ! Remember that !

A great singer, a great dancer, a great actress—she's not just a voice, a pair of nimble feet, a face—she's all these, *plus* personality.

And you're in show business too—the greatest show on earth—the show of life !

LESSON TWELVE

Part C

Your Perfume

PERFUME is the magic touch which transforms a charming woman into an enchanting one. It has a subtle allure, an undeniable appeal to every man's emotions. A suggestion of subtle perfume will be the final touch to your glamour.

Every perfume was made for an individual type of woman. The scent which is enthralling on an olive-skinned brunette becomes ridiculous when used by an ash-blonde. Yes, perfume is as personal as your silk underthings. There is heady fascination in just a dab of it behind the ears.

Do not confuse perfumes with the Colognes and day-time perfume, which are used for everything from general scenting to after-bath fragrance.

There are really three main types of perfume. First, the concentrated perfume which contains rich essences of many different types skilfully blended together to give a sophisticated, stimulating or exciting note. These should be used discreetly to give a most attractive and charming effect.

You must never drench yourself with it. A woman should perfume her hands, throat, the inside of her elbows, and behind her ears. For evening excursions she can add a touch to her shoulders, back and bosom. If it is the right scent, it will lend her an allure comparable to no other beauty aid.

Since, frankly, a woman usually wears a lovely fragrance to attract a man, she should early ascertain whether or not her particular brand appeals to him. Men are allergic to some odours—it makes them restless, irritable. No matter how highly you prize a perfume, no matter how expensive it is, no matter if you know it's absolutely right for your type, don't wear it

if your loved one does not care for it. Try something else—he'll be sure to find at least one of your experimental fragrances enchanting. That is the one to use.

Then there is the second type of perfume, lighter in character and greater in volume. It is a perfume ideally suited to daytime wear as it can be used plentifully, being at no time overpowering. It is made up of the same lovely essences as the concentrated perfume but is more diffuse in character—such perfumes are Atkinson's Daytime perfumes Bal des Fleurs and Lightheart. They are modern in character and very light and appealing.

The third type of perfume is the toilet water which, as its name implies, is intended to be used for toilet purposes to refresh and give fragrance at the same time. You can use it as a body friction or sprinkled in cold water as a stimulating rinse, on the hair for a quick setting lotion and all the innumerable purposes for which you require a fragrant lotion. Atkinson's Gold Medal Eau de Cologne and English Lavender are supreme in this field, for they are stimulating with a certain satisfying sweetness.

It is a mistake to think of toilet waters as a " poor relation " of essence perfumes. They are, in point of fact, just as carefully blended and the ingredients are of the same quality.

HOW TO CHOOSE AND USE PERFUMES

When selecting a perfume it is necessary to know how to smell fragrance. Our sense of smell is very acute but it tires easily and after smelling three or four different types of scent, it is difficult to form an accurate idea of quality and strength. The different perfume notes become confused and may blend together. This frequently leads to the perfume favoured and chosen so carefully in the perfume shop being very disappointing when smelt later. Try to test not more than three different perfumes at once, and then your choice is likely to be much more accurate because they will not be confused in your mind.

The correct way to make this test is to place a drop of the liquid on the wrist or back of the hand, allow the alcohol to dry off (the wait need not be more than half a minute) and then savour the tone note of the perfume which should be released. The warmth of the skin will bring out the undertones of the perfume as well as the obvious notes, and your own skin, which has an individual action, will make the perfume *your own*.

It is worth remembering that some people turn perfumes very sweet—they should, therefore, select perfumes with a sharp, dry note, so that the result is not sickly or overpowering.

Other people can turn perfumes aromatic, almost bitter ; they, in contrast, should aim for the sweeter warmer notes, to which they will give subtlety and roundness.

Again, some women may exhaust quickly the potency of a scent, while others will seem to accentuate its sharpness and will retain it for a much longer time. One of the reasons for this curious reaction is that a perfume attracts other odours to it, and is in turn modified by them. Therefore, a woman should renew her perfume during the day and evening hours. The most convenient way to do this is to carry a little dram vial of her favourite scent with her in her handbag.

And now, having chosen your perfume cleverly, use it correctly :

Concentrated Perfumes should be used as we have said very sparingly ; a drop behind the ear, on the wrists, in the fold of the arm at the elbow, or saturating a tiny wad of cotton wool tucked in the neck of the dress, so that the warmth of the skin may bring the fragrance to life.

Daytime Perfumes use more lavishly. Spray on to the body as a skin perfume, spray the lining of coats, the hem of the skirt or the inside of the handbag. But remember that all good perfumes tend to stain or may take colour from delicate fabrics, so never place where stains might spoil the effect. Place perfume also on the band of your hat or on a fur necklet, for in all these ways the scent will be given the chance to diffuse and so give that aura of fragrance which is the correct way to wear perfume.

Toilet Waters use as perfumes, if so desired, and in addition sprinkle in the bath, use as a setting lotion for the hair, diluted as a refresher and cleanser on wads of cotton wool when travelling, as a body friction or foot lotion to remove fatigue, in sachets in the linen cupboard or " undies " drawer. In other words, whenever a waft of fragrance would delight you or your companion. Be ingenious and contrive a method of placing it there—not too strongly but subtly and with distinction.

Just as many men dislike seeing a woman make up in public, so they prefer not to see perfume being applied. Of course, a man is well aware of the fact that you use perfume, but it gives him a pleasant feeling to regard it as a natural fragrance emanating from your person. It never pays to be cynical and disillusioning about these things, for in the illusion is harboured the very soul of romance. There is still another reason why the utmost delicacy must be employed in the application of a scent—why it must never be blatantly and obviously used.

Perfumes exercise a very desirable psychological effect upon a woman. Let her use a dainty, alluring scent and somehow it lends her a confidence, a sureness of her own beauty, which in turn endows her with added power to attract men. If she really has loveliness of features, it dramatises them, lending them an even greater magnetism. Above all, it is one of the voices of love.

There have been many kinds of perfumes made since the early beginning of this art. Primitive women garlanded themselves with flowers which gave off a rich and lovely fragrance. Sweet gums, such as frankincense and myrrh, were early perfumes, sometimes burned, sometimes carried on the person to impart a pleasing aroma. Perfumes made from oils are a discovery centuries old. Synthetic perfumes from vegetable and mineral sources are a discovery of the last century.

Modern perfumes are manufactured from a great number of fragrant sources. Oil of orange blossoms, roses, jasmine, violets—all are bases for lovely perfumes. The iris root, the rind of lemons, musk from a variety of Asiatic deer, castor from beavers, ambergris from the Indian Ocean—all these raw materials are brought from the far corners of the earth, along with many others, to make the perfumes found on the dressing-tables of the most glamorous women.

The Riviera is a potent source of perfume materials. Acres upon acres of fertile land are sown with flower seeds, from which grow violets, mignonette, jasmine, narcissus, tuberoses, and other flowers from which the precious scent is extracted. Not that they are generally distilled and marketed in this fashion—your alluring modern perfume is most often an intricate and secret process of combining and blending a dozen varied scents.

CHANGE YOUR SCENT NOW AND THEN

It is a truism that a perfume loses its drawing power if used constantly. If you move in the same set and consistently use one perfume, you will find that your friends no longer notice it. In other words, they have become accustomed to the fragrance, and it no longer registers. For this reason, a woman should vary her perfume. This doesn't mean that she should change it drastically—every woman is a distinctive type, so the types of perfumes which suit her will all be similar in fragrance. But there should be enough difference so that outsiders, the man you love in particular, are stimulated by it and made aware of its insinuating loveliness.

If a perfume is right for you, it will add zest and excitement to your spirit. It will inspire you, thrill you, make you feel confident of yourself and of your beauty.

MATCH PERFUME TO YOUR PERSONALITY

Choose perfumes that represent your type. If you're refined, delicate, shy, then select a perfume that emphasises these qualities and accents them.

Atkinson's Flower Perfumes such as Lily of the Valley or Freesia would be ideal for you.

The strident, unsubtle, sexy perfume would be horrid on you. If you're a healthy athletic type, *Atkinson's* " Lightheart " would be delightful for you. Whereas the career girl would favour for daytime use **Bal des Fleurs.**

It will pay you to know perfumes, to know the different kinds sold and the odour of each. When you have learned this, then classify yourself as to personality, and find your favourite fragrance in the group of perfumes suitable for your particular kind of person.

Perfumes are so definite a part of the charming woman's costume that, like her hats, shoes, or coiffures, they change with the times. For example, the mere mention of a fragrance such as Rosemary immediately brings to mind a picture of quaint old world gentility. In our own generation we have streamlined everything, given women equal rights, and by the same token bestowed upon them burdens equal to those of the male sex. Nevertheless, there is still very much alive in the heart of every woman, and more so in the heart of every man, the necessity for women to possess the femininity that Rosemary suggests.

And so names like "Bal des Fleurs," " Mirage," " Golden Age," " Shocking," "Jabot," " Tweed," should become as much a part of the charming woman's vocabulary as any words she uses in her everyday language.

329

LESSON TWELVE

Part D

Fifty Beauty Hints

IN this Lesson I have set down the following fifty general beauty hints that many women have found extremely valuable. When you have learned them all, you will have found a number of roads which lead to greater personal attractiveness.

These suggestions are short cuts to beauty, little ways of becoming better groomed, more tidy and clean-cut in appearance. Study these and you will have a much better understanding of what it takes to improve your looks and make yourself more glamorous.

1. A broken nail may be covered with an artificial one, purchased quite inexpensively at chemists or hairdressers.

2. If you smoke a great deal, keep your fingers white with nicotine remover. This eliminates both stain and odour.

3. If your breath is bad, carry breath pastilles. There are various causes for bad breath, but it is most important that you should not offend. An antiseptic mouth wash and frequent cleanings of your teeth are also recommended.

4. If your feet perspire, a dash of deodorant powder in your shoes is a thing you will do well to remember.

5. Winter does not excuse you for having a " fuzz " on your legs. Sheer hose do not hide it. Use a depilatory.

6. Polish your elbows once a week with a mixture of oatmeal and cleansing cream, making certain that the resultant product is still rough enough to create friction. This will whiten and soften them beautifully.

7. Hair on your arms is ugly. It can be made almost invisible by bleaching.

8. If you shave your arms or legs, sprinkle baby powder on first. This prevents friction chapping.

9. Does cold weather cause your legs to become rough and mottled ? A solution of castor oil in alcohol will do much to remedy this defect.

10. Remember that well-manicured nails and a dainty perfume are two outstanding essentials of good grooming for women.

11. Eat to live—don't live to eat.

12. Before applying your mascara, dip the eyelash brush in boric acid solution and then brush your lashes and brows—it will lend them a lustre.

13. How to exercise is as important as if you exercise. Don't expect results unless you do your workout with verve, eagerness and enthusiasm.

14. Plenty of milk and green leafy vegetables will help keep your nails in condition and help prevent them from becoming brittle.

15. Use the right make-up. If you can't select it yourself, trust the salespeople in the better-class stores.

16. Dermatologists have proved that the skin can be helped and kept in good condition by nourishing creams. But it is fed and made lovely by the blood stream, so watch what you eat.

17. Certain skin lubricants will not cause new tissue to grow. All they can do, and this is of value, is to keep your existing tissue in good condition.

18. Start each day fresh—forget yesterday's troubles.

19. Before starting any dieting or exercising programme, be sure to consult your family doctor.

20. The Lesson on skin informs you how to eliminate blackheads. Do this the right way, or you will seriously infect one of your finest beauty assets.

21. If you use a complexion brush for stirring up the circulation of your skin, it must be of the very softest bristles.

22. For reducing weight, see that about fifty per cent of your food consists of raw fruits and vegetables.

23. If you're heavy, stick largely to liquid breakfasts, for food has been found to be more fattening before noon.

24. A glass of hot water in the morning will pay you dividends.

25. If your energy runs low at midday, try some honey on a cracker. This is a potent producer of warmth and vitality.

26. Water is good for your system—drink at least one quart daily.

27. Don't gorge food—always leave the table not, quite full.

28. Don't drink water with your meals. Chew your food thoroughly ; let the saliva help you get it down, instead of flooding it down with water, and delivering it half-masticated to your over-worked stomach.

29. Wear high heels for dress only, as they tend to cause lower back curvatures.

30. Vitamin D, which is sunshine, makes for strength of bone, beautiful teeth, wholesome blood, and a lovely skin. Get plenty of it.

31. Vitamins are not " hocus-pocus " foods, but vital substances for the body.
Find out which foods contain the different vitamins—then see that you get plenty of them.

32. Always use an under-arm deodorant and shields if necessary, to prevent perspiration stains.

33. If you do a lot of reading, relieve the strain on your eyes by rolling them around in your head, and then fixing them on varied objects.

34. Lie on your back and let your head hang from the edge of the bed a few moments each

day. This has three purposes : (1) It tightens muscles under the chin. (2) It brings a sudden rush of blood to the head and face which helps tone the tissues of the face. (3) It gives nourishment and stimulation to the hair follicles.

35. Brush your hair every day and massage the scalp at frequent intervals. A healthy head of hair, well-groomed, is indubitably a woman's " crowning glory."

36. In brushing the hair, part it in the middle of the back of your head, and brush away from the parting, first up, then down. Repeat this all over the head—it is splendid for stimulating circulation of blood through the scalp.

37. Castor oil is a wonderful aid to the growth of your hair.

38. Sleep " knits the ravelled sleeve of care." If you're tired, despondent, nervous, try getting an extra hour's sleep at night. It will do wonders for you.

39. Don't wear shoes two sizes too small because it is the fashionable thing to do. Be sure your shoes fit you, in order to avoid corns, bunions and calluses.

40. See a chiropodist for all serious foot ailments, and don't cut corns, or bunions yourself with a razor—the resultant infection might be extremely serious.

41. Take extra stockings with you if your feet perspire. This will prevent irritations and bad odours, both detriments to beauty.

42. Walk at least an hour every day. It improves your circulation, tones up your system, and gives you a better appetite at meal times.

43. Remember, if you're constipated, your skin will suffer. Train yourself to a regular bowel movement. The first thing in the morning, the last thing at night are good times for bowel action.

44. Regulate your diet, substituting laxative fruits for rough laxatives, for these have only temporary value and injure the membranous lining of the intestines.

45. Do not eat if you are tired or angry—a case of indigestion will thus be avoided, and you will benefit by postponing the meal.

46. Avoid over-indulgence in strong liquor. It is bad for your system and bad for beauty.

47. If you work indoors, in an office or factory, do some simple exercise before an open window before retiring for the night. Inhale through the nose, exhale through the mouth.

48. Be poised. Learn to use your hands gracefully, not jerkily and abruptly. Make every gesture mean something.

49. Wear a smile—it's natural. Be animated and interested in life and living.

50. Learn to be generous, open-minded, kindly, decent in your attitude towards others. These emotions will eventually be reflected in your face and will attract people to you.

LESSON TWELVE

Part E

Woman Through A Man's Eyes

" To men a man is but a mind.
Who cares what face he carries
or what form he wears ? But
woman's body is the woman."
—The Devil's Dictionary.

REMEMBER that there are as many types of beauty as there are women. You're one type and there will always be an audience—perhaps a world, perhaps one man—who will prefer you to all others, if you make an effort.

There is no more fitting introduction to the subject of this Lesson. While most of the famous authorities who give advice to the lovelorn are women, perhaps it is a worth-while idea to hear a man's viewpoint.

" All my life," Mr. Everyman says, " I've thought of one thing in regard to women—and that is, I want to be terribly proud of the woman I marry."

Yes, he wants her to be, in his eyes, the most beautiful, the most intelligent, and the most charming of women. He wants everyone to be properly impressed with his wife, with her physical loveliness, with her good taste in matters of dress, with her mentality.

Now let us break this down into practical details. Let's see what qualities his ideal woman should possess to cause him not only to fall in love with her, but to remain enamoured.

First of all, a woman would have to be physically appealing—that's important. " She wouldn't have to be a raving beauty," Mr. Everyman says. " I'd probably be afraid to fall in love with such a woman. But she'd have to have some physical attraction for me to fall in love with her."

What makes a woman physically attractive ? Clarity of skin, shining eyes and hair, a lovely figure, vibrancy and vitality, good taste in the matters of dress, well-kept nails, unobtrusive make-up which subtly enhances her best points —all these are important.

" Animation is important, too," says Mr. Everyman. He is bored stiff by a blank-faced girl who shows no interest in his conversation, in the things which appeal to him, in his everyday activities.

" A lively spirit lends zest and gaiety to everything a girl does, adds piquancy to life with her, makes every moment spent in her presence exciting.

" Daintiness and femininity are highly desirable. Leave it to the men to be rough, hardy, masculine. Oh, that doesn't mean a girl may not be athletic, that she cannot play a bang-up game of tennis or golf, or be a splendid swimmer. But in the evening, men become sentimental and like a woman to be soft and tempting to the eye and touch. At such times, matter-of-factness and cynicism are out of place—this is a time for gentle allure, delicate loveliness · of appearance, and other typical feminine qualities."

MR. EVERYMAN ON CONVERSATION

" My ideal woman is a good listener," says Mr. Everyman. " A girl who wants to get on with men can do well to remember the old maxim : ' A man says what he knows, a woman says what will please.' To interrupt every conversation with whatever rattlebrained observation pops into her head, is one sure way to discourage any future conversation.

" If she cares about a man, she should study the subjects around which his interests and work centre, so that she can listen and discuss them intelligently. Nothing flatters a man so much

335

as the knowledge that the girl loves the same things he does. It makes him feel that they possess a community of interests which augurs well for their future life together.

" Men are the natural wage-earners of a family. They must go out into the business and financial worlds and earn a living for themselves and the ones they love. The woman who cares about her man and wants him to succeed, will do everything she possibly can to foster in him a sense of power, a sense of adequacy, a sense of fitness for his job. Her unquestioning faith and belief in him will reassure him of his ability to make good. Men need to wear the trousers in any family, and it is a wise woman who sees to it that her husband does wear them, who does not try to rob him of this privilege.

" Many women who have successful marriages actually manage them, but their firm hand is encased in a glove of softest velvet, so that their direction of the family's affairs is never humiliating to the husband. There are men who are naturally less equipped than their wives to handle the finances of the family, to budget their incomes, or decide where money should be spent. These men are usually glad to permit their wives to make decisions, but it would hurt their pride to have the rest of the world know about it. The wise wife is content with the power, letting the title go."

Apropos of this is the following story :

The woman was a top-flight scenarist at one of the major film studios earning an exceptionally large salary. She fell in love with and married a struggling writer who had not yet established himself. He loved his wife desperately, but was awed by her money, her important friends, the impressive setting necessary to her position. This woman understood the situation thoroughly, however, and did everything in her power to overcome it. Their earnings were pooled in a single bank account, and although she ran the household the husband signed all cheques. At social gatherings in her home, she adroitly brought him into every conversation and listened to his opinions with interest and respect. Constantly she made him feel the integrity of his character and the quality of his abilities.

Inspired by this love and devotion, he wrote a really worth-while book, a best seller. Today his name is as important as that of his wife in the scenario field, and their marriage is considered ideal in a town where but one marriage in ten succeeds.

MR. EVERYMAN CONTINUES . . .

" The man who works for a living has only so much time to play," says Mr. Everyman. " If he goes with a girl who isn't interested in his pet diversions, then, sooner or later, they are bound to be at loggerheads. For this reason, a man naturally gravitates toward the girl who loves to do the same things he does. And if a woman is interested in a man, she should be sure that the pastimes he favours are not unpleasant to her, and make it a point to become proficient in them.

" The man who is crazy about golf, or bowling, or tennis, loves to have his wife participate in these sports with him. Nothing causes disruption in a marriage as quickly as the indifference of the wife to the man's hobbies. A good bridge player can be driven crazy by a wife who plays sloppily and unthinkingly. An ardent philatelist is angered to fever pitch by his wife's statement that she can't see how he can fool around with those silly little stamps. A man with a desk job, who has a passion for exploring the countryside in his car on Sundays—to see the woods, the mountains, the ocean—comes actually to dislike a wife who continuously complains, ' Oh, dear, we're not going again ! '

" Every human being needs a certain amount of privacy, a time when he can go into a room by himself to think out a problem, to sulk or to play. Let him have a small portion of his life which he can call his own. Don't insist on doing everything with him, on knowing and discussing his innermost thoughts, unless he himself invites such participation. If he wants to go off for a stag evening with some of the boys, or to a lodge meeting, don't stand in his way—the change will do you both good.

" Never, never nag a man if you want to keep his love. Don't keep reminding him of his shortcomings, of the things he should have done or has failed to accomplish. Don't pester and nag him until he explodes and says things you will both later regret. Try to give him joy and pleasure, so that your company will be something he looks forward to eagerly, with anticipation. Make being with you a treat, not a trial. Inspire him, thrill him, amuse him, intrigue him—but don't pester, don't harass, don't heckle a man—and he always will adore you.

" A man and his woman should be two against the world, fighting side by side for a common goal. She must be his companion, his pal, his critic and confidante and his inspiration, as well as his love. It is a really happy union when this is truly so."

These are what Mr. Everyman wants and looks for in a woman. They are vital to marital happiness.

A man needs a woman as much as a woman needs a man. To lapse into a lighter vein for a moment, I recall my grandfather once voicing an objection to the latter part of this statement. " What do we need women for anyway ? " he wanted to know.

" If there were no women in the world," my grandmother pointed out defensively, " who'd sew the buttons on your pants ? "

" If there were no women in the world," the old boy retorted, " who'd need pants ? "

Notes:

Self-Test Questions Based On Lesson Twelve

This Lesson is a challenge—especially to the older woman—to make the most of what she has. Even the plain woman can be different, can cultivate personality and be charming. Try out the suggestions in this Lesson and you will be amazed at the way they work. You can be attractive. Decide to alter NOW. Start Living !

After you have studied this Lesson, you should be able to answer the following questions. If you have any difficulty in doing so, refer to the Lesson for further study and revision. Your answers should not be sent to the publishers of this Course.

1. Have you examined yourself along the lines suggested in this Lesson ?

   Do you look your age ?

   If you are over thirty—have you neglected yourself ?

   Could you improve your appearance as suggested in this and previous Lessons ?

   (a) Are you happily married or could you possibly improve your happiness ?

   (b) Are you still single with dreams of marriage ? What have you done about these dreams ?

2. Do you wish to put your career first ? If so, could you be more successful in your work and socially by following advice given throughout this Course ?

3. What type of person are you ? Analyse yourself as suggested on page 8 and make a list of your faults and virtues.

4. Have you begun to overcome your faults, and to develop your personality as suggested in the Lesson ?

5. What emotions must you cultivate in order to help you acquire an attractive personality ?

6. What should guide you in your choice of perfumes ?

7. Quote three ways in which you may protect and beautify your eyes.

8. Besides physical attractiveness what else must a woman cultivate if she wishes to win and hold her man ?

9. What is a common fault among wives which often ruins married life, though men, too, sometimes indulge in it ?

10. Sum up shortly what a woman should strive to be to her man.

If you wish to determine the progress you are making, give yourself 10 points for each question you answer correctly. If the total comes to 90 or more, it is excellent; 80 or more, good; 70 or more, fair.

Personal Progress Chart

Record your weight and measurements without clothes, in the Personal Measurement Chart here. A model is measured, dressed, minus her coat. Weigh and measure yourself once a week.

Be sure you measure in the same spot each time, because even a half-inch variation might make a considerable difference. No use fooling yourself! Keep the information to yourself! Here is how the experts measure you:

Height, without shoes.
Chest, under armpits.
Bust, largest part.
Waist—waist-line should be level with elbows, but measure so many inches from the floor.
Abdomen, over navel.
Upper hips, level with tip of hip-bone.
Lower hips, largest part of buttocks.

Thigh, largest part; measure from floor.
Knee, over knee-cap.
Calf, largest part.
Ankle, above ankle-bone.
Wrist, below wrist-bone.
Arm; measure halfway between shoulder and elbow.
Neck, level with bottom of chin.

Make A Note Every Week Of Your Weight And Measurements

	Weight	Neck	Bust	Waist	Wrist	Abdomen	Hips	Thigh	Calf	Ankle	Arm
Present Weight and Measurements											
1st Week											
2nd ''											
3rd ''											
4th ''											
5th ''											
6th '' '											
Weight and Measurements After 3 Months											
After 6 Months											

If you want drastically to reduce or gain weight, we recommend your consulting your doctor.

Part A of Lesson Seven also contains a copy of this Chart and gives more detailed information about the ideal figure.

Weight and Measurement Chart

IS there a woman who isn't interested in her size? So many skills involved in being your loveliest can be read about and applied without much effort. But reducing or putting on weight is another matter.

You'll want to know how your weight, measurements and proportions compare with the average. Study the Weight and Measurement Chart here, and then measure yourself. Even if your weight is exactly as the average indicates, remember that you are working with the AVERAGE weight.

The weights and measurements in this Chart have been compiled from records of my students who are actresses, models and others whose professional work demands they keep extra slim and shapely. In addition, they diet entirely under my supervision, and with the approval of a doctor.

The normal average woman must in no wise undertake drastic slimming without first consulting a doctor.

Height	Age	Weight	Neck	Bust	Waist	Wrist	Abdomen	Hips	Thigh	Calf	Ankle	Arm
5′ 0″	15–35	7 st. 2 lbs.	11¾	31⅛	23⅝	5⅜	28	31½	18⅞	11⅝	7⅛	9⅜
	35–60	7 st. 6 lbs.	11⅞	31¾	24	5½	28½	32¼	19⅛	11⅞	7⅜	9⅝
5′ 1″	15–35	7 st. 7 lbs.	11⅞	32⅛	23¾	5½	28¼	32	19	12	7¼	9½
	35–60	7 st. 11 lbs.	12	32⅝	24½	5⅝	28¾	32½	19¼	12⅛	7¾	9¾
5′ 2″	15–35	7 st. 12 lbs.	12⅛	32¼	23⅞	5½	28½	32¼	19⅛	12⅛	7½	9⅝
	35–60	8 st. 2 lbs.	12¼	32¾	24¾	5⅝	28⅞	32¾	19½	12⅜	7⅝	9⅞
5′ 3″	15–35	8 st. 3 lbs.	12¼	32½	24	5⅝	29	33	19½	12¼	7⅝	9¾
	35–60	8 st. 7 lbs.	12⅜	33	24⅞	5¾	29½	33¾	19¾	12½	7¾	10
5′ 4″	15–35	8 st. 8 lbs.	12⅜	33¼	24⅛	5¾	29¼	33½	19⅞	12⅜	7¾	10
	35–60	8 st. 12 lbs.	12½	33¾	25	5⅞	29¾	34½	20¼	12⅝	7⅞	10¼
5′ 5″	15–35	8 st. 13 lbs.	12⅝	33¾	24¼	5⅞	29½	34¼	20⅛	12½	7⅞	10¼
	35–60	9 st. 3 lbs.	12¾	34	25¼	6	30	35¼	20½	12⅞	8	10½
5′ 6″	15–35	9 st. 4 lbs.	12¾	34½	25½	6	30	35½	20¼	12⅝	8	10½
	35–60	9 st. 8 lbs.	12⅞	34¾	25⅞	6¼	30¾	35¾	20⅝	13	8⅛	10¾
5′ 7″	15–35	9 st. 9 lbs.	12¾	35	26	6⅛	31	36	20¾	12¾	8⅛	10¾
	35–60	9 st. 13 lbs.	13	35½	26½	6⅜	31¾	36½	21	13⅛	8¼	11
5′ 8″	15–35	10 st. 0 lbs.	13⅛	36	27	6¼	32	37	21¼	13⅛	8½	10⅞
	35–60	10 st. 4 lbs.	13¼	36½	27½	6½	32¾	37¼	21⅝	13½	8⅝	11¼
5′ 9″	15–35	10 st. 5 lbs.	13½	36⅛	27¼	6⅜	33	37¼	21¾	13½	8⅝	11⅛
	35–60	10 st. 9 lbs.	13¾	37	27¾	6⅝	33¾	37¾	22¼	13¾	8⅞	11½
5′ 10″	15–35	10 st. 10 lbs.	13⅞	37½	27¾	6½	33½	37½	22⅛	13⅞	8¾	11⅜
	35–60	11 st. 0 lbs.	14¼	38	29	6¾	34¼	38½	22¾	14¼	9	11¾

These measurements and weights are for the modern "streamlined" actress or model figure. For heavier-than-average bone structure allow about seven pounds more and an inch for torso measurements. For very small bone structure, deduct five to ten pounds. For a well-proportioned figure, the bust and hip measurements should be about the same and the waist-line about ten inches less. Within an inch or two—either way—is good.

Part A of Lesson Seven also contains a copy of this Chart and gives more detailed information about the ideal figure.

Index to the Course "Glorify Yourself"

346

351

New, Easy Way to Charm and Beauty

he techniques and secrets you get in e twelve amazing Lessons of "Glorify ourself" are refreshingly different from nything you have ever seen. In this ecially compiled Course on Beauty, harm and Personality, the author akes no extravagant claims of changg you into a ravishing beauty overght.

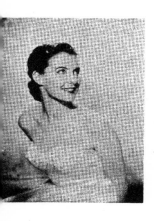

rom the knowledge that one is looking one's best mes all the confidence and poise in the world— thout this knowledge you cannot be gay and laxed.

hat the author does give to you are ghly successful techniques and beauty crets that she has developed over any years in acting as Beauty Consultt to famous Film Stars and in personly teaching thousands of women of all ges and in all walks of life how to be ore charming and more beautiful.

ere in this unique Course of Lessons ou have the much-wanted beauty hints permanent form — always on hand to elp to keep you looking your best.

n this Course, "Glorify Yourself," you ave a practical guide by an authority hose name is synonymous with a oman's concept of beauty and charm unique features that have earned for er the confidence of thousands of omen in all walks of life. Emphasis

throughout the Lessons of this Course is on how, in the privacy of your own home and during your leisure moments, you can put Eleanore King's tried and tested formulas to work for you.

Guide to Glamour

Eleanore King tells you in this Home Study Course how to make the most of your face, figure and personality; how to retain youth and beauty irrespective of whether you are fifteen or fifty. Her corrective exercises and diets have shown many other people besides Film Stars and other celebrities the way to health, beauty and happiness.

This fascinating Course reveals certain sure methods of effectively streamlining the waist, bust, hips and thighs, and gives the same expert advice and specific instruction that you would receive if you were to go to the author's Studio for personal tuition.

One of the first requisites for attaining the heights of beauty and charm, is glowing, vibrant health, and by following the tested and proven methods outlined in this Course, you can acquire a healthy, beautiful body which is one of the essentials of true glamour.

Each of the twelve Lessons is profusely illustrated by sketches and photographs. The sketches, in particular, are linked to the text of the Lessons in such a way that every sentence is crystal clear. Every step you take through the Course will be fascinating—no tedious drudgery. Just master each Lesson as slowly or as quickly as you desire. You waste no time, but concentrate on the things that will help you most.

No matter what your age may be, irrespective of whether you are married or single, or whether you are employed in office, factory, shop or at home, this wonderful Home Study Course reveals to you how to become more attractive, more charming, more self-confident— easily — quickly — surely. " Glorify Yourself " is the Magic Key to true

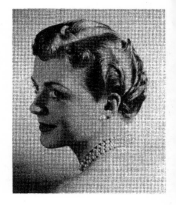

Beautiful hair—the sweet aroma which emanates from it, the gleaming, shining highlights, the soft, velvety sheen—is certainly among woman's most magnificent assets.

loveliness — and you now have it in your own hands!

Binder for Lessons

The Binder is for the permanent filing of the Lessons. When this is done, the material will be available at all times for future reading and reference.

There is no need for you to study and complete the Self-Test Questions inside each Lesson unless you prefer to do so. The Questions have only been included for the use of those Students who want to keep a strict check on the progress they make with each Lesson. The Lessons themselves contain all you need to know about Charm, Beauty, Glamour and Personality.